Cardiovascular PET

Notice

Cardiovascular PET
Current Concepts

Editors

Gary V. Heller, MD, PhD, FACC, MASNC

Gagnon Cardiovascular Institute
Morristown Medical Center
Morristown, New Jersey

Timothy M. Bateman, MD

Clinical Professor of Medicine
University of Missouri—Kansas City School of Medicine
Saint Luke's Cardiovascular Consultants
Kansas City, Missouri

James A. Case, PhD

University of Missouri, Columbia
Cardiovascular Imaging Technologies
Kansas City, Missouri

Parthiban Arumugam, MD

Clinical Director and Lead in Nuclear Cardiology
Nuclear Medicine Centre
Manchester Royal Infirmary
Manchester, United Kingdom

Mc Graw Hill Education

New York Chicago San Francisco Athens London Madrid Mexico City
Milan New Delhi Singapore Sydney Toronto

Cardiovascular PET: Current Concepts

1 2 3 4 5 6 7 8 9 DSS 23 22 21 20 19 18

ISBN 978-1-259-86048-5
MHID 1-259-86048-5

This book was set in Minion Pro by Thomson Digital.
The editors were Karen G. Edmonson and Robert Pancotti.
The production supervisor was Catherine H. Saggese.
Project management was provided by Shikha Pahuja, Thomson Digital.
The text designer was Eve Siegel; the cover designer was W2 Design.

Library of Congress Cataloging-in-Publication Data

Names: Heller, Gary V., editor.
Title: Cardiovascular PET : current concepts / editors, Gary V. Heller, MD, PhD, FACC, MASNC, Gagnon Cardiovascular Institute, Morristown Medical Center, Morristown, New Jersey [and three others].
Description: New York, NY : McGraw-Hill Education, [2019]
Identifiers: LCCN 2018043984| ISBN 9781259860485 (hardback) | ISBN 1259860485 (hardback)
Subjects: LCSH: Heart–Radionuclide imaging. | BISAC: MEDICAL / Cardiology.
Classification: LCC RC683.5.R33 C39 2019 | DDC 616.1/207575–dc23
LC record available at https://lccn.loc.gov/2018043984

CONTENTS

CONTRIBUTORS

Ali Alenazy, MD
Department of Medicine, University of Ottawa
Division of Cardiology, University of Ottawa Heart Institute, Ottawa, Ontario, Canada

Parthiban Arumugam, MD
Clinical Director and Lead in Nuclear Cardiology, Nuclear Medicine Centre, Manchester Royal Infirmary, Manchester, United Kingdom

May Aung, CNMT
Molecular Function and Imaging Program, the National Cardiac PET Centre, Division of Cardiology, Department of Medicine, The University of Ottawa Heart Institute, Ottawa, Ontario, Canada

Timothy M. Bateman, MD
Clinical Professor of Medicine, University of Missouri—Kansas City School of Medicine
Saint Luke's Cardiovascular Consultants, Kansas City, Missouri

Rob S. Beanlands, MD
Molecular Function and Imaging Program, the National Cardiac PET Centre, and the Cardiac Imaging Program, Division of Cardiology, Department of Medicine, The University of Ottawa Heart Institute, Ottawa, Ontario, Canada

Daniel S. Berman, MD
Departments of Imaging and Medicine, Burns and Allen Research Institute, Cedars-Sinai Medical Center, Los Angeles, California

Dennis A. Calnon, MD, FACC, FASE, MASNC, FSCCT
Director, Cardiac Imaging, Riverside Methodist Hospital, Columbus Ohio

James A. Case, PhD
University of Missouri, Columbia, Cardiovascular Imaging Technologies, Kansas City, Missouri

Wengen Chen, MD, PhD
Associate Professor, Departments of Diagnostic Radiology and Nuclear Medicine, University of Maryland School of Medicine
Director, Nuclear Medicine Residency Program, University of Maryland Medical Center, Baltimore, Maryland

Robert A. deKemp, BASc, MSc, PhD, PEng, PPhys
Molecular Function and Imaging Program, the National Cardiac PET Centre, Division of Cardiology, Department of Medicine, The University of Ottawa Heart Institute, Ottawa, Ontario, Canada

Vasken Dilsizian, MD
Departments of Diagnostic Radiology and Nuclear Medicine, University of Maryland School of Medicine, Baltimore, Maryland

Sharmila Dorbala, MD, MPH
Cardiac Amyloidosis Program, Division of Cardiology, Department of Medicine, Heart & Vascular Center
Division of Nuclear Medicine and Molecular Imaging, Department of Radiology
Brigham and Women's Hospital and Harvard Medical School, Boston, Massachusetts

Fernanda Erthal, MD
Department of Medicine, University of Ottawa
Division of Cardiology, University of Ottawa Heart Institute, Ottawa, Ontario, Canada

Gary V. Heller, MD, PhD, FACC, MASNC
Gagnon Cardiovascular Institute, Morristown Medical Center, Morristown, New Jersey

S. Massalha, MD
Cardiac Imaging Program, Division of Cardiology, Department of Medicine, The University of Ottawa Heart Institute, Ottawa, Ontario, Canada

Matthew Memmott, MSc
Chemical Engineering Department, Brigham Young University, Provo, Utah

Hiroshi Ohira, MD, PhD
First Department of Medicine, Hokkaido University, Sapporo, Japan

Jennifer Renaud, MSc
Molecular Function and Imaging Program, the National Cardiac PET Centre, Division of Cardiology, Department of Medicine, The University of Ottawa Heart Institute, Ottawa, Ontario, Canada

Dillenia Rosica, MD
Division of Nuclear Medicine and Molecular Imaging, Department of Radiology, Geisinger Medical Center, Danville, Pennsylvania

Alan Rozanski, MD
Department of Cardiology, Mount Sinai St. Luke's Hospital and Mount Sinai Heart, New York, New York

Terrence D. Ruddy, MD
Molecular Function and Imaging Program, the National Cardiac PET Centre, Division of Cardiology, Department of Medicine, The University of Ottawa Heart Institute, Ottawa, Ontario, Canada

Piotr J. Slomka, PhD
Departments of Imaging and Medicine, Cedars-Sinai Medical Center, Los Angeles, California

Gary R. Small, MB, BCh, BSc, PhD, MRCP
Cardiac Imaging Program, Division of Cardiology, Department of Medicine, The University of Ottawa Heart Institute, Ottawa, Ontario, Canada

Seth Uretsky, MD
Department of Cardiology, Morristown Medical Center, Morristown, New Jersey

PREFACE

On behalf of the editors, we welcome you to the First Edition of *Cardiovascular PET: Current Concepts*. This book comes as a result of the tremendous worldwide clinical growth in Cardiovascular PET Imaging. Cardiac PET has revolutionized myocardial perfusion imaging, as well as the detection of myocardial viability, sarcoidosis, and device/lead infection. In addition, new tracers and instrumentation that will be entering the cardiac PET arena will drive new indications and patient management pathways as well as new camera systems that will continue to improve image quality. This book represents a comprehensive compilation of all aspects related to contemporary cardiovascular PET Imaging. Our intent is to present current knowledge and practical aspects of clinical cardiovascular PET, rather than taking a comprehensive textbook approach.

This book is divided into sections that are relevant to the clinical practice of PET. The first section vividly describes the scientific advances that have driven the growing value of cardiovascular PET. The second section describes the practical clinical and technical aspects of PET myocardial perfusion imaging as well as adjunctive evaluation of calcium during the CT acquisition. Special attention is given to the growing field of absolute myocardial blood flow quantitation. This technique is now an integral and essential part of a cardiac PET program and for this reason we have devoted an entire section to this subject including clinical data, quality control, and interpretation. A crucial driver of these advancements is the new technical developments and instrumentation that have become available. We provide an overview of these advancements and their practical value to the practicing clinician. Myocardial viability assessment with FDG PET is an underutilized component of this modality. This section describes the compelling PET literature supporting a metabolic approach to viability and describes practical methods important for patient preparation, data acquisition, and, finally, interpretation. The final two sections are devoted to the rapidly emerging applications of PET to nontraditional diseases and disease states that are becoming essential nuclear cardiology services: namely, inflammation and infection imaging. These exciting arenas are expanding the value of cardiac PET to healthcare providers not generally familiar with nuclear cardiology. We have added a brief discussion at the end of each chapter entitled "Editor's Perspective" to emphasize and enhance the clinical value of the chapter based upon the editor's clinical experience in PET.

We are honored to include as chapter authors some of the most respected members of the cardiovascular PET community who have often contributed to the literature that is being cited. Their contributions offer the most up-to-date understanding of the current research and practices as well as unique insight into the direction of cardiac PET. We are extremely grateful for their important contributions. In each section we have also focused on practical aspects which include descriptions of the performance of these procedures and, just as important, the interpretation skills necessary for each modality.

It is our profound hope that this book will provide you with important insights into the growing development of clinical cardiovascular PET and show you how to implement state-of-the-art cardiac PET in your own clinical practice. Your input after reading this book would be greatly appreciated and crucial in developing future editions.

Gary V. Heller
Timothy M. Bateman
James A. Case
Parthiban Arumugam

SECTION 1

CURRENT CONCEPTS OF CARDIOVASCULAR PET IMAGING: THE NEW PARADIGM

Timothy M. Bateman

An important evolutionary advancement in the field of nuclear cardiology has been the introduction of cardiovascular positron emission tomography (PET) into mainstream clinical care. An extensive peer-reviewed literature spanning almost 30 years virtually shouts out a role for cardiac PET in a substantial proportion of patients historically assessed with single-photon emission computed tomography (SPECT) or not previously evaluable by nuclear cardiology techniques. The substantial and growing evidence base has led to several pivotal multisocietal guidelines,[1] position statements,[2] and consensus documents[3,4] on the role of PET imaging in cardiovascular disorders. The theme of this Introduction is that a contemporary nuclear cardiology laboratory will not be SPECT-only or PET-only, but that these two modalities will coexist, at least for the foreseeable future.[5] The published data and clinical need together are moving toward a concept in which SPECT or PET will be a preferred test for definable presentations and clinical descriptors.

In the coming chapters of this book, all of the various applications of cardiovascular PET will be thoroughly explored. The purpose of the current section is to provide a vision for how SPECT and PET should and can coexist in a culture of high-quality patient-centered imaging while achieving space and workforce efficiencies.

A BRIEF HISTORICAL OVERVIEW OF THE ROLE OF SINGLE PHOTON IMAGING IN THE ASSESSMENT OF CORONARY ARTERY DISEASE

Cardiac radionuclide imaging had its birth in an era in which cardiologists were primarily focused on coronary artery disease (CAD). By the 1970s, multicenter studies had shown that patients with triple-vessel, left main, and proximal left anterior descending disease fared better if treated with revascularization compared to medical therapies available at the time.

However, it was difficult to identify among the large number of patients with symptoms potentially indicating CAD those who needed invasive evaluation. Cardiac radionuclide imaging addressed that need, evolving newer and better approaches in hardware (first with rectilinear scanners,[6] then with planar cameras,[7] and by the mid-1980s with SPECT),[8] tracers (thallium-201 followed by Tc-99m sestamibi and tetrofosmin), and quantitative software. With an almost singular focus on CAD, a voluminous literature established the value of SPECT myocardial perfusion imaging (MPI) as a gatekeeper to the catheterization laboratory for many patients with nonacute known or suspected CAD. SPECT MPI also found daily use for diagnosing CAD, for risk stratification, and for assessing likelihood of viability of dysfunctioning myocardium. Figure S1-1 illustrates schematically how SPECT became positioned as a pivotal test for almost all patients except those who could perform a diagnostic-level treadmill exercise test that was adequate for decision making or who were deemed to be appropriate for direct referral to coronary angiography. Levin et al[9] used only Medicare data to show that SPECT MPI grew from 63.4 tests per 1000 beneficiaries in 2001 to 88 tests per 1000 beneficiaries in 2006, an impressive rate of growth that propelled SPECT MPI to become one of the top 10 annual Medicare expenditures. As expected, focus on SPECT MPI raised questions about the appropriateness and safety of so much testing. Table S1-1 highlights some of the major criticisms.

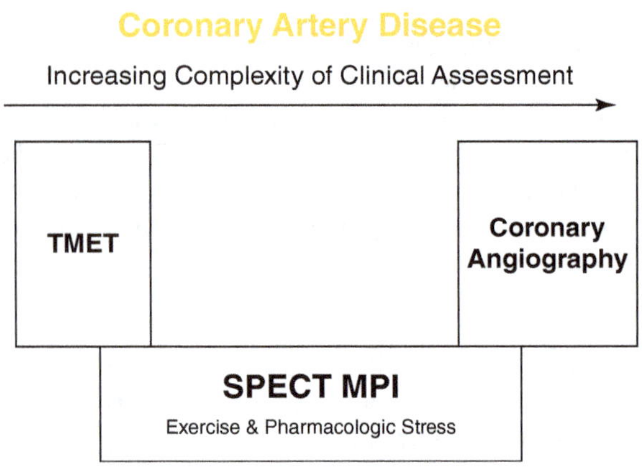

FIGURE S1-1 The pivotal role of planar followed by SPECT MPI from the early 1980s through approximately 2010. Over that long time span, nuclear MPI was a test of choice for most patients presenting with symptoms suggestive of nonemergent CAD. The exceptions were patients with normal ECGs capable of a treadmill exercise test, or those whose symptoms were so compelling that direct referral to coronary angiography was warranted. Note that this paradigm included low-risk, less complicated scenarios through to high-risk, more complicated presentations.

Table S1-1

Common Concerns about SPECT MPI That Have Been Expressed in Numerous Professional and Lay Publications

Expense
Test duration
Safety (radiation exposure)
Frequent false-positives
Underdetection of multivessel CAD
Overutilization
Low frequency of prognostically concerning ischemia

CHALLENGES TO THE STATUS QUO IN AN INCREASINGLY COMPETITIVE ENVIRONMENT

The past 15 years have seen increasing focus from payers, the public, from professional medical societies, and from the Institute of Medicine on the concept of patient-centered imaging.[10] The Centers for Medicare and Medicaid Services defines patient-centered imaging as effective, efficient, equitable, and safe.[11] In this paradigm, it becomes challenging to advocate that a single imaging procedure and protocol for the wide array of patients (Table S1-2) presenting for CAD assessment will be optimal for all. The SPECT community has been slow to address the concerns expressed in Table S1-1. While SPECT MPI has proved to be highly valuable, the reader will appreciate that for many of the criticisms, there is a common theme centering on expense, risk (radiation exposure), and the length of the test.

1. SPECT MPI is expensive relative to other tests for evaluating presence, extent, and severity of CAD. In fact, the 2018 Medicare fee schedule for

Table S1-2

The Varied Clinical and Physical Descriptors of Patients Referred for Myocardial Perfusion Imaging Challenge the Concept that One Protocol Can Address the CMS Mandate of Being Patient-Centered, Effective, Efficient, Safe, and Equitable

Men and women
Small, medium, large, and immense people Can/cannot lie still
Low likelihood for CAD, known CAD
Simple and complex CAD
Normal LV function; severe COM
NSR, atrial fibrillation, pacemakers, PVCs
Able to exercise; require pharmacologic stress
No versus multiple comorbidities

NSR = normal sinus rhythm; PVCs = premature ventricular contractions

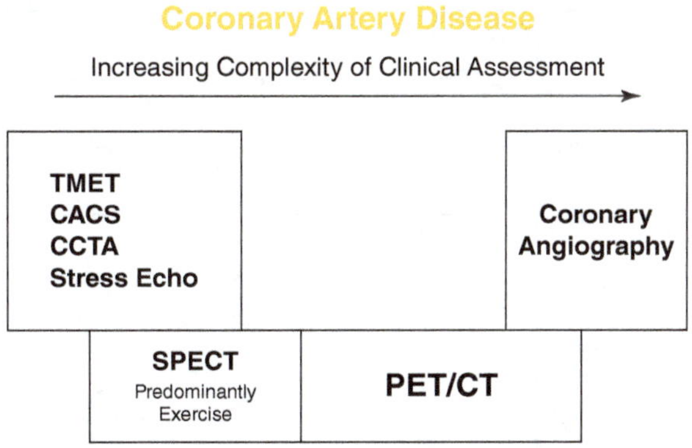

FIGURE S1-2 The adoption of PET MPI for more complex patients and those unable to undergo exercise stress; and of less expensive and less time-consuming tests, and arguably as useful for lower-likelihood patients (exercise treadmill testing without imaging, coronary CT angiography, stress echo) has resulted in a conceptual shifting of the role of SPECT MPI (compare Figure S1-2 with Figure S1-1). To compete successfully for the lower likelihood population, SPECT needs to improve accuracy, shorten image and test times, reduce radiation exposure, and consume less resource.

the technical performance of a rest/stress SPECT MPI is more than 4 times that of coronary CT angiography, and almost as much as a rest/stress PET MPI (Table S1-3). For lower at-risk patients, SPECT now competes with several modalities that are less expensive to payers and to patients (Figure S1-2). Figure S1-2 also shows how PET has claimed superiority for higher-risk patients, such that if SPECT is to survive, it must embrace principles of faster throughput (eg, stress-only imaging when appropriate), less risk (lower radiation associated with stress-only studies; lower dosages when CZT cameras are used), and higher accuracy (fewer false-positives when attenuation correction is employed). To successfully compete for the lower-risk patients, the typical large field of view cameras that necessitate high tracer dosages and long imaging times will be at a major disadvantage.

2. Studies show that the prevalence of an abnormal SPECT MPI has become low, suggesting that the test is being used in a progressively lower risk population[12–14] (Figure S1-3). As discussed previously, if SPECT is to compete with lower-cost alternatives for lower-risk patients, it must adapt to a value proposition that includes faster throughput, lower radiation, and fewer false-positive studies due primarily to bodily attenuation.
3. Because of its frequent and widespread use, SPECT MPI became identified as a significant source of population-based radiation exposure.[15] Despite efforts from major professional medical societies,[16] the provider community as a whole has failed to adopt radiation-saving protocols such as stress-only imaging when appropriate.[17] Newer CZT technology with the capability of major

Table S1-3

2018 Technical Payments Under the Hospital Out-Patient Prospective Payment System (HOPPS) for Medicare Patients

Test	Technical Payment
TMET	$249
CCTA (coronaries)	$253
Stress Echo	$450
Stress MR	$682
Stress-Only SPECT	$1203
Rest/Stress SPECT MPI	$1203
Rest/Stress PET MPI	$1377

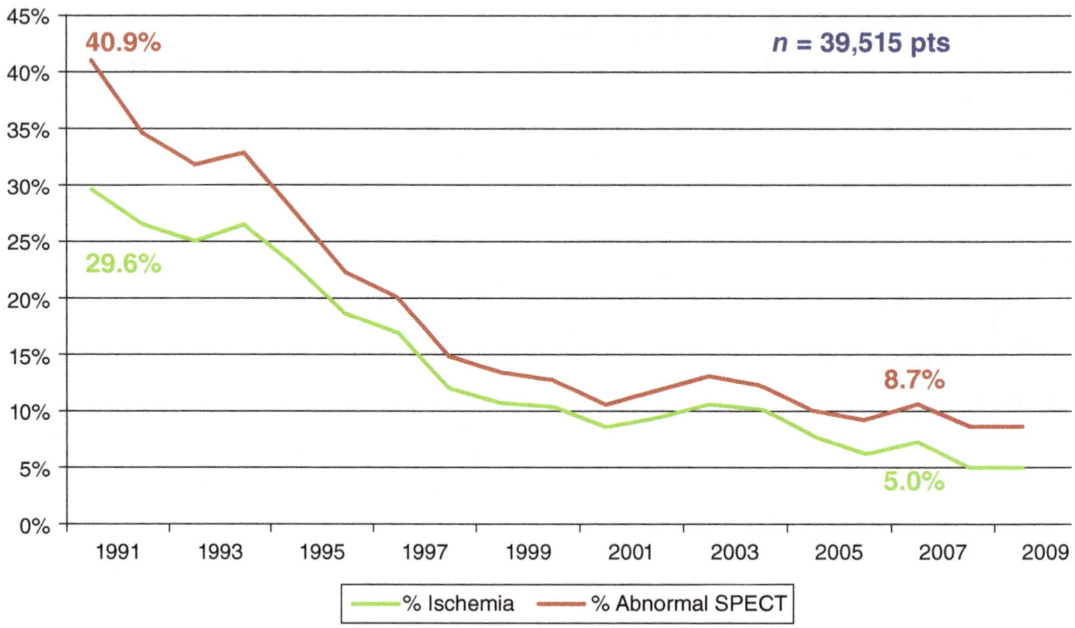

FIGURE S1-3 A graph from one of several studies showing the marked decline in the % of abnormal SPECT myocardial perfusion studies over time. (Modified with permission from Rozanski A, Gransar H, Hayes SW, et al. Temporal trends in the frequency of inducible myocardial ischemia during cardiac stress testing: 1991 – 2009, J Am Coll Cardiol 2013 Mar 12;61(10):1054-1065)

reductions in radiation exposure[18] has been slow to be adopted, as providers choose to retain older Anger-based systems that require longer procedures and higher dosages of tracer and, hence, radiation exposure in order to provide sufficient count density for diagnostic quality images.[19]

4. A major step forward for the SPECT MPI field was the introduction of intravenous vasodilators for "stressing" those patients unable to undergo a diagnostic level of treadmill exercise. Unfortunately, numerous studies and subsequent meta-analyses showed that such patients could never be categorized as being at low risk for events, even when the SPECT scan was normal.[20] Furthermore, for any MPI result, the events were higher after vasodilator stress than after exercise stress to an adequate end-point.[21] In addition, the "warranty period" of a normal SPECT MPI was much shorter after vasodilator stress versus exercise stress.[22] Many providers and clinicians began to look for more definitive assessments as focus changed from population-based to individual-based metrics.
5. The spatially relative nature of SPECT MPI and the inherent limitations of the most often used radionuclides (Tc-99m sestamibi or Tc-99m tetrofosmin) carry limitations for identifying multivessel or left main disease.[23,24] This well-publicized reality has seriously limited the ability of SPECT MPI to be an optimal gatekeeper to the catheterization laboratory. All clinicians fear the possibility that SPECT MPI may be missing the most serious of high-risk CAD patients: those with multivessel or left main CAD. One study showed that fewer than 40% of patients with three-vessel disease had any more than a single vessel SPECT perfusion defect.[23] Another demonstrated that less than 10% of 99 patients with significant left main CAD had even a small localized perfusion defect.[24]
6. Finally, there is an inherent inefficiency to the traditional yet commonly utilized rest/stress protocol that requires some 4–6 hours from patient arrival until departure from the testing facility. This is a large inconvenience as well as societal cost to the elective outpatient. For hospital inpatients, it can often make for an extra day or two of hospitalization, limiting the ability to accommodate late-day add-ons or to complete testing early enough to

allow same-day coronary angiography when indicated by MPI results.

SPECT technology has been evolving and through important advances can address some of these challenges. However, the necessity of incorporating cardiac PET into the milieu of a nuclear cardiology laboratory places constraints on SPECT advancements, especially in regard to the costs of upgrading hardware and software while volumes are being reduced owing to sharing the patient volume with PET. Once a practice or a hospital incorporates cardiac PET as an essential component of the cardiovascular service line, it becomes more challenging to allocate funding to cardiac SPECT.

STRENGTHS OF PET AND PET/CT FOR MPI

Table S1-4 enumerates the major advantages of rest/stress PET for MPI. Meta-analyses consistently show that PET has higher diagnostic accuracy than SPECT.[25–28] Image quality is superior to SPECT when performed in the same patients[29] and because all data are routinely corrected for tissue attenuation and scatter, image quality and interpretive certainty are relatively unaffected by patient gender, body size, or body shape.[30,31] Scan acquisition times are shorter versus traditional SPECT, in the range of 5 minutes versus 15–25 minutes. The shorter acquisition times make the test more equitable for acutely ill patients and for those who find it difficult to lay still. A full rest/stress study using rubidium-82 can be completed in 30 minutes, compared to several hours for a rest/stress SPECT, facilitating decisions about discharge versus same-day invasive procedures. Radiation exposures are in the range of 2–4 mSv for a rest/stress rubidium-82 PET MPI,[32–34] a fraction of the 12-13 mSv associated with typical rest/stress SPECT exposures and well below levels associated with risk for adverse effects. The lower radiation is important because most patients with chronic CAD will undergo a number of radiation-associated diagnostic and therapeutic procedures over their lifetimes. Finally, many PET scanners include a computed tomography (CT) component. For MPI studies, the CT is usually set at low tube current and voltage settings because the scans are used primarily for attenuation correction. These CT scans expose patients to only about 0.2 mSv of radiation but are adequate to visualize presence of coronary calcium and accurately estimate its Agatston score[35] while also permitting recognition of pericardial and pleural effusions, thoracic aortic aneurysms, chamber sizes, valve calcifications, and pulmonary pathologies. Studies such as those of Dorbala et al[36] have demonstrated independent and incremental improvements in risk stratification when PET-derived indices are considered in addition to myocardial perfusion patterns.

Table S1-4

Important Properties of Myocardial Perfusion PET

High diagnostic accuracy: • High sensitivity and specificity • Peak hyperemic vs rest regional wall motion and LVEF • Coronary artery calcium • Myocardial blood flow reserve
Consistent high-quality images regardless of body habitus: • High myocardial counts • High spatial and contrast resolution • High signal-to-noise ratio • Accurate correction for scatter and bodily attenuation
Low radiation exposure Quantification of myocardial blood flow Strong prognostic power Short image acquisitions and ~30 minute complete rest/stress studies

(Data from Bateman TM, Dilsizian V, Beanlands RS,et al: American Society of Nuclear Cardiology and Society of Nuclear Medicine and Molecular Imaging Joint Position Statement on the Clinical Indications for Myocardial Perfusion PET, J Nucl Med 2016 Oct;57(10):1654-1656)

QUANTIFICATION OF MYOCARDIAL BLOOD FLOW: A UNIQUE CAPABILITY OF PET MYOCARDIAL PERFUSION IMAGING

SPECT myocardial perfusion imaging is a spatially relative technique. It depends on differential perfusion of vascular territories in order to recognize functionally significant CAD, raising the potential to underdetect multivessel CAD. Investigations have established that in patients with catheterization-proved left main or 3-vessel CAD, only a minority of patients have perfusion defects that would suggest the presence of high-risk CAD. With vasodilator stress, balanced flow reduction can go completely undiagnosed. Cardiac PET is currently the only modality that permits routine quantification of myocardial blood flow, providing a patient-centric assessment of perfusion. Because myocardial blood flow is dependent on the functional integrity of the epicardial coronary arteries as well as the microvasculature, this measurement adds incrementally to perfusion defect analysis for risk stratification. In daily practice, myocardial blood flow quantification assures adequacy of vasodilator stress, improves recognition of multivessel CAD, rules out multivessel CAD, and often results in different and more cost-effective management than would have occurred if this only depended on perfusion defect detection.[37–41]

BEYOND PERFUSION: THE EXPANDING APPLICATIONS OF PET/CT FOR CARDIAC PATIENTS

In most cardiology programs, a PET/CT camera finds diverse uses beyond MPI. For example, a PET/16-slice CT can be used for coronary artery calcium scoring, thoracic and abdominal aortic studies, runoff studies, left atrial imaging prior to atrial fibrillation ablation procedures, identification of cardiac sarcoidosis, and workup of device infections. PET/64 and PET/128-slice scanners can be used for coronary artery, carotid artery, and renal artery studies. Experience shows that when a lab has both a cardiac-dedicated SPECT and a cardiac-dedicated PET camera, the PET camera will be used far more frequently than the SPECT camera, moving beyond MPI alone. It is important to reflect on the fact that MPI has thrived because cardiologists who cared for CAD patients required it for assistance in diagnosis, risk stratification, and strategizing management. In the current era, heart failure and electrophysiology subspecialists need the power of radionuclide imaging to address their evolving issues. These needs require the unique advantages of PET, and their path toward better care algorithms will be impeded if PET is not available.

A MODERN-DAY CLINICAL CARDIOLOGY NUCLEAR LABORATORY

Design of a modern-day clinical nuclear cardiology laboratory needs to consider the diversity of patients needing nuclear cardiovascular imaging procedures. The paradigm of one camera and one protocol for all MPI needs has passed (Figure S1-1). An ideal laboratory today (Figure S1-4) will have a cardiac-dedicated SPECT camera for low-intermediate CAD-likelihood patients who need an MPI but can exercise. Such a device might be a solid-state camera with high sensitivity and high resolution, such that microdosages of tracer can be used. The same laboratory will have a PET/CT for more complicated patients as described earlier, predominantly those requiring vasodilator stress. A recently published position statement[2] provides guidance on the types of patients optimally imaged with PET. Because of the high efficiency of the PET/CT, numerous other imaging applications will be possible each day.

While it might be argued that a SPECT camera in a cardiology department and a PET/CT in a radiology/nuclear medicine department could accomplish the same end-point as a revised nuclear cardiology laboratory that included both SPECT and a PET/CT, this would, however, require duplication of stress-testing facilities and stress-test clinical teams and would impede ability of the imaging teams making rapid decisions regarding best test after actually seeing the referred patient. An example might be recognizing on presentation that a patient admitted from the emergency department overnight had a caffeinated beverage 8 hours earlier and is unable to exercise. In this situation, only a PET study with blood flow quantification would be able to determine if a normal scan can be trusted or if the patient's A2a receptors did

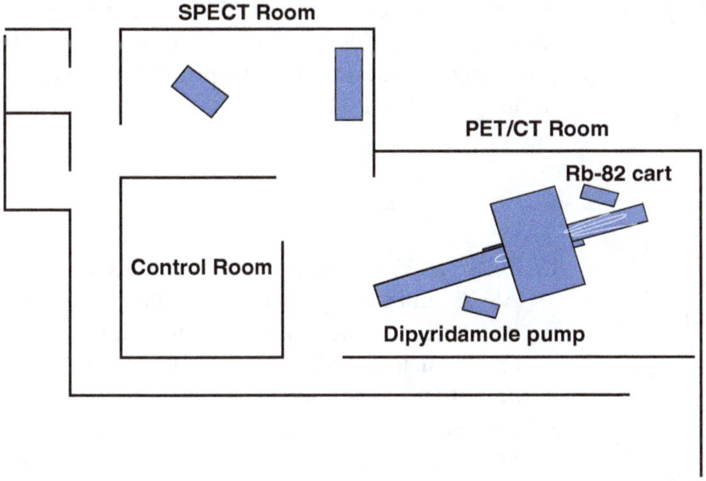

FIGURE S1-4 A highly efficient lab design to accommodate both cardiac SPECT and PET. The physical layout permits both modalities to operate with one nuclear technologist, one RN, one stress physiologist, and 0.5 of a CT technologist.

not respond to vasodilation stress. Thus, this scenario is enhanced by having the PET/CT situated within the stress-test area that includes SPECT. The PET/CT can easily be assigned throughout the day, via either block scheduling or interspersed with cardiac indications, for oncologic or central nervous system studies. Figure S1-5 compares the applications of a PET/CT camera with those of a SPECT camera and demonstrates why a contemporary lab needs both SPECT and PET.

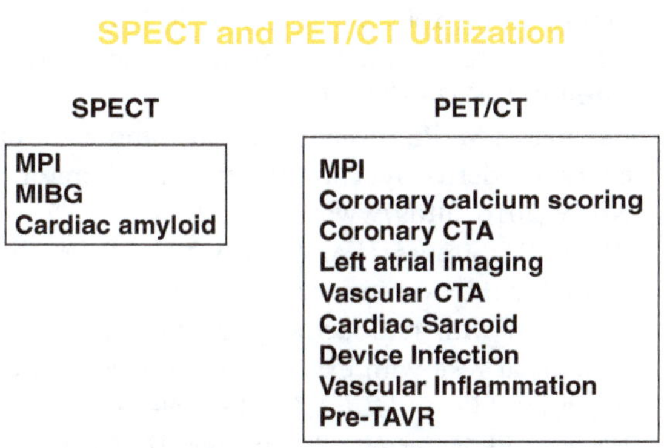

FIGURE S1-5 The varied applications of a PET/CT camera compared to a traditional SPECT camera within a space dedicated to cardiovascular imaging shows why the PET/CT camera has strikingly higher daily utilization. The figure also demonstrates why a contemporary lab has a need for both SPECT and PET, as there are SPECT-specific applications as well as PET-specific applications.

ECONOMIC CONSIDERATIONS

Imaging technology is expensive to purchase and maintain, and provision of PET radionuclides adds additional cost. However, PET/CT has a much greater potential than SPECT to add value and reduce the costs of care. Its rapid acquisition times and ability to complete studies in ~30 minutes makes it ideal for improving the efficiency of diagnosing inpatients and those in chest pain units, facilitating timely discharges or same-day coronary angiograms depending on the findings. The costs are largely fixed, such that costs do not rise in proportion to volume as with SPECT. The radionuclide most commonly used, rubidium-82, is on-site and immediately available, as opposed to the technetium-99m-based SPECT tracers that from time of order may take an hour or more to arrive on-site. Greater diagnostic certainty by virtue of several markers not available from SPECT, such as peak stress versus rest global and regional function, coronary calcium presence and extent, attenuation correction, scatter compensation, and blood flow quantification can all expedite correct diagnoses and limit unnecessary downstream testing. This will provide an opportunity to inform both patients and referring physicians in a far more comprehensive way about the state of myocardial perfusion. As indicated, opportunities for shared usage are enabled by the rapid acquisition protocols; SPECT imaging takes longer and the rest/stress protocols are longer, making economically feasible sharing of a camera more challenging.

WITH ALL THE ADVANTAGES, WHY DO MANY CARDIOLOGY PROGRAMS STILL NOT HAVE ACCESS TO CARDIAC PET?

Few nuclear cardiologists today would argue that cardiac SPECT alone is sufficient to address the radionuclide imaging needs of a contemporary cardiology practice. In time, virtually all sizable programs will need to have access to cardiac PET imaging to adequately serve their patients and referring health-care providers. The impediments are financial, educational, and political. The economic barrier to entry is high for small practices but not so for larger programs, for which the high utilization for diverse purposes makes it more attractive than SPECT. Providers (technologists, physicians, and nurses) do need opportunities for both education and training because PET tracers and instrumentation differ significantly from SPECT. PET scanners are widely available in the United States. In some settings, a PET scanner can and should be shared for oncologic and cardiac imaging. In others, the scanner might be dedicated for cardiac imaging. A cardiology program in an advanced center that does not have access to cardiac PET is most likely laboring under political constraints concerning interspecialty cooperation that is standing in the way of best patient care. The reader is encouraged to browse two recent joint publications[1,2] of the American Society of Nuclear Cardiology and the Society of Nuclear Medicine and Molecular Imaging to understand the professional societal viewpoint on the role of PET in the contemporary care of cardiac patients.

CONCLUSIONS

While cardiac PET is not "new" technology, its entrance into mainstream clinical practice is a relatively new paradigm. This section and subsequent chapters endeavor to provide sufficient detail such that clinicians and imagers can clearly see its role vis-à-vis SPECT or other imaging modalities. Further, because some cardiology training programs still do not have access to cardiac PET, it is hoped that trainees reading this book will be provided a solid grounding in understanding the principles and applications of cardiac PET.

REFERENCES

1. Dilsizian V, Bacharach SL, Beanlands RS, et al. ASNC imaging guidelines/SNMMI procedure standard for positron emission tomography (PET) nuclear cardiology procedures. *J Nucl Cardiol.* 2016;23:1187–1226.
2. Bateman TM, Dilsizian V, Beanlands RS, DePuey EG, Heller GV, Wolinsky DA. American Society of Nuclear Cardiology and Society of Nuclear Medicine and Molecular Imaging joint position statement on the clinical indications for myocardial perfusion PET. *J Nucl Med.* 2016;57:1654–1656.
3. Murthy VL, Bateman TM, Beanlands RS, et al. Quantification of myocardial blood flow using positron emission tomography: a joint position paper of the Cardiovascular Council (CVC) of the Society of Nuclear Medicine and Molecular Imaging (SNMMI) and the American Society of Nuclear Cardiology (ASNC). *J Nucl Cardiol.* 2018;25:269–297.
4. Chareonthaitawee P, Beanlands RS, Chen W, et al. Joint SNMMI-ASNC expert consensus document on the role of F-FDG PET/CT in cardiac sarcoid detection and therapy monitoring. *J Nucl Cardiol.* 2017;24:1741–1758.
5. Bateman TM. PET as an essential component of every modern-day clinical nuclear laboratory. Nov 9, 2016. http://www.acc.org.
6. Zaret BL, Strauss HW, Martin ND, Wells HP, Flamm MD. Noninvasive regional myocardial perfusion with radioactive potassium. Study of patients at rest, with exercise and during angina pectoris. *N Engl J Med.* 1973;288:809–812.
7. Wackers FJ, Fetterman RC, Mattera JA, Clements JP. Quantitative planar thallium-201 stress scintigraphy: a critical evaluation of the method. *Semin Nucl Med.* 1985;15:46–66.
8. Holly TA, Abbott BG, Al-Mallah M, et al. Single photon emission computed tomography. *J Nucl Cardiol.* 2010; doi:10.1007/s12350-010-9246-y.

9. Levin DC, Parker L, Halpern EJ, Rao VM. Recent trends in imaging for suspected coronary artery disease: what is the best approach? *J Am Coll Radiol.* 2016;13:381–386.
10. DePuey EG, Mahmarian JJ, Miller TD, et al. Patient-centered imaging. *J Nucl Cardiol.* 2012; doi:10.1007/s12350-012-9523-z.
11. Centers for Medicare and Medicaid Services. Clinical quality measures basics. https://www.cms.gov/regulations-and-guidance/legislation/ehrincentiveprograms/clinicalqualitymeasures.html.
12. Rozanski A, Gransar H, Hayes SW, et al. Temporal trends in the frequency of inducible myocardial ischemia during cardiac stress testing: 1991-2009. *J Am Coll Cardiol.* 2013;61:1054–1065.
13. Jouni H, Askew JW, Crusan DJ, Miller TD, Gibbons RJ. Temporal trends of single-photon emission computed tomography myocardial perfusion imaging in patients without prior coronary artery disease: a 22-year experience at a tertiary academic medical center. *Am Heart J.* 2016;176:127–133.
14. Jouni H, Askew JW, Crusan DJ, Miller TD, Gibbons RJ. Temporal trends of single-photon emission computed tomography myocardial perfusion imaging in patients with coronary artery disease: a 22-year experience from a tertiary academic medical center. *Circ Cardiovasc Imaging.* 2017;10:127–133.
15. Chen J, Einstein AJ, Fazel R, et al. Cumulative exposure to ionizing radiation from diagnostic and therapeutic cardiac imaging procedures. *J Am Coll Cardiol.* 2010;56:702–711.
16. Cerqueira MD, Allman KC, Ficaro EP, et al. Recommendations for reducing radiation exposure in myocardial perfusion imaging. *J Nucl Cardiol.* 2010;17:709–718.
17. Jerome SD, Tilkemeier PL, Farrell MB, Shaw LJ. Nationwide laboratory adherence to myocardial perfusion imaging radiation reduction practices. *J Am Coll Cardiol Imaging.* 2015;8:1170–1176.
18. Einstein AJ, Blankstein R, Andrews H, et al. Comparison of image quality, myocardial perfusion, and left ventricular function between standard imaging and single-injection ultra-low-dose imaging using a high-efficiency SPECT camera: the MILLISIEVERT study. *J Nucl Med.* 2014;55:1430–1437.
19. Patil HR, Abdallah M, Bateman TM. Correlates between camera age, patient volume, and laboratory accreditation: a snapshot of equipment utilization in the practice of nuclear cardiology in the U.S. *J Nucl Med.* 2013;54:156P.
20. Navare SM, Mather JF, Shaw LJ, et al. Comparison of risk stratification with pharmacologic and exercise stress myocardial perfusion imaging: a meta-analysis. *J Nucl Cardiol.* 2004;11:551–561.
21. Rozanski A, Gransar H, Hayes SW, Friedman JD, Hachamovitch R, Berman DS. Comparison of long-term mortality risk following normal exercise vs adenosine myocardial perfusion SPECT. *J Nucl Cardiol.* 2010;17:999–1008.
22. Hachamovitch R, Hayes S, Friedman JD, et al. Determinants of risk and its temporal variation in patients with normal stress myocardial perfusion scans: what is the warranty period of a normal scan? *J Am Coll Cardiol.* 2003;41:1329–1340.
23. Lima RSL, Watson DD, Goode AR, et al. Incremental value of combined perfusion and function over perfusion alone by gated SPECT myocardial perfusion imaging for detection of severe three-vessel coronary artery disease. *J Am Coll Cardiol.* 2003;42:64–70.
24. Berman DS, Kang X, Slomka PJ, Gerlach J, de Yang L, Hayes SW. Underestimation of extent of ischemia by gated SPECT myocardial perfusion imaging in patients with left main coronary artery disease. *J Nucl Cardiol.* 2007;14:521–528.
25. Nandular KR, Dwamena BA, Choudhri AF, Nandalur SR, Reddy P, Carlos RC. Diagnostic performance of positron emission tomography in the detection of coronary artery disease: a meta-analysis. *Acad Radiol.* 2008;15:444–451.
26. McArdle, BA, Dowsley TF, deKemp RA, Wells GA, Beanlands RS. Does rubidium-82 have superior accuracy to SPECT perfusion imaging for the diagnosis of obstructive coronary disease? A systematic review and meta-analysis. *J Am Coll Cardiol.* 2012;60:1828–1837.
27. Parker MW, Iskandar A, Limone B, Perugini A, et al. Diagnostic accuracy of cardiac positron emission tomography versus single photon emission computed tomography for coronary artery disease: a bivariate meta-analysis. *Circ Cardiovascular Imaging.* 2012;5:700–707.

28. Danad I, Rajimakers PG, Driessen RS, et al. Comparison of coronary CT angiography, SPECT, PET, and hybrid imaging for diagnosis of ischemic heart disease determined by flow fractional reserve. *JAMA Cardiol.* 2017. Epub ahead of print.
29. Yoshinaga K, Chow BJ, Williams K, et al. What is the prognostic value of myocardial perfusion imaging using rubidium-82 positron emission tomography? *J Am Coll Cardiol.* 2006;48:1029–1039.
30. Harnett DT, Hazra S, Maze R, et al. Clinical performance of Rb-82 myocardial perfusion PET and Tc-99m-based SPECT in patients with extreme obesity. *J Nucl Cardiol.* 2017. Epub ahead of print.
31. Bateman T, Heller GV, McGhie I, et al. Diagnostic accuracy of rest/stress ECG-gated rubidium-82 myocardial perfusion PET: comparison with ECG-gated Tc-99m-sestamibi SPECT. *J Nucl Cardiol.* 2006;12:24–33.
32. Senthamizhchelvan S, Bravo PE, Lodge MA, Merrill J, Bengel FM, Sgouros G. Radiation dosimetry of 82Rb in humans under pharmacologic stress. *J Nucl Med.* 2011;52:485–491.
33. Hunter CR, Hill J, Ziadi MC, Beanlands RS, deKemp RA. Biodistribution and radiation dosimetry of (82)Rb at rest and during peak pharmacological stress in patients referred for myocardial perfusion imaging. *Eur J Nucl Med Mol Imaging.* 2015;42:1032–1042.
34. ICRP. Radiation dose to patients from radiopharmaceuticals: a compendium of current information related to frequently used substances. *ICRP Publication 128.* 2015;Ann ICRP 44(2S):143.
35. Einstein AJ, Johnson LL, Bokhari S, et al. Agreement of visual estimation of coronary artery calcium from low-dose CT attenuation correction scans in hybrid PET/CT and SPECT/CT with standard Agatston score. *JACC.* 2010;56:1941–1921.
36. Dorbala S, Hachamovitch R, Curillova Z, et al. Incremental prognostic value of gated Rb-82 positron emission tomography myocardial perfusion imaging over clinical variables and rest LVEF. *J Am Coll Cardiol Imaging.* 2009;2:846–854.
37. Herzog BA, Husmann L, Valenta I, et al. Long-term prognostic value of 13N-ammonia myocardial perfusion positron emission tomography added value of coronary flow reserve. *J Am Coll Cardiol.* 2009;54:150–156.
38. Murthy VL, Naya M, Foster CR, et al. Improved cardiac risk assessment with noninvasive measures of coronary flow reserve. *Circulation.* 2011;124:2215–2224.
39. Ziadi MC, Williams KA, Guo A, et al. Impaired myocardial flow reserve on rubidium-82 positron emission tomography imaging predicts adverse outcomes in patients assessed for myocardial ischemia. *J Am Coll Cardiol.* 2011;58:740–748.
40. Naya M, Murthy VL, Taqueti VR, et al. Preserved coronary flow reserve effectively excludes high-risk coronary artery disease on angiography. *J Nucl Med.* 2014;55:248–255.
41. Ziadi MC, Williams K, Guo A, et al. Does quantification of myocardial flow reserve using rubidium-82 positron emission tomography facilitate detection of multivessel coronary artery disease? *J Nucl Cardiol.* 2012;19:670–680.

SECTION

2

CLINICAL OVERVIEW OF CONTEMPORARY MYOCARDIAL PERFUSION IMAGING WITH CARDIAC PET

Clinical Overview of Contemporary Myocardial Perfusion Imaging with Cardiac Positron Emission Tomography (PET)

CHAPTER 1

Parthiban Arumugam, Matthew Memmott, and Gary V. Heller

INTRODUCTION

Cardiac PET myocardial perfusion imaging has gained considerable acceptance in the clinical world of Nuclear Cardiology for many reasons. One driving force has been the substantial expansion of PET oncology, which has led to widespread availability of PET scanners in hospital settings. However, the burgeoning literature has also provided a demonstration of the incremental clinical value of cardiac PET, which has resonated in the marketplace and resulted in a gradual but steady growth of this modality into office-based and hospital settings. Finally, the sustained availability of radiotracers in the form of generator-produced ^{82}Rb and cyclotron-produced ^{13}N-ammonia has provided a stable milieu for the growth of cardiac PET myocardial perfusion imaging. This chapter describes the latest documentation of the important aspects of cardiac PET that makes this a compelling story for the present and future of nuclear cardiology. Sections include: brief history of cardiac PET, description of available tracers, diagnostic accuracy, image quality, unique aspects of PET MPI data, including myocardial blood flow (MBF), risk stratification, radiation exposure, protocols, and patients best suited for evaluation and tracers in development.

History of PET/CT Scanners

William Sweet and Frank Wren used positron-emitting radionuclides in the 1950s to localize brain tumors.[1,2] This was achieved by using two opposing gamma-ray detectors. Subsequently, in the 1970s, using multidetector systems, Burnham et al[3] were able to map out a 2-dimensional distribution of positron-emitting radionuclides. The first PET scanner for use in humans was developed by Michael Phelps and Ed Hoffman in 1976.[4] Short-lived radionuclides, such as carbon-11, nitrogen-13, and oxygen-15, however, were used mainly in neurology.

Detectors used in PET scanners changed from Bismuth Germinate (BGO) in 1985[5] to a new scintillation material called lutetium oxyorthosilicate (LSO). The faster decay time of LSO meant that it could handle higher count rates, which allowed dynamic image acquisition. The first commercial scanner with LSO crystals was introduced in 2001 by Siemens. Initially, attenuation correction (AC) on PET systems was performed using a radioactive source. It was only during the early 21st century that CT was integrated into PET systems that led to more accurate AC, which enabled accurate quantification of tracer distribution and along with LSO crystal technology made quantifying myocardial perfusion in mL/gm/min feasible.

It was not long after thallium-201 was seen as a viable myocardial perfusion tracer for gamma camera imaging in the mid- to late 1970s, that ^{13}N-ammonia was among the first radioactive tracers to be investigated for use in myocardial PET (Figure 1-1). In 1979, Schelbert et al[6] demonstrated images of myocardial perfusion in humans, with the quantitation of MBF in normal volunteers at stress and rest in 1989.[7] The use of ^{13}N-ammonia for cardiac imaging, however,

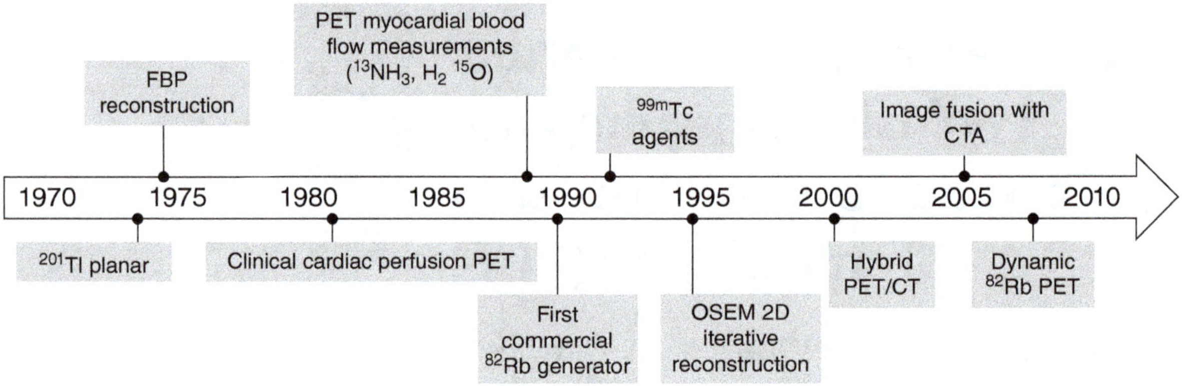

FIGURE 1-1 Timeline demonstrating significant milestones in the evolution of nuclear cardiology over the last 50 years.

was only approved by the US Food and Drug Administration (FDA) in 2007.

Around the same time of developments with ^{13}N-ammonia, the use of ^{82}Rb in PET myocardial perfusion imaging was reported by Selwyn et al.[8] Soon after this publication, larger clinical studies took place using generator-produced ^{82}Rb chloride[9], leading to FDA approval of the first commercial strontium-82/^{82}Rb generator in 1989 and reimbursement within the United States in 1995.[10] In 2016, a second commercial generator also received FDA approval. Initially for only perfusion imaging, or flow determination using external detectors[11], the advent of current generation PET scanners and application of compartmental models to dynamically acquired ^{82}Rb images has more recently allowed the tracer to be used to quantify MBF.[12] The optimization of fluorodeoxyglucose FDG imaging for several nonperfusion applications, such as myocardial viability, infection, and inflammation imaging has added breadth to cardiovascular PET.

TRACERS USED FOR CARDIAC PET PERFUSION

Cardiac PET tracers used in clinical practice are produced in a cyclotron or by a generator. Cyclotrons are particle accelerators that can produce positron-emitting isotopes by bombarding a target with rapidly accelerating charged particles. ^{13}N-ammonia (^{13}N NH_3), O-15 water (^{15}O-H_2O) and fluorine-18 fluorodeoxyglucose (^{18}F–FDG) are cyclotron-produced PET tracers. The former two are perfusion tracers and the latter is used in viability and infection/inflammation imaging. Table 1-1 shows the characteristics of the two most commonly used tracers, ^{82}Rb and ^{13}N-ammonia.

Rubidium-82 (^{82}Rb)

^{82}Rb is a potassium analog radiopharmaceutical that is produced with commercially available generators that can be delivered on-site. It is the result of the decay of strontium-82 (^{82}Sr), which has a half-life of 25.5 days. Thus, the generator life in the laboratory is 4–6 weeks depending on the camera system used. Once produced, ^{82}Rb has a half-life of 76 seconds. The extraction fraction of ^{82}Rb is estimated to be 65%-75%[13,14], substantially higher than SPECT technetium agents.

The use of ^{82}Rb is provided by an on-site generator and delivery system, which can be stored conveniently in the camera room. The generator is supplied at a fixed cost, independent of the number of studies performed. Because of the cost involved with the generator, consideration for PET use in a facility should include adequate patient volumes, generally considered 3–4 patients a day or more. When in use, the generated rubidium is replenished quickly, within 10 min via ^{82}Sr to ^{82}Rb decay. This permits minimal downtime between stress and rest imaging, allowing efficient utilization of the generator. The protocol for stress imaging requires the use of a pharmacologic stress agent because of the short half-life of ^{82}Rb. Protocols are described in more detail later in this chapter.

Table 1-1

Comparison of Routinely Used Radioactive Tracers for PET Myocardial Perfusion Imaging

	^{13}N ammonia	^{82}Rb
Half-life (minutes)	9.96 minutes	76 seconds
Imaging duration	10–20 min	6–10 min
Administered activity (3D scanner)	740 MBq (20 mCi)	740-1480 MBq (20-40 mCi)
Production	Cyclotron	Generator
Typical distances to annihilation event in tissue (FWHM)	0.26–0.62 mm	0.56–1.43 mm
Image resolution	Moderate	Low
First-pass extraction fraction	80%	65%
Perfusion defect contrast	Moderate	Low
Pharmacological stress	Routine	Routine
Treadmill exercise	Possible (static/ gated only)	Technically challenging

Advantages of ^{82}Rb include the ability to have rapid acquisition times for rest and stress imaging and continuous availability. The acquisition time is generally 7 minutes after injection of tracer. There are also disadvantages to ^{82}Rb imaging. Because of the half-life of ^{82}Sr, the same generator is used for a month to 6 weeks. Depending on the density of surrounding tissue the annihilation event occurs typically 0.56–1.43 mm from the emission[15], producing lesser quality images although still superior to SPECT. The short half-life of rubidium limits its use to pharmacologic stress and not exercise, and mandates an on-site generator, rather than regional "per dose" distribution. Thus, adequate patient volume is very important for financial feasibility.

^{13}N Ammonia ($^{13}N\ NH_3$)

$^{13}N\ NH_3$ is one of the earliest PET tracers that was used for myocardial perfusion imaging. $^{13}N\ NH_3$ undergoes several enzymatic metabolic changes to ^{13}N glutamine and is retained in the myocardium and liver. Implementation requires the presence of an on-site or close-by cyclotron because it has a half-life of 9.96 min. ^{13}N has an extraction fraction of approximately 80%.[16] Advantages of ^{13}N-ammonia include the high tomographic counts and a clear blood-to-myocardial delineation. In comparison to rubidium, the annihilation event is much closer to the emission (0.26–0.62 mm)[15] and, therefore, image quality is considered superior. Because of the longer half-life, exercise is possible, in contrast to rubidium. Limitations include the finding that even in normal subjects, the retention of ^{13}N in the lateral wall is 10% less than other segments creating false-positive results.[17] Prominent liver activity in some studies can make interpretation of the inferior wall difficult.[18] Finally, the necessity for on-site or close proximity cyclotron availability because of short half-life limits its implementation. This has severely limited its use, with perhaps 15–20 laboratories using this agent in the United States. This may change with the availability of a relatively small cyclotron designed for ^{13}N-ammonia production, which can be placed onsite.

^{15}O-water ($^{15}O\text{-}H_2O$)

$^{15}O\text{-}H_2O$ is a perfusion tracer that is not approved by FDA. It is mainly used for research purposes and in clinical practice in some European centers and is only briefly discussed. $^{15}O\text{-}H_2O$ is a cyclotron-produced tracer with short half-life of 2.07 minutes. It is a freely diffusible agent with very high (95%-100%) myocardial extraction[19] and, hence, a near linear relationship to MBF. It has no myocardial retention because of rapid equilibration with extracellular tissue and is independent of MBF. The linearity to MBF makes it the most physiological radiopharmaceutical and is the gold standard for noninvasively measuring MBF. However, myocardial perfusion imaging is not possible owing to poor myocardial retention as well as retained blood pooling with resultant poor image quality. Despite this limitation, the use of MBF has been used to validate the use of cardiac PET in comparative studies with other modalities, to be discussed later in this chapter.

DIAGNOSTIC ACCURACY OF CARDIAC PET

The diagnostic accuracy of cardiac PET perfusion imaging has been assessed with multiple studies. However, most studies are small and selected, and the same patients not used for comparison between modalities. The "gold standard" has been that of anatomic findings at cardiac catheterization, which has its own issues for judging accuracy. That said, there is a growing literature for cardiac PET, although fewer than for SPECT. Generally results are from ^{82}Rb and line source AC although a few studies also assess ^{13}N-ammonia and PET/CT systems. Most evaluations have used the meta-analysis format to provide the best assessment of diagnostic accuracy for PET and in particular comparison to SPECT.

With regard to independent literature of the diagnostic accuracy for cardiac PET perfusion, several studies report high sensitivity and specificity. Nandalur performed a meta-analysis of more than 1400 patients who underwent PET imaging and reported a sensitivity of 93% and a specificity of 83%.[20] Beanlands, several years later, evaluated the literature of PET alone, reporting on 18 studies and found a weighted sensitivity of 90% with a specificity of 89% similar to that of Nandalur.[21] In a single center study, Sampson et al[22] reported a high sensitivity and specificity for rubidium PET/CT imaging, a newer technique for cardiac PET growing in use and often replacing dedicated PET cameras for AC.

Jaarsma et al[23] reported a meta-analysis comparing the diagnostic accuracy of myocardial perfusion imaging using SPECT, PET, and CMR. A total of 166 studies were included in their analysis (114 SPECT, 15 PET, and 37 CMR). However, this review included studies with both SPECT tracers (thallium and technetium) and nonstandard imaging protocols (predominantly nonattenuation corrected studies and no reference to ECG gating, as well as retrospective studies). The PET studies included mostly ^{82}Rb as the tracer (1/15 with Copper-62) and only three were with PET/CT while the rest of the studies used line source for AC. The authors concluded that all three modalities have similar sensitivity. PET had better specificity and overall best diagnostic accuracy among the three modalities. However, this study had limitations, some of which are highlighted earlier. An important limitation was in allowing retrospective studies to be included in the analysis.

A more contemporary comparative meta-analysis of only SPECT and PET technology was undertaken by McArdle et al.[24] Inclusion criteria included prospective, observational, and retrospective studies as well as case series using either ^{82}Rb PET, or ^{99m}Tc SPECT with both ECG-gating and AC using either CT or radionuclide sources. Coronary angiogram was used as the reference standard for diagnosis of obstructive CAD. Fifteen PET comprising 1344 patients and 8 SPECT studies with 1755 patients, met their inclusion criteria. Using weighted averages proportional to the patient population size, sensitivities for PET and SPECT was 90% (CI 0.88–0.92) and 85% (CI 0.82–0.87), respectively, and specificities of 88% (CI 0.85–0.91) and 85% (CI 0.82–0.87), respectively, and ROC curve was 0.95 and 0.90 for PET and SPECT, respectively (P <0.0001) (Figure 1-2). Despite some limitations caused by referral bias and heterogeneity in the study population, this is an important study that confirmed that PET perfusion imaging is more accurate in detecting CAD despite technological advances in SPECT.

Another meta-analysis was reported by Parker et al.[25] The authors included only prospective studies and excluded any that explicitly stated that it was retrospective. Additionally, they used a bivariate random effects model, rather than pooled sensitivity and specificity from individual studies. They identified 117 studies, including 108 evaluating SPECT MPI, 4 evaluating PET MPI, and 5 evaluating both modalities. Bivariate meta-analysis demonstrated a significantly higher pooled mean sensitivity with PET [92.6% (95% confidence interval 88.3%-95.5%)] compared with SPECT [88.3% (95% confidence interval 86.4%-90.0%)] (P = 0.035). While the specificity for PET was higher than SPECT, the differences did not reach statistical significance [81.3% (95% confidence interval 66.6%-90.4%)] and SPECT [75.8% (95% confidence

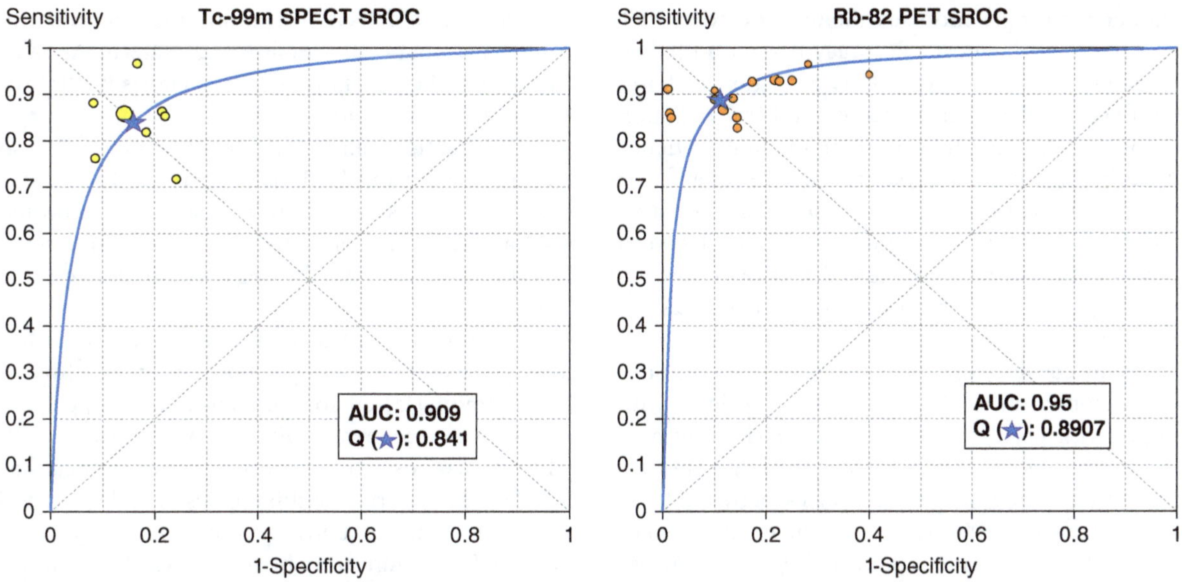

FIGURE 1-2 Summary receiver operating characteristic curves demonstrating superior diagnostic performance of MPI PET over SPECT. (Reproduced with permission from Mc Ardle BA, Dowsley TF, deKemp RA: Does rubidium-82 PET have superior accuracy to SPECT perfusion imaging for the diagnosis of obstructive coronary disease? A systematic review and meta-analysis, J Am Coll Cardiol. 2012 Oct 30;60(18):1828-37)

interval 72.1%-79.1%)] (P = 0.39). Thus, two major studies reported higher sensitivity for PET and improved overall diagnostic accuracy (Figure 1-3). The more general study of Parker reflecting current SPECT practice reported higher specificity as well although it did not reach statistical significance.

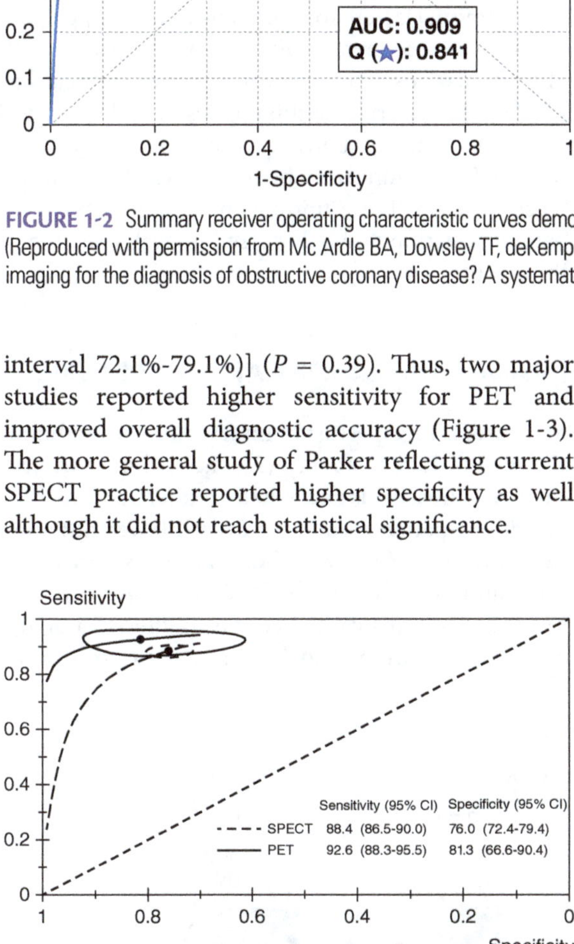

FIGURE 1-3 Summary receiver operating characteristic curves demonstrating superior diagnostic performance of MPI PET over SPECT. (Reproduced with permission from Parker MW, Iskandar A, Limone B: Diagnostic accuracy of cardiac positron emission tomography versus single photon emission computed tomography for coronary artery disease: a bivariate meta-analysis, Circ Cardiovasc Imaging 2012 Nov;5(6):700-707)

Using ^{13}N-ammonia PET/CT, a prospective study[26] was undertaken to assess the added diagnostic value of MPR independent to findings on relative perfusion images for predicting CAD (luminal narrowing ≥50%) using invasive coronary angiography as the reference standard. The study included 73 patients who underwent a standard adenosine protocol. The pretest likelihood of CAD was high in this patient group (73%). Per patient, the sensitivity, specificity, positive predictive value, negative predictive value, and accuracy of MPI for detecting significant CAD were 79%, 80%, 91%, 59%, and 79%, respectively. With a cutoff of less than 2.0 for global MPI to relative perfusion images findings improved the values to 96% (P <0.005), 80%, 93%, 89% (P <0.005), and 92% (P <0.005), respectively. The authors demonstrated that quantification of global MPR with ^{13}N-ammonia provides a substantial added diagnostic value, particularly improvement in sensitivity for detection of CAD, in a selective group of patients.

The diagnostic accuracy of cardiac PET has not been systematically evaluated in subgroups of patients, such as diabetic patients, women, and body habitus. However, a recent article by Taqueti and

Dorbala[27] strongly endorsed the use of cardiac PET in women for diagnostic accuracy based on the two meta-analysis studies as well as reduction of false-positives, excellent image quality and low radiation exposure, particularly important in these patients. In addition, a meta-analysis by Iskander et al[28] as a subevaluation of the study by Parker et al[25] found no difference in SPECT diagnostic accuracy between genders. Thus, it may be inferred that the improved accuracy reported by both Parker et al and McArdle et al applies to women.[24,25]

Many consider PET useful in obese patients only. In a comparison of PET and SPECT patients with similar risk profiles undergoing clinically indicated coronary angiography, Bateman et al did address gender and body weight accuracies between these two tests.[29] With 70% stenosis in one or more major vessels at catheterization, these authors reported significantly greater diagnostic accuracy for cardiac PET than SPECT regardless of gender (male and female) and body habitus (BMI >30 or <30). These findings are illustrated in Figure 1-4. Another important comparison in this study was the ability to correctly identify multivessel CAD at catheterization.[29] Bateman et al found that PET was significantly better at identifying two or greater vessel CAD than SPECT (71% vs 48%, P <0.001). An example of this is shown in Figure 1-5 of a patient who underwent a rest/stress SPECT and rest/stress PET study on the same day prior to catheterization. In Panel A is the rest/stress SPECT study demonstrating a reversible infero/lateral perfusion abnormality suggesting single vessel disease, while in Panel B the PET study demonstrated TID and reversible defects in the inferior, anterior, and lateral distributions, a multivessel pattern. At catheterization the patient had >70% stenosis in all three major vascular territories.

Diagnostic accuracy with cardiac PET can also be improved using MBF data, particularly in minimizing CAD likelihood. In a small study reported by Nava et al[30], the presence of normal MBF reserve (in this study >1.93), the negative predictive value was 97%.

In summary, the diagnostic accuracy of cardiac PET perfusion imaging with both tracers of ^{82}Rb and ^{13}N-ammonia is high for both sensitivity and specificity. In two large meta-analyses comparing PET with SPECT, diagnostic accuracy was higher with cardiac PET. Data supports that this applies to both male and female patients, is body habitus-independent, and that PET is significantly better at identifying multivessel disease. These findings have implications for patient selection, to be discussed in a later section of this chapter.

IMAGE QUALITY OF CARDIAC PET MPI

Myocardial PET perfusion imaging utilizes radionuclides with higher energy (511 keV), but with very short half-lives. This necessitates higher administered activity to patients but with overall lower radiation exposure owing to very short half-lives and better acquisition characteristics. PET imaging procedures result in high myocardial counts, higher spatial and contrast resolution, and high signal-to-noise ratio.

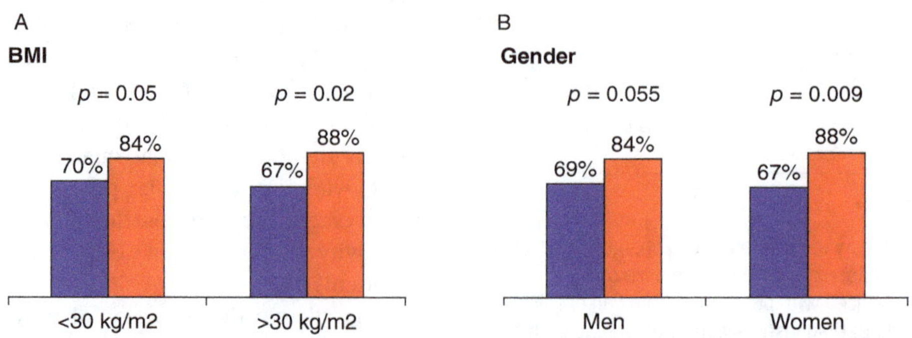

FIGURE 1-4 Comparison of sensitivities for PET (red) and SPECT (blue) in the subgroup analysis of Bateman et al[32] for BMI (A) and gender (B) demonstrating superior performance of PET MPI over SPECT in both subgroups.

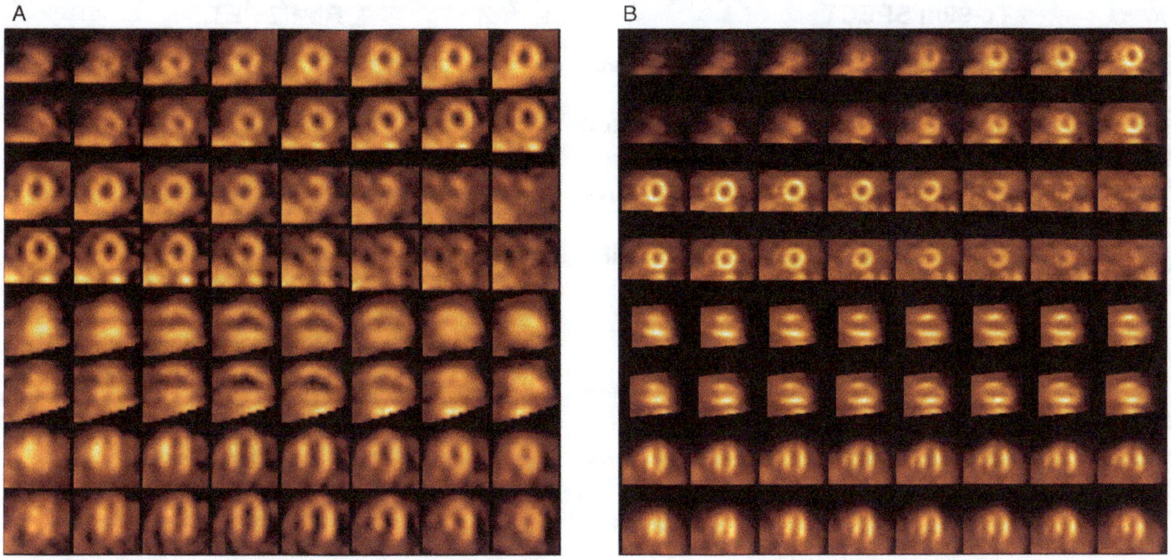

FIGURE 1-5 Patient who underwent a rest/stress SPECT and rest/stress PET study on the same day prior to catheterization; the (A) rest/stress SPECT study demonstrating a reversible infero/lateral perfusion abnormality suggesting single vessel disease, (B) PET study demonstrating TID and reversible defects in the inferior, anterior, and lateral distributions, a multivessel pattern. At catheterization the patient had >70% stenosis in all three major vascular territories.

Thus one would anticipate superb image quality. This was demonstrated by Yoshinaga et al[31] in which patients with equivocal SPECT studies were referred for ^{82}Rb cardiac PET imaging. In a very high percentage of patients, the PET study resulted in good to excellent image quality compared to the equivocal findings of SPECT. Using a comparison of similar but matched patients undergoing SPECT or PET, Bateman et al[32] also reported a significant improvement in image quality with PET over SPECT, with fewer equivocal reports.

The routine use of AC plus higher energy levels of PET tracers substantially reduces attenuation artifacts in images, in turn reducing the potential for false-positive studies for interpretation. This may be particularly useful in obese patients. It should be noted that obesity should not be a prerequisite for a cardiac PET examination. In a study by Bateman et al[32] the specificity of PET was significantly higher in comparison to SPECT, regardless of body habitus, including obese patients; see Figure 1-4. Similarly, in this study, patients who had equivocal SPECT studies were found to have diagnostically useful PET studies in 98% of the referred patients; this is exemplified in Figure 1-6 where an equivocal area of reduced perfusion on the ^{99m}Tc-SPECT/CT study is much more apparent on the ^{82}Rb PET/CT study. Additionally, the incidence of gut activity affecting interpretation was significantly and substantially reduced with PET in relation to pharmacologic SPECT. An example of image quality between SPECT and PET in the same patient is shown in Figure 1-7. As noted, considerably less gut and liver activity is observed in the PET study as well as uniformity in counts in the myocardium.

These results were also confirmed by Flotats et al.[33] In this study the imaging results were compared in 27 patients who underwent both rest/stress SPECT and PET. In a blinded read format, the image quality, interpretive certainty, and catherization results were all statistically significantly better with PET than SPECT.

In conclusion, image quality of cardiac PET studies in comparison to SPECT is significantly better for both rest and stress imaging. While this holds true for obese patients, it is not confined to those alone, particularly with regard to diagnostic confidence and, therefore, consideration should be given to the use of cardiac PET in any patient who is a candidate for either study.

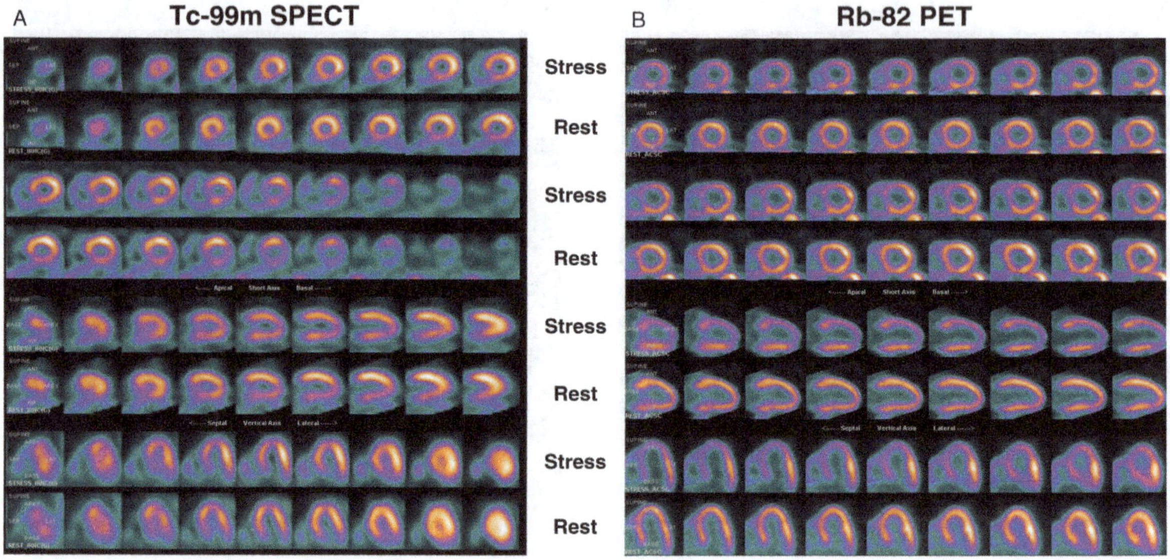

FIGURE 1-6 An example of increased diagnostic confidence when using PET over SPECT in a male patient with normal BMI. An equivocal antero-septal reversible defect on ^{99m}Tc SPECT (A) was more clearly visualized on the 82Rb PET study (B).

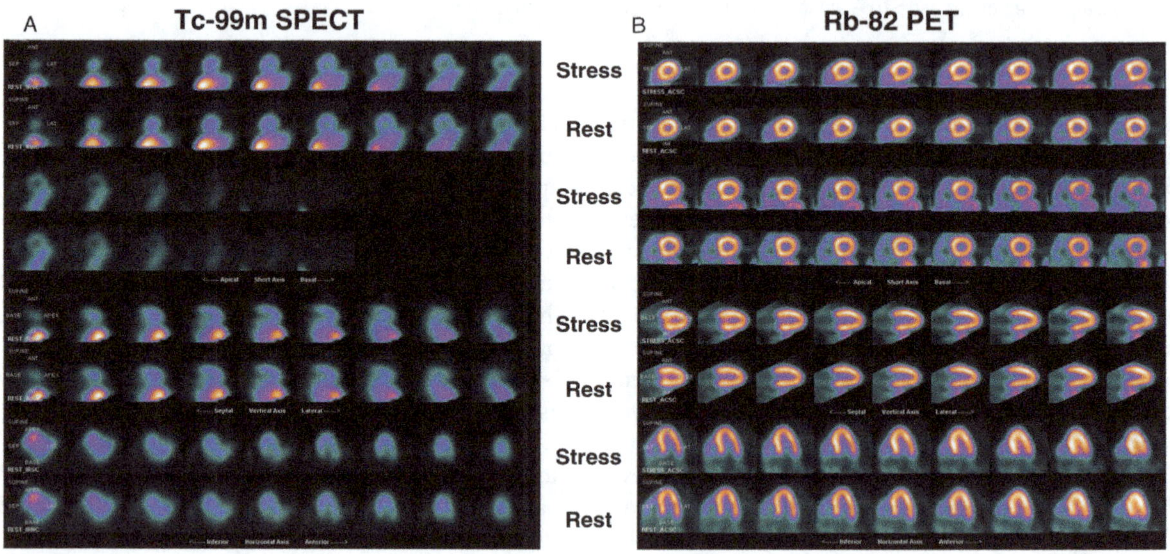

FIGURE 1-7 An example of image quality difference between SPECT (A) and PET (B) in the same patient. Considerably less gut and liver activity is noted in the PET study as well as improved uniformity in the myocardium.

UNIQUE ASPECTS OF CARDIAC PET

The acquisition of data with cardiac PET perfusion imaging is performed shortly after injection of tracer, particularly with ^{82}Rb, owing to short half-lives. For example, as described in the protocol section, acquisition of ^{82}Rb perfusion data is 90–120 seconds after tracer injection in contrast to SPECT acquisition, which occurs 45–60 minutes later. The implication of this is that data acquisition is accomplished under the hyperemic phase of both dipyridamole, and regadenoson infusion and shortly thereafter

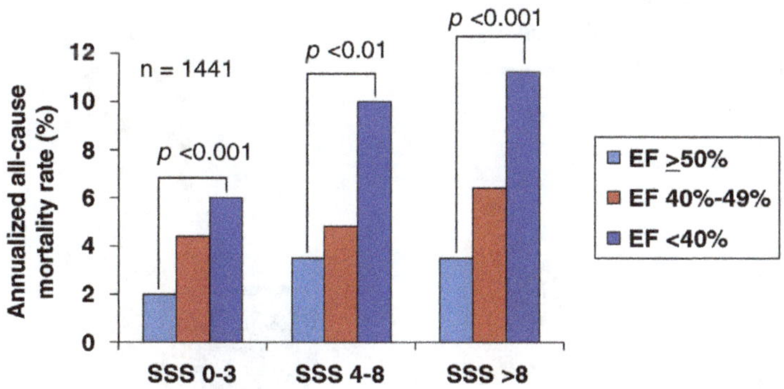

FIGURE 1-8 Incremental prognostic value of functional data derived from rubium-82 MPI studies. Patients with the worse outcomes had markedly abnormal perfusion and function. (Modified with permission from Lertsburapa K, Ahlberg AW, Bateman TM, et al: Independent and incremental prognostic value of left ventricular ejection fraction determined by stress gated rubidium 82 PET imaging in patients with known or suspected coronary artery disease, J Nucl Cardiol 2008 Nov-Dec;15(6):745-53)

adenosine. This has implications for such information as transient ischemic cavity dilation (TID) and stress-induced wall motion abnormalities and changes in ejection fraction (EF).

Transient ischemic cavity dilation (TID) with PET differs from SPECT in that the acquisition of data is still in a hyperemic phase of pharmacologic influence, particularly with the tracer ^{82}Rb. The protocol for ^{82}Rb begins collection of perfusion data 90–120 seconds after tracer injection. Thus, there could be true stress-induced cavity dilation, which is separate from subendocadial ischemia. Observational data have identified the presence of TID with both ^{82}Rb and ^{13}N-ammonia to be relatively common, perhaps more so than with SPECT. The presence of TID with PET is strongly associated with CAD, very uncommon without disease, and associated with both single vessel and multivessel conditions. As with SPECT, PET TID can be both visual and quantitative. Two studies have established that a TID ratio of 1.13–1.15 +/- 2 SD to be upper limits of normal.[34,35] In these studies, the presence of TID was associated with more extensive perfusion abnormalities and left ventricular dysfunction[35]; however, it was noted to be found in patients with single vessel ischemia as well as single vessel CAD at catherization.[34] Both studies concluded that TID was specific, but not necessarily sensitive. The differences between SPECT and PET TID need to be elucidated in future studies. Thus, the clinical value of TID is in supporting the diagnosis of CAD and may be an indication of more severe disease.

As with SPECT, left ventricular functional evaluation in the form of wall motion and overall EF has clinical value. It is generally accepted that in normal subjects, the PET EF rises about 5% during stress in relation to rest. Traditional examination of stress EF with cardiac PET has been shown to have prognostic value in more than 1600 patients and is complementary to perfusion data.[36] As shown in Figure 1-8, from that study, patients with the worse outcomes had markedly abnormal perfusion and function. Stress-induced wall motion abnormities as well as a fall in EF during stress are occasionally noted in SPECT but is more commonly observed with cardiac PET studies. The frequency of this finding in PET, as well as previously noted with TID most likely results from the rapid acquisition of data following tracer injection, thus in the hyperemic phase of the pharmaceutical drug. One of the first studies to note a relationship between change in EF between rest/stress cardiac PET and perfusion abnormalities was reported by Brown et al.[37] They reported an inverse relationship between negative change in LVEF between rest and stress and the presence and severity of PET perfusion abnormalities as well as reversibility. Dorbala and colleagues developed the concept of EF reserve, and drew an association between EF reserve <0 and severe reversibility and multivessel disease, while a less dramatic fall in EF was correlated with mild-moderate reversibility in more than 900 patients.[38] In a subsequent study, the same group examined the prognostic value of EF reserve.[39] In the latter study, they reported that an EF reserve of <0 (stress EF lower than rest) was associated with a significantly higher risk of all-cause mortality and cardiac death (Figure 1-9).

In summary, TID and wall motion/EF are both important aspects of cardiac PET MPI. Both differ in frequency and significance from SPECT, and have very important independent value in cardiac PET MPI.

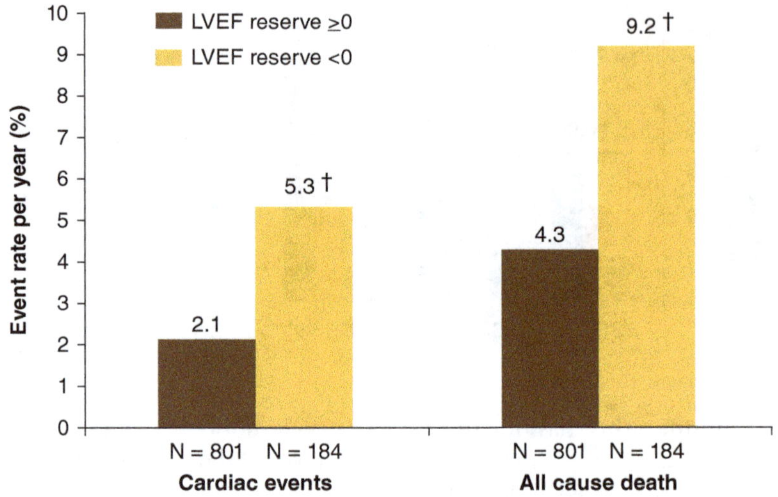

FIGURE 1-9 Adverse cardiac event rate and all cause death in patients with normal and abnormal LVEF reserve. Event rates were significantly lower for those patients with reserve <0%. (Reproduced with permission from Dorbala S, Hachamovitch R, Curillova Z et al: Incremental Prognostic Value of Gated Rb-82 Positron Emission Tomography Myocardial Perfusion Imaging over Clinical Variables and Rest LVEF, JACC Cardiovasc Imaging. 2009 Jul;2(7):846-854)

MYOCARDIAL BLOOD FLOW

MBF is discussed in detail in Chapters 4 and 5. This section is intended to give a brief introduction to this concept and its potential role in diagnosis and risk stratification complimentary to myocardial perfusion data with cardiac PET.

Myocardial perfusion SPECT and PET images are read in the clinical setting using nonlinear color display scaled to the highest uptake or counts in the myocardium within the data set (stress and rest images) and is often referred to as "relative images." The highest uptake does not equate to normal coronary blood flow because this is a semiquantitative measure. Hence, when reading relative perfusion images, there is a potential to miss balanced ischemia or underestimating relatively milder degree of stenosis in patients with multivessel disease. This can be overcome by measuring MBF in absolute terms, that is, in mL/g/min.

Dynamic list mode image acquisition during PET enables measuring myocardial blood input. Precise AC using CT or radionuclide source during PET and excellent scatter correction makes accurate estimation of myocardial uptake feasible. Hence, with the input and uptake measures, commercially available software is able to calculate absolute measurement of MBF at rest and during peak stress without the need for additional scanner time or radiation dose to the patient. Generally, the acquisition of the blood flow data is during the first 2 minutes after injection of tracer.

PET imaging is considered to be the most accurate noninvasive means to quantify MBF and myocardial perfusion reserve (MPR—the ratio of stress MBF and rest MBF). MBF is a composite measure of blood flow of the epicardial coronary vessels and the microvasculature. Hence, it can be affected by both coronary artery disease and microvasculature dysfunction. Whereas fractional flow reserve (FFR) is influenced by epicardial disease only, both focal and diffuse, and, hence, FFR and MBF/MPR reflect potentially different pathophysiological processes.

While ^{15}O has a linear relationship between myocardial uptake and blood flow, ^{13}N-ammonia is regarded as the more practical "gold standard" for measuring MBF. Generator-produced ^{82}Rb is the most convenient tracer to perform routine clinical myocardial perfusion studies as well as to measure MBF. Various commercial software systems are available for analysis of absolute MBF using ^{82}Rb PET, and results have compared favorably against other well-validated methods for MBF quantitation. Normal ranges for stress and rest MBF varies with the tracer and the rest MBF is dependent on heart rate, systolic blood pressure, and vascular resistance. The MBF values for ^{82}Rb tend to be lower than that of ^{13}N-ammonia and ^{15}O-water.

The clinical value of MBF assessment is for both diagnosis and prognosis. With regard to diagnosis, there is value in both the normal and abnormal blood flow in conjunction with PET perfusion data.[40] For diagnosis, the presence of both normal perfusion and normal MBF further reduces the likelihood of CAD. Some authors state the negative predictive value to be 97%-99%.[41] While the absolute number still needs to be confirmed, it is reasonable to state that the likelihood of "balanced ischemia" is substantially reduced in contrast to perfusion data alone in which the likelihood of CAD is higher (10%). The presence of abnormal blood flow with normal perfusion may indicate either small vessel disease or CAD and needs further evaluation. A final scenario of normal perfusion is that of blood flow data indicating no change between rest and stress. This indicates failure of augmentation of the pharmacologic stress and invalidates the study. Such a patient should be restudied after careful evaluation for causes, often relating to caffeine consumption. Abnormal blood flow in the presence of a perfusion abnormality is confirmatory, and at times can aid in the identification of more severe disease beyond the perfusion data alone. The technical aspects of MBF are presented in Chapter 4, while the clinical situations are further discussed in Chapter 5.

Prognostic data for cardiac PET blood flow are also available. A prospective study by Ziadi et al[42] evaluated nearly 700 patients who underwent ^{82}Rb PET and were split into normal and abnormal based on traditional summed stress scores. In each group, patients with abnormal MPR had a worse prognosis at 1-year follow-up when compared to patients with normal MPR. In addition, all cardiac deaths occurred in patients with abnormal MPR of less than 1.5. Reduced MPR in a single vascular territory was associated with a higher hard cardiac event rate when compared to patients with a normal global MPR. A larger study by Murthy et al[43] comprising 2783 patients who underwent ^{82}Rb PET were followed up for a median of 1.4 years. Compared to an MPR >2, an intermediate MPR (1.5< MFR <2) was associated with a 5.7-fold increased risk of cardiac death and an MPR <1.5 was associated with a 16-fold increased risk. These two studies confirmed the value of routinely incorporating blood flow measurement in clinical practice because it provided incremental prognostic information to relative perfusion images. MPR of less than 2 carries an adverse prognosis even in the presence of a normal or mildly abnormal perfusion scan and, hence, helps better risk stratification of patients and thus potentially change patient management and a MPR of less than 1.5 is associated with higher incidence of cardiac death.

Gupta et al evaluated the prognostic value of hyperemic MBF and MPR in a prospective study comprising 4029 patients with a mean follow-up of 5.6 years.[44] Based on a threshold for impaired hyperemic MBF of 1.8 $mL \cdot g^{-1} \cdot min^{-1}$ and MPR of greater than 2, they subdivided the patients into four groups based on concordant or discordant values of the two blood flow parameters. Based on univariate analysis, those patients with concordantly impaired hyperemic MBF and MPR had the highest cardiovascular mortality (3.3%). The event rate was 0.9% with preserved MPR but impaired hyperemic MBF and 0.4% in those with preserved MPR and hyperemic MBF. Using multivariate analysis, impaired MPR was the main determinant of cardiovascular mortality risk gradient across the four groups and was independent of impairment in maximal MBF. The authors concluded that MPR is a better predictor of cardiovascular mortality than hyperemic MBF.

In conclusion, the combination of myocardial perfusion data with MBF is powerful and is now being implemented into many laboratories performing cardiac PET. Blood flow data is helpful in reducing the likelihood of CAD, discovering when the pharmacologic stress is not effective in assisting in diagnosis of CAD, and an independent predictor of outcomes. Chapter 5 discusses MBF in greater detail.

RISK STRATIFICATION OF CARDIAC PET MYOCARDIAL PERFUSION IMAGING

The prognostic value of SPECT MPS has been established in many thousands of patients demonstrating that the size and severity of a perfusion abnormality is related to outcomes. Conversely, a normal scan is associated with an annual hard cardiac event rate of less than 1% for patients undergoing exercise, but approximately 2-fold higher with pharmacologic stress. While not as extensive as the SPECT, data are now accumulating supporting the prognostic value of cardiac PET.[1–5] The number of patients included in the PET MPS data is currently in the thousands and shows similar relationships to SPECT. Of note, the hard cardiac event rate in a setting of a normal PET MPS is less than 1%, despite being in the setting

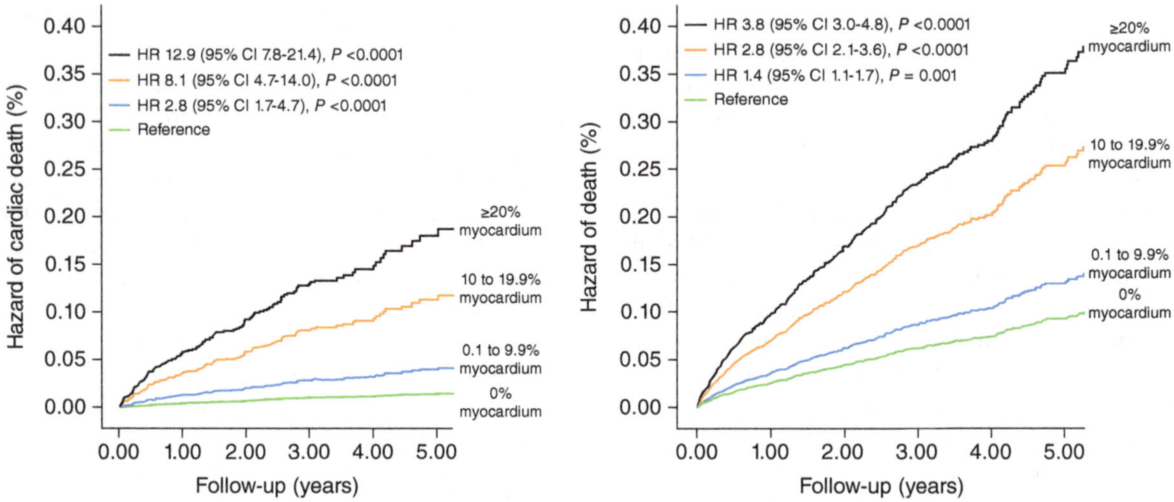

FIGURE 1-10 Risk-adjusted hazard of cardiac death by extent of abnormal myocardium on ^{82}Rb stress PET. PET MPS reclassified risk of cardiac death in 11.6% of patients when compared with risk factors as cited in the text and hence potentially changed patient management. (Data from Marwick TH, Shan K, Patel S et al: Incremental value of rubidium-82 positron emission tomography for prognostic assessment of known or suspected coronary artery disease, Am J Cardiol. 1997 Oct 1;80(7):865-870)

of pharmacologic stress.[45,46] This may have clinical importance for downstream evaluation, perhaps being less necessary than after pharmacologic SPECT.

A multicenter trial of more than 7000 patients to determine the prognostic value of Rb PET MPS was published in 2013 by Dorbala et al.[46] The mean follow-up was 2.2 years. The extent and severity of ischemia and scar added incremental prognostic value when compared with traditional CAD risk factors like age, female sex, BMI, hypertension, diabetes, dyslipidemia, smoking, angina, beta blocker use, prior revascularization, and resting heart rate. PET MPS reclassified risk of cardiac death in 11.6% of patients when compared with risk factors cited earlier and, hence, potentially changed patient management (Figure 1-10). This study classified risk on the basis of myocardium at risk (0% to >20%) and demonstrated clear separation of outcomes by several categories. Thus, these data suggest not only very low risk for normal studies, but gradations to help caretakers make clinical decisions. It should be noted that the mean radiation exposure to a patient in this study was approximately 3 mSv, considerably lower than a comparable SPECT study.

PET MPS has superior imaging characteristics including the use of scatter and AC when compared to SPECT and hence has improved specificity and diagnostic accuracy particularly in patients with high BMI. Chow et al investigated the prognostic value of pharmacological ^{82}Rb PET MPI in normal, overweight, and obese patients.[47] Seven thousand sixty-one patients were entered in a multicenter observational registry. The patients were followed for cardiac death and all-cause mortality for a median of 2.2 years. Based on body mass index (BMI), patients were categorized as normal (<25 kg·m2), overweight (25–29.9 kg·m2), or obese (>30 kg·m2). The mean BMI was 30.5 ± 7.4 kg·m2. A normal PET MPI conferred an excellent prognosis with very low annual cardiac death rates –0.38% in those patients with a normal BMI, 0.43% in overweight patients, and 0.15% in obese patients. In addition, in the moderately and severe obese patients, a normal PET MPI had excellent prognosis (0.20% and 0.10%, respectively). The net reclassification improvement of PET was 0.46 (95% confidence interval [CI] 0.31–0.61) and appeared similar in the moderately and severe obese patients, which were 0.44 (95% CI 0.12–0.76) and 0.63 (95% CI 0.27–0.98), respectively. This study demonstrates the incremental prognostic value of Rb PET irrespective of the patient's BMI. These findings are also supported by a more recent smaller study by Harnett et al[48] who investigated 108 patients with BMI ≥40 kgm^{-2} undergoing either SPECT (n = 57) or ^{82}Rb PET (n = 51) imaging, with angiographic following within 6 months. They found that PET gave more definite normal or abnormal results when compared to SPECT (83.3% vs 60.5%, respectively, P <0.01) and offered greater diagnostic accuracy in this extreme obesity cohort.

The previous studies reported on general populations. The prognostic value of cardiac MPI PET in women was recently reported by Kay et al.[49] They included a total of 6037 women and men were enrolled in the PET Prognosis Multicentre Registry. Patients were followed up for cardiac death with a median follow-up of 2.2 years.

The 5-year mortality was 3.7% for women and 6.0% for men (P <0.0001). Unadjusted CAD mortality ranged from 0.9% to 12.9% for women (P <0.0001) and from 1.5% to 17.4% for men (P <0.0001) for 0% to ≥15% abnormal myocardium at stress. In multivariable models, the percentage of abnormal stress myocardium was independently predictive of CAD mortality in women and men. An interaction term of gender by the percentage of abnormal stress myocardium was nonsignificant (P = 0.39). The categorical net reclassification improvement (NRI) when ^{82}Rb PET data were added to a clinical risk model was 0.12 for women and 0.17 for men. Only two cardiac deaths were reported in women <55 years of age; accordingly, the percentage of abnormal myocardium at stress was of borderline significance (P = 0.063), but it was highly significant for women ≥55 years of age (P <0.0001), with an increased NRI of 0.21 (95% confidence interval: 0.09–0.34), including 17% of CAD deaths and 3.9% of CAD survivors that were correctly reclassified in this older female subset.

Data are also available with risk classification based on both perfusion data and ventricular function. In the study by Lertsburapa et al[36] of more than 1600 patients undergoing PET perfusion and function, the highest risk category was that of low EF and large perfusion abnormalities (see Figure 1-8). Rest-only ^{82}Rb PET has been demonstrated to also have value in the early risk stratification for STEMI patients undergoing PCI. In a small study, Ghotbi et al[50] demonstrated that the segmental extent of hypoperfusion was significantly associated with the infarct size at 3 months, demonstrated by late gadolinium enhancement cardiac-MR.

There has recently been interest in the literature regarding the application of a hybrid approach to cardiovascular imaging. It has been demonstrated that PET perfusion imaging used in a sequential hybrid strategy along with coronary CTA improves risk stratification of patients with suspected obstructive coronary artery disease (CAD). Maaniitty et al[51] investigated 864 consecutive patients with intermediate probability of CAD. All patients underwent coronary CTA in the first instance, of which 47% had suspected obstructive CAD and underwent a PET perfusion study using $H_2{}^{15}O$. Subsequently, 49% of those undergoing PET perfusion imaging had normal perfusion and a significantly lower annual rate of adverse events compared to those with abnormal perfusion (0.5% vs 2.5%, P = 0.004), and close to the annualized rate for patients with normal and nonobstructive coronary CTA results (0.4%). However, because the "normal-CTA" cohort underwent no further investigation, the diagnostic accuracy of the combined approach could not be assessed because the number of false-negatives was not determined.

Furthermore, the aforementioned authors only investigated PET as a secondary modality to CTA and, hence, did not evaluate the performance of PET alone, with the earlier results only highlighting the high sensitivity and poorer specificity of CTA. On a per-patient basis, Danad et al[52] demonstrated that $H_2{}^{15}O$ PET indeed has similar sensitivity (87% vs 90%) but higher specificity (84% vs 60%) when compared to CTA alone, using FFR as the gold standard. When analyzing a combined approach, the authors found that while specificity increased, there was a reduction in sensitivity of the hybrid approach owing to an increase in false-negative findings. Thus, the authors argue, a hybrid approach would affect clinical decision making in an unfavorable manner. This conclusion is supported by a recent editorial affirming the importance of physiology over a hybrid approach.[53]

Thus, accumulating data demonstrate that rest/stress PET provides significant and clinically meaningful effective risk stratification of women and men, supporting this modality as an alternative to comparative imaging modalities. PET findings were particularly helpful at identifying high-risk, older women.

RADIATION EXPOSURE DATA

In the United States alone, myocardial perfusion imaging is the greatest contributor to public medical exposures, accounting for a fifth of the total effective dose from all procedures performed between 2005 and 2008.[54] When compared to other regions across the world, Latin and North America contribute the greatest radiation burden for myocardial perfusion imaging, with median effective doses of 12.1–12.8 mSv, nearly 40% higher than in Europe, 8.8 mSv.[55] Appropriate selection of patients, technology, and radiopharmaceutical, therefore, are vital in reducing public radiation exposure, along with occupational doses received by staff performing the examinations. Radiation exposure with cardiac PET to both patients and personnel is substantially lower than with standard SPECT.

Patient Radiation Exposure With Cardiac PET

The effective radiation dose to the patient inherently depends on the protocol and radiopharmaceutical used. Traditionally, ^{99m}Tc-based SPECT has been the method of choice, implementing either a one- or two-day protocol. The guideline administered activities for these procedures are relatively high, ranging from 8 to 45 mCi per administration for a one-day protocol and 20–40 mCi for a 2-day ^{99m}Tc-tetrofosmin protocol[54], resulting in combined effective doses of 8.5–12.7 mSv.[57] In comparison, radiation doses from current, state-of-the-art technologies such as ^{82}Rb and ^{13}N-ammonia myocardial perfusion PET are substantially lower. Depending on the generation and technology (2D vs 3D) of the scanner used, activities administered for ^{82}Rb are generally 20–60 mCi; resulting in a combined stress and rest effective dose of 1.9–5.4 mSv.[58] These findings were confirmed by Hunter et al in a single-center study in which the PET radiation exposure was calculated to be as low as 1–3 mSv.[59] For ^{13}N-ammonia administered activities of 10–20 mCi result in a similar effective dose of 2.0–4.0 mSv.[60] For overall cardiac PET radiation exposure in the United States, a recent study by Desiderio et al confirmed that radiation exposure to patients using either ^{82}Rb or NH_3 ammonia was on average 3.59 mSv in 122 accredited laboratories by the Intersocietal Accreditation Commission.[61] The effective dose to the patient for all the earlier examinations would be increased by approximately 0.5 mSv if low-dose CT is used for AC purposes.

Staff Radiation Exposure With Cardiac PET

A consequence of lower radiation exposure to patients is a reduction in the occupational exposure to members of staff. It has been demonstrated that radiation exposures to staff during routine ^{82}Rb myocardial perfusion PET, when following good radiation protection practice, such as maximizing distance and reducing contact times, are in the order of 0.4 μSv per procedure.[62,63] This is significantly lower than for routine ^{99m}Tc SPECT studies, with procedural doses reported to be almost an order of magnitude higher at 3.3 μSv.

In conclusion, there is a growing literature for radiation exposure to patients and staff using cardiac PET. The radiation exposure for both patients and staff are considerably lower than with standard SPECT protocols.

PROTOCOLS FOR PET MYOCARDIAL PERFUSION IMAGING

Acquisition protocols for PET/CT MPI are dependent on the isotope used as well as whether line-source or CT AC is applied. The two main cardiac PET isotopes routinely used for MPI are the short-lived ^{82}Rb, ^{82}Rb, with half-life of 76 seconds, and the longer-lived nitrogen-13 in the form of ^{13}N-ammonia, with a half-life of 9.96 minutes. Time must be allowed for sufficient decay of the isotope between sequential acquisitions so that later images are not contaminated with residual activity; for ^{82}Rb this is typically around 10 minutes, whereas longer delays of 30–40 minutes are required for ^{13}N-ammonia. This period is short enough to allow both rest and stress acquisitions to be performed in one appointment without removing the patient from the imaging couch. Figure 1-11 shows typical acquisition protocols for ^{82}Rb and ^{13}N-ammonia.

Attenuation Correction

Two methods exist for the correction of attenuation in PET imaging depending on the generation of technology; these either use rotating rod sources containing germanium-68 or cesium-127 to acquire a transmission scan, or implement an integrated CT subsystem.

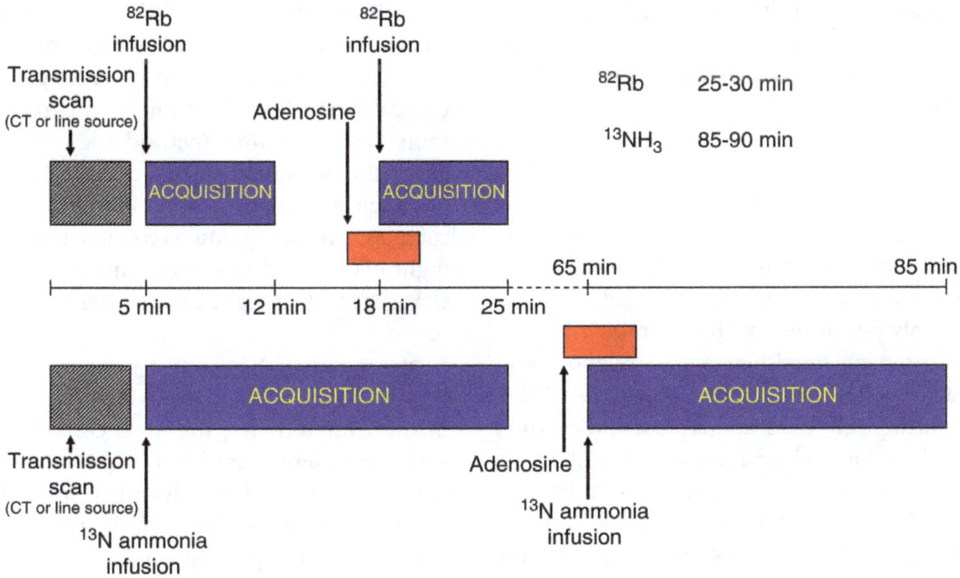

FIGURE 1-11 Comparison of rest-stress acquisition protocols for ^{82}Rb (top) and ^{13}N-ammonia (bottom), both using adenosine as the pharmacological stressing agent.

Transmission scans have the advantage that the attenuation and emission energies are matched and, therefore, no scaling or conversion takes place. However, depending on count-rate, the transmission scan can add between 60 seconds and 10 minutes onto the emission study and they do not offer an accurate portrayal of the underlying anatomy. For these reasons, they have been largely superseded in modern commercial systems by the use of CT.

For CT-based AC, an initial topogram is used to define the limits of the PET and CT acquisitions. To facilitate dynamic acquisitions, this is generally restricted to one PET field-of-view (FoV). On some modern scanners, with several detector rings, this allows data to be acquired from the carina to the superior aspect of the diaphragm, with the myocardium positioned centrally where the sensitivity of the PET scanner is most uniform. A low-dose CT, typically less than 0.5 mSv, is acquired (10–20 mAs, 120 kV) for purposes of AC and immediately followed by the PET acquisition to ensure accurate anatomical registration.

Careful quality control of the registration between the CT and emission data is required to ensure accurate quantitative reconstruction. The majority of misalignments tend to be small and translational in nature; hence, they can be compensated for by software-based registration. More complex patient motion, such as rotation, or gross misalignment, would require a repeat of the AC scan. Because of the short delay between rest and stress imaging, therefore, the need for a repeat AC scan is infrequent.

Rest

Administered activity depends on the sensitivity and generation of the scanner. For ^{82}Rb, higher activities of around 1480–2040 MBq (40–60 mCi), are recommended for 2-dimensional scanners. For higher sensitivity 3-dimensional scanners, activities can be reduced to 1110–1480 MBq (30–40 mCi) for system utilizing (LSO) detectors, or further to 370–740 MBq (10–20 mCi) for bismuth germinate (BGO).[64] Caution is advised for high count-rate situations, however, because saturation of the detector blocks can occur[65], causing inaccuracies in the estimation of quantitative parameters.[66] For ^{13}N-ammonia, the administered activity is lower, around 370–740 MBq (10–20 mCi), with 3-dimensional scanners permitting scanning at the lower range of activities.[67] Guidelines for maximal activities and corresponding performance metrics (including peak prompts, singles, and dead-time factors) have been reported in the literature for ^{82}Rb and ^{13}N-ammonia[66] for a range of commercial scanners and can be used as a guide to reduce bias in quantitation when implementing clinical protocols.

Stress

Administered activities follow the same protocol as for the rest acquisition, although pharmacological stressing with adenosine, dipyridamole, or regadenoson is most commonly performed, with the tracer infusion timed to occur at maximal hyperemia. Adenosine is infused at a rate of 140 μg kg^{-1} min^{-1} for between 4 and 6 minutes, starting 120–150 seconds prior to the radioactive tracer infusion and data acquisition. Although potentially more tolerable for patients, the termination of the shorter durations within the acquisition window can lead to increased patient motion.[68] Regadenoson injection follows the recommended protocol at a standardized dose of 400 μg over 10–20 seconds followed by a 10-second saline flush, with the tracer administration and data acquisition beginning 50 seconds after the start of the regadenoson injection. Exercise stress, although technically challenging because of the half-lives of the isotopes used, can be performed for both ^{82}Rb and ^{13}N-ammonia[69,70]; however, only static and gated images can be reconstructed owing to the delay from infusion at peak stress to positioning and starting the PET acquisition.

Reconstruction

Acquisition is preferably performed in list-mode, starting at the point at which activity enters the camera field of view, and lasting for 7 minutes (^{82}Rb) or 15–20 minutes (^{13}N-ammonia). This allows for dynamic reconstructions to be performed, capturing the tracer kinetics, along with the traditional static and gated reconstructions. The latter reconstructions should incorporate a delay of typically around 150 seconds to allow for clearance of the tracer from the blood pool. A quality control image can also be reconstructed based on the initial data, which allows for CT registration to be checked and adjusted, prior to the subsequent reconstructions. Ordered-subset expectation maximization (OSEM) reconstruction is preferred, although filtered back projection (FBP) can be used for reconstruction of the data. It is recommended that for ^{82}Rb studies, data are reconstructed with compensation for prompt gamma emission. When deriving kinetic parameters for clinical evaluation, it is important to note that the same reconstruction methodology should be used as for the derivation of reference values. However, it has been demonstrated that incorporating methods, such as prompt gamma compensation[71], time-of-flight (TOF), and resolution modeling[72], can lead to changes in the dynamic parameters derived.

Pharmacologic Stress Agents

In the United States, the most common pharmacologic stress agent used is regadenoson, followed by dipyridamole, and finally adenosine. Recent data suggest that for regadenoson the ideal time to inject tracer to capture peak hyperemia is 90–120 seconds, in contrast to the company-recommended 30 seconds.[73] This is true for dipyridamole stress as well.

INDICATIONS FOR CARDIAC PET PERFUSION IMAGING

Cardiac PET perfusion studies offer high diagnostic accuracy and image quality, short protocols, low radiation exposure, and now additional information from MBF data. Thus, this test provides considerable value to the patient who qualifies and for the reasons mentioned earlier supersedes current SPECT procedures. The decision for performing cardiac PET rather than another noninvasive imaging study should reflect those advantages to the patient. In general, thought processes favoring PET have been in the direction of patients unable to exercise, because of short half-lives of PET tracers. Until very recently, there has been little guidance from professional societies, because neither recommendations for Appropriate Use Criteria nor ASNC/ACC Guidelines made distinctions between imaging procedures. This has now changed, because a joint position statement[74] was endorsed and published by the American Society of Nuclear Cardiology (ASNC) and the Society of Nuclear Medicine and Molecular Imaging (SNMMI) that addressed the patient choices between cardiac PET and other noninvasive options. These professional societies stated that PET was the "preferred test" for patients recommended

Table 1-2

Joint ASNC/SNMMI Position Statement on Patients Suitable for Cardiac PET Perfusion Imaging

	Preferred	Recommended
Unable to complete an ETT	✓	
Prior poor-quality stress imaging		✓
Anticipated significant attenuation artifact		✓
High-risk patients in whom diagnostic errors carry even greater clinical implications		✓
Anticipated repeated radiation exposure, to minimize exposure		✓
Patients in whom myocardial blood flow quantification is identified by clinicians to be a needed adjunct to the image findings		✓

(Data from Memmott MJ, Tonge CM, Saint KS et al: Impact of pharmacological stress agent on patient motion during rubidium-82 myocardial perfusion PET/CT, J Nucl Cardiol. 2017 Jan 4)

for pharmacologic stress imaging in both patients with suspected or known coronary artery disease that met proper indications. The societies also extended their position on PET as a "recommended test" for several patient conditions beyond pharmacologic stress alone, as noted in Table 1-2 and discussed in the next sections.

Preferred: Rest-stress myocardial perfusion PET is a first-line preferred test for patients with suspected or known CAD who meet the appropriate criteria, are unable to complete a diagnostic exercise test, and for pharmacological stress imaging (pharmacological vasodilator) should be considered for cardiac PET.

Recommended: This group of patients are those with known or suspected CAD who meet the appropriate criteria for stress imaging and fall into one of the subgroups listed below. These patients may be able to complete an exercise stress but for the following reasons are still to be considered for PET:

a. Patients with previous equivocal or inconclusive stress imaging study owing to poor image quality or affected by artefacts, or in those patients for whom the findings are discordant with clinical impressions or other diagnostic test results including findings at coronary angiography.
b. Patients with body characteristics that commonly affect image quality; examples include dense or large breasts, breast implants, obesity, protuberant abdomen, and potential truncation artefacts caused by limited SPECT and CT attenuation field of view such as arm positioning.
c. High-risk patients and those with high pretest likelihood of CAD in whom accurate diagnosis is critical. Some examples are those with advanced kidney disease (CKD Stage 3,4,5), diabetic patients; known or suspected potentially high-risk CAD, such as left main stem, multivessel, or proximal LAD disease, previous coronary artery bypass grafting and percutaneous coronary intervention; those with suspected ischemic LV dysfunction, suspected cardiac transplant vasculopathy; and those for whom revascularization carries an increased morbidity and mortality. Several of these patients would potentially benefit from MBF quantitation in addition to relative PET perfusion images to better risk stratify them.
d. Young patients with established CAD who are anticipated to need repeated exposures to radiation-associated cardiac imaging procedures (who are not suitable to undergo functional imaging modalities that do not expose patients to radiation), in order to minimize accumulated lifetime exposure.
e. Patients in whom MBF quantification is identified by clinicians to be a needed adjunct to the image findings, to better identify or exclude multivessel CAD, for improved risk stratification, and when assessment of microcirculatory function is needed for clinical decision making.

This document elucidates the current patients in whom cardiac PET would be most useful. If longer acting agents for PET perfusion such as F-18 (2-hour half-life) are developed, this may be extended. It is also understood that, in other countries, exercise may be seen as of lesser consideration for the diagnostic procedure and therefore a pharmacologic stress PET may be preferred even in patients who have reasonable exercise capacity. In those laboratories utilizing NH_3 ammonia, this may also be an option even in the United States.

NEW PERFUSION TRACERS FOR CARDIAC PET

This chapter has described the strengths and benefits of the current practice of cardiac PET. An important aspect of this modality is what investors call the "pipeline." Industry has turned to cardiac PET as a potential market for development of new tracers, including those for myocardial perfusion imaging. Agents in development include neuronal imaging, ischemic memory, and myocardial perfusion imaging potential. Because this book focuses on current PET, we felt that it was beyond the scope of this chapter to present conceptual data on several agents that are far from approval. An exception is that of F-18 Flurpiridaz. This agent has completed the first Phase 3 FDA study and the company responsible, Lantheus Medical Imaging, just announced an agreement with GE Healthcare to complete the Phase 3 requirements and apply for approval. Given that this agent may arrive in the clinical area within the next few years, this tracer in development is discussed briefly.

Fluorine F-18 as a Cardiac PET Myocardial Perfusion Imaging Tracer

At present, cardiac PET myocardial perfusion imaging is limited to two primary agents, ^{82}Rb and NH_3-ammonia. The latter, ^{13}N-ammonia, has not gained wide acceptance primarily because of the cyclotron production and necessity for close proximity to the PET laboratory. ^{82}Rb is limited by its very short half-life of 76 seconds, necessitating an on-site generator and applicability only to pharmacologic stress. These factors have limited the growth of cardiac PET because a critical volume of patients is necessary and patients who are able to complete exercise remain in the realm of SPECT imaging. A Fluorine F-18 tracer may change that equation considerably.

Fluorine F-18 has a half-life of 110 minutes and is cyclotron-produced. In the United States, F-18 has been extensively used for PET oncology in the form of FDG F-18 imaging. Cyclotrons are available throughout the country for this purpose. Because of the longer half-life, there are several opportunities not available to ^{82}Rb for use in cardiology. First, production can be several hours away, providing regional production and distribution. Second, because of this longer half-life, it can be ordered as a "unit dose" for the number of patients to be studied on a given day, in contrast to the monthly on-site generator of ^{82}Rb. Thus, a laboratory can control costs on the basis of the number of studies being performed. Finally, any ^{18}F tracer developed for PET myocardial perfusion imaging can be utilized not only for pharmacologic stress but for exercise as well. If data for an F-18 perfusion were to become available demonstrating superiority to other imaging options, this would open PET imaging to a much larger patient group and allow "stress-only" imaging as well.

F-18 Flurpiridaz as a PET Myocardial Perfusion Imaging Tracer

There are several F-18 myocardial perfusion imaging agents in developmental stage. The only one with FDA Phase 1, 2, and 3 data is that of F-18 Flurpiridaz. Flurpiridaz, chemical name 18F-BMS747158-02, is an analog of the insecticide, pyridaben, an inhibitor of mitochondrial complex I (MC-1), and has been shown to be nontoxic. Of considerable importance for any tracer is its relationship to MBF. In an animal study reported by Yu et al[75], a study of a wide range of blood flow, there was near linearity of this agent up to over 4.5 mL/min/g, the peak of hyperemic range for available pharmacologic stress compounds (Figure 1-12).

This was particularly striking in comparison to two SPECT agents, thallium-201 and Tc-99 m sestamibi, in which nonlinearity occurred well within the exercise and pharmacologic stress range (2–4 mL/min/g. In addition, these authors reported excellent myocardial retention while liver counts dropped over time. These results indicate excellent characteristics for identification of CAD in humans. A Phase 1 study reported the safety and image analysis of the product in humans.[76] A Phase 2 trial evaluated 132 patients who underwent cardiac catheterization following both a rest/stress Tc-99 m study as well as a

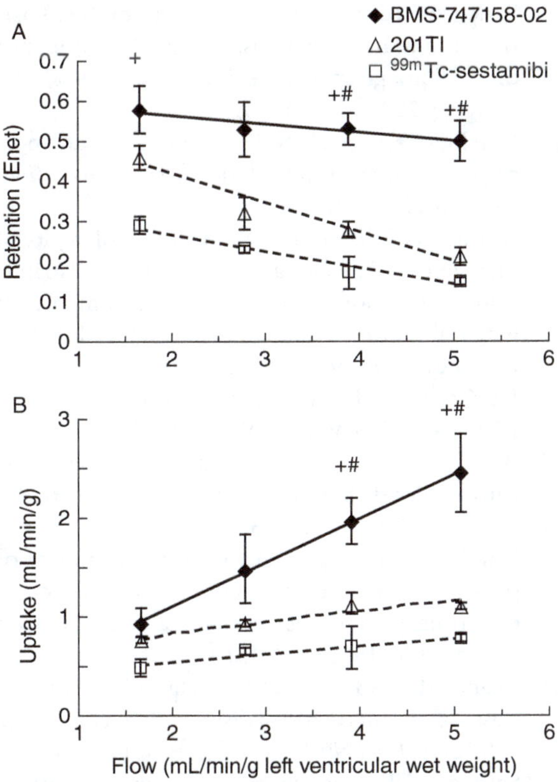

FIGURE 1-12 Comparison of retention (A) and uptake (B) of BMS-747158-02, Tl-201 and Tc99m-Sestamibi at increasing flow rates in an isolated perfused rabbit heart. (Data from Chow B.J., Ananthasubramaniam K, deKemp R.A. et al: Comparison of Treadmill Exercise versus Dipyridamole Stress with Myocardial Perfusion Imaging Using Rubidium-82 Positron Emission Tomography, J Am Coll Cardiol. 2005 Apr 19;45(8):1227-1234)

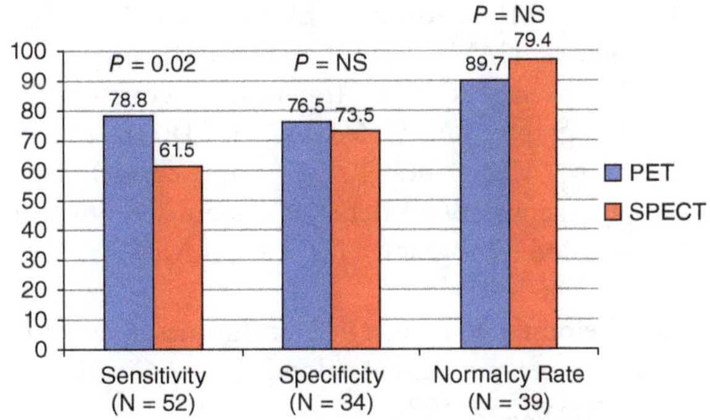

FIGURE 1-13 Comparison of sensitivity and specificity for F18-flurpiridax PET MPI and SPECT MPI in the detection of CAD.

rest/stress F-18 Flurpiridaz study.[77] An additional 39 patients underwent both evaluations and were considered low likelihood patients. Berman et al[77] reported statistically significantly higher image quality and diagnostic certainty. The diagnostic accuracy of Flurpiridaz was also significantly higher (sensitivity 79% vs 61% favoring Flurpiridaz; Figure 1-13).

Phase 3 data have been presented in abstract form only but confirm the striking improvement in sensitivity in a much larger population of 795 patients who also underwent both imaging protocols and cardiac catheterization.[78] The larger trial confirmed the high diagnostic accuracy differences in important subsets of patients: women, obese patients, and patients undergoing exercise for both protocols.[78] In conclusion this promising F-18 myocardial perfusion imaging agent has excellent flow characteristics that appear significantly better than those of existing SPECT agents as well as very promising data on image quality, diagnostic certainty, and diagnostic accuracy. It is anticipated that the second Phase 3 trial will begin in the calendar year of 2017.

CONCLUSIONS: CARDIAC PET MYOCARDIAL PERFUSION IMAGING

Cardiac PET myocardial perfusion imaging has become an increasingly popular method of assessing patients with known or suspected CAD. This chapter has outlined the potential benefits of this procedure for appropriate patients, such as high diagnostic accuracy, high image quality, fast procedures, low radiation exposure, unique data gained, and beneficial risk stratification. The chapter also provides insights into the best patients for cardiac PET MPI based on new recommendations from professional societies.

REFERENCES

1. Wrenn FR Jr, Good ML, Handler P. The use of positron-emitting radioisotopes for the localization of brain tumors. *Science.* 1951;113(2940):525–527.
2. Brownell GL, Sweet WH. Localization of brain tumors with positron emitters *Nucleonics.* 1953;11(30).
3. Burnham CA, Aronow S, Brownell GL. A hybrid positron scanner. *Phys Med Biol.* 1970;15(3):517–528.

4. Phelps ME, Hoffman EJ, Mullani NA, Ter-Pogossian MM. Application of annihilation coincidence detection to transaxial reconstruction tomography. *J Nucl Med.* 1975;16(3):210–224.
5. Casey ME, Nutt R. A multi-crystal two-dimensional BGO detector system for positron emission tomography. *IEEE Trans Nucl Sci.* 1985; NS33:460–463.
6. Schelbert HR et al. N-13 ammonia as an indicator of myocardial blood flow. *Circulation.* 1981;63:1259–1272.
7. Krivokapich et al. 13N ammonia myocardial imaging at rest and stress with exercise in normal volunteers. *Circulation.* 1989;80(5):1328–1337.
8. Selwyn AP, Allan RM, L'Abbate A et al. Relation between regional myocardial uptake of rubidium-82 and perfusion: absolute reduction of cation uptake in ischemia. *Am J Cardiol.* 1982;50(1):112–121.
9. Gould KL, Goldstein RA, Mullani NA et al. Noninvasive assessment of coronary stenoses by myocardial perfusion imaging during pharmacologic coronary vasodilation. VIII. Clinical feasibility of positron cardiac imaging without a cyclotron using generator-produced rubidium-82. *J Am Coll Cardiol.* 1986;7(4):775–789.
10. Yoshinaga K, Klein R, Tamaki N et al. Generator-produced rubidium-82 positron emission tomography myocardial perfusion imaging: from basic aspects to clinical applications. *J Nucl Cardiol.* 2010;55(2):163–173.
11. Mullani NA et al. Myocardial perfusion with rubidium-82. I. Measurement of extraction fraction and flow with external detectors. *J Nucl Med.* 1983;24:898–906.
12. Lortie M, Beanlands RS, Yoshinaga K, DeKemp RA. Quantification of myocardial blood flow with Rb-82 dynamic PET imaging. *Eur J Nucl Med Mol Imaging.* 2007;34(11):1765–1774.
13. Mullani NA et al. Myocardial perfusion with rubidium-82. I. Measurement of extraction fraction and flow with external detectors. *J Nucl. Med.* 1983;24:898–906.
14. Goldstein RA et al. Myocardial perfusion with rubidium-82. II. Effects of metabolic and pharmacologic interventions. *J Nucl Med.* 1983;24:907–915.
15. Sanchez-Crespo A, Andreo P, Larsson SA. Positron flight in human tissues and its influence on PET image spatial resolution. *Eur J Nucl Mol Imaging.* 2004;31(1):44–51.
16. Schelbert HR et al. N-13 ammonia as an indicator of myocardial blood flow. *Circulation.* 1981;63:1259–1272.
17. Beanlands RSB et al. Heterogeneity of regional nitrogen 13-labeled ammonia tracer distribution in the normal human heart: comparison with rubidium 82 and copper 62-labeled PTSM. *J Nucl Cardiol.* 1994;1(3):225–235.
18. Di Carli et al. Clinical myocardial perfusion PET/CT. *J Nucl Med.* 2007;48:783–793.
19. Bergmann et al. Quantification of regional myocardial blood flow in vivo with $H_2{}^{15}O$. *Circulation.* 1984;70(4):724–733.
20. Nandalur KR et al. Diagnostic performance of positron emission tomography in the detection of coronary artery disease: a meta-analysis. *Acad Radiol.* 2008;15(4):444–451.
21. Beanlands RSB, Youssef G. Diagnosis and prognosis of coronary artery disease: PET is superior to SPECT: *Pro J Nucl Cardiol.* 2010;17(4):683–695.
22. Sampson UK et al. Diagnostic accuracy of rubidium-82 myocardial perfusion imaging with hybrid positron emission tomography/computed tomography in the detection of coronary artery disease. *J Am Coll Cardiol.* 2007:49(10):1052–1058.
23. Jaarsma et al. Diagnostic performance of noninvasive myocardial perfusion imaging using single-photon emission computed tomography, cardiac magnetic resonance, and positron emission tomography imaging for the detection of obstructive coronary artery disease: a meta-analysis. *J Am Coll Cardiol.* 2012;59(19):1719–1728.
24. McArdle et al. Does rubidium-82 PET have superior accuracy to SPECT perfusion imaging for the diagnosis of obstructive coronary disease? A systematic review and meta-analysis. *J Am Coll Cardiol.* 2012;60(18):1828–1837.
25. Parker et al. Diagnostic accuracy of cardiac positron emission tomography versus single photon emission computed tomography for coronary artery disease: a bivariate meta-analysis. *Circ Cardiovasc Imaging.* 2012;5(6):700–707.

26. Fiechter M, Ghardri JR, Gebhard C et al. Diagnostic value of ^{13}N-ammonia myocardial perfusion PET: added value of myocardial flow reserve. *J Nucl Med.* 2012;53(8):1230–1234.
27. Taqueti VR, Dorbala S. The role of positron emission tomography in the evaluation of myocardial ischemia in women. *J Nucl Cardiol.* 2016;23(5):1008–1015.
28. Iskander A, Limone B, Parker MW et al. Gender Differences in the diagnostic accuracy with SPECT myocardial perfusion imaging: a bivariate meta-analysis. *J Nucl Cardiol.* 2013;20(1):53–63.
29. Bateman T, Heller GV, McGhie I et al. Diagnostic accuracy of rest/stress ECG-gated rubidium-82 myocardial perfusion PET: comparison with ECG-gated Tc-99m-sestamibi SPECT. *J Nucl Cardiol.* 2006;(12):24–33.
30. Nava M, Murthy VL, Taqueti VR et al. Preserved coronary flow reserve effectively excludes high-risk coronary artery disease on angiography. *J Nucl Med.* 2014;55(2):248–255.
31. Yoshinaga K et al. What is the prognostic value of myocardial perfusion imaging using rubidium-82 positron emission tomography? *J Am Coll Cardiol.* 2006;48(5):1029–1039.
32. Bateman T, Heller GV, McGhie I et al. Diagnostic accuracy of rest/stress ECG-gated rubidium-82 myocardial perfusion PET: comparison with ECG-gated Tc-99m-sestamibi SPECT. *J Nucl Cardiol.* 2006;13(1):24–33.
33. Flotats A, Bravo PE, Kukushima K et al. Rb-82 PET myocardial perfusion imaging is superior to Tc-99m-labeled agent SPECT in patients with known or suspected coronary artery disease. *Eur J Nucl Med Mol Imaging.* 2012;39(8):1233–1239.
34. Shi H, Santana CA, Rivero A et al. Normal values and prospective validation of transient ischemic dilation index in 82 Rb PET myocardial perfusion imaging. *Nucl Med Commun.* 2007;28(11):859–63
35. Rischpler C, Higuchi T, Kukushima K et al. Transient ischemic dilation ration in 82 Rb PET myocardial perfusion imaging: normal values and significance as a diagnostic and prognostic marker. *J Nucl Med.* 2012;53(5):723–730.
36. Lertsburapa K, Ahlberg AW, Bateman TM et al. Independent and incremental prognostic value of left ventricular ejection fraction determined by stress gated rubidium 82 PET imaging in patients with known or suspected coronary artery disease. *J Nucl Cardiol.* 2008;15(6): 745–753.
37. Brown, TL, Merrill J, Volokh L, Bengel FM. Determinants of the response of left ventricular ejection fraction to vasodilator stress in electrocardiographically gated 82 rubidium myocardial perfusion PET. *Euro J Nucl Med Molec Imag.* 2008;35(2):336–342.
38. Dorbala S, Vangala D, Sampson U et al. Value of vasodilator left ventricular ejection fraction reserve in evaluating the magnitude of myocardium at risk and the extent of angiographic coronary artery disease: an 82Rb PET/CT study. *J Nucl Med.* 2007;48(3):349–358.
39. Dorbala S, Hachamovitch R, Curillova Z et al. Incremental Prognostic Value of Gated Rb-82 Positron Emission Tomography Myocardial Perfusion Imaging over Clinical Variables and Rest LVEF. *JACC Cardiovascular Imaging.* 2009; 2(7):846–854.
40. Bateman MB, Gould KL, Di Carli MF. Proceedings of the Cardiac PET Summit, 12 May 2014, Baltimore, MD: Quantitation of myocardial blood flow *J Nucl Cardiol.* 2015;(22):571–578.
41. Nava M, Murthy VL, Taqueti VR et al. Preserved coronary flow reserve effectively excludes high-risk coronary artery disease on angiography. *J Nucl Med.* 2014;55(2):248–255.
42. Ziadi, Maria C et al. Impaired myocardial flow reserve on rubidium-82 positron emission tomography imaging predicts adverse outcomes in patients assessed for myocardial ischemia. *J Am Coll Cardiol.* 2011;58(7):740–748.
43. Murthy, VL et al. Comparison and prognostic validation of multiple methods of quantification of myocardial blood flow with 82Rb PET. *J Nucl Med.* 2014;55(12):1952–1958.
44. Gupta A et al. Integrated noninvasive physiological assessment of coronary circulatory function and impact on cardiovascular mortality in patients with stable coronary artery disease. *Circulation.* Dec 12 2017; 136(24):2325–2336.

45. Marwick TH, Shan K, Patel S et al. Incremental value of rubidium-82 positron emission tomography for prognostic assessment of known or suspected coronary artery disease. *Am J Cardiol.* 1997;80(7):865–870.
46. Dorbala S, Di Carli MF, Beanlands RS et al. Prognostic value of stress myocardial perfusion positron emission tomography: results from a multicenter observational registry. *J AM Coll Cardiol.* 2013;61(2):176–184.
47. Chow B, Dorbala S, Di Carli MF et al. Prognostic value of PET myocardial perfusion imaging in obese patients. *JACC Cardiovasc Imaging.* 2014;7(3):278–287.
48. Harnett DT et al. Clinical performance of Rb-82 myocardial perfusion PET and Tc-99m based SPECT in patients with extreme obesity. *J Nucl Cardiol.* 2017. Epub ahead of print.
49. Kay J, Dorbala S, Goyal A et al. Influence of sex on risk stratification with stress myocardial perfusion Rb-82 positron emission tomography: Results from the PET (Positron Emission Tomography) prognosis multicenter registry. *J Am Coll Cardiol.* 2013;62(20):1866–1876.
50. Ghotbi et al. Early risk stratification using rubidium-82 positron emission tomography in STEMI patients. *J Nucl Cardiol.* 2017. Epub ahead of print.
51. Maaniitty et al. Prognostic value of coronary CT angiography with selective PET perfusion imaging in coronary artery disease. *JACC: Cardiovasc Imaging.* 2017;10(11):1362–1370.
52. Danad et al. Comparison of coronary CT angiography, SPECT, PET, and hybrid imaging for diagnosis of ischaemic heart disease determined by fractional flow reserve. *JAMA Cardiol.* 2017;2(10):1100–1107.
53. Gould KL, Johnson NP. Coronary CT angiography with PET perfusion imaging: hybrid or hype? *JACC: Cardiovasc Imaging.* 2017;10(11):1371–1373.
54. Fazel et al. Exposure to low-dose ionizing radiation from medical imaging procedures. *N Eng J Med.* 2009;361:849–857.
55. Einstein et al. Current worldwide nuclear cardiology practices and radiation exposure: results from the 65 country IAEA nuclear cardiology protocols cross-sectional study (INCAPS). *Eur Heart J.* 2015;36(26):1689–1696.
56. Holly et al. ASNC imaging guidelines for nuclear cardiology procedures: single photon emission computed tomography. *J Nucl Cardiol.* 2010;17(5):941–973.
57. Stabin MG. Radiopharmaceuticals for nuclear cardiology: radiation dosimetry, uncertainties, and risk. *J Nucl Med.* 2008;49(9):1555–1563.
58. Senthamizchelvan et al. Human biodistribution and radiation dosimetry of ^{82}Rb. *J Nucl Med.* 2010;51(10):1592–1599.
59. Hunter CR, Hill J, Ziadi MC et al. Biodistribution and radiation dosimetry of (82) Rb at rest and during peak pharmacological stress in patients referred for myocardial perfusion imaging. *Eur J Nucl Med Mol Imaging.* 2015;42(7):1032–1042.
60. Dorbala et al. SNMMI/ASNC/SCCT guideline for cardiac SPECT/CT and PET/CT 1.0. *J Nucl Med.* 2013;5498:1485–1507.
61. Desiderio MC, Lundbye JB Saucier S et al. Is there regional variability of radiation exposure amongst cardiac PET laboratories in the United States? Abstracts of Original Contributions ASNC2016 the 21st Annual Scientific Session of the American Society of Nuclear Cardiology, September 22–25, 2016, Boca Raton, FL. *J Nucl Cardiol.* 2016;23(4):899–937.
62. Schleipman et al. Occupational radiation dose associated with Rb-82 myocardial perfusion positron emission tomography imaging. *J Nucl Cardiol.* 2006;13(3):378–384.
63. Tout et al. Comparison of occupational radiation exposure from myocardial perfusion imaging with Rb-82 PET and Tc-99m SPECT. *Nucl Med Commun.* 2014;35(1):1032–1037.
64. Dorbala S et al. SNMMI/ASNC/SCCT guideline for cardiac SPECT/CT and PET/CT 1.0. *J Nucl Med.* 2012;54(8):1485–1507.
65. Tout D, Tonge CM, Muthu S, Arumugam P. Assessment of a protocol for routine simultaneous myocardial blood flow measurement and standard myocardial perfusion imaging with rubidium-82 on a high count rate positron emission tomography system. *Nucl Med Comms.* 2012;33(11):1202–1211.
66. Renaud J.M. et al. Characterization of 3-dimensional PET systems for accurate

quantification of myocardial blow flow. *J Nucl Med.* 2017;58(1):103–109.

67. Dilsizian V et al. PET myocardial perfusion and metabolism clinical imaging. J Nucl Cardiol. *Imaging Med.* 2009;5(1):35–46.
68. Memmott MJ, Tonge CM, Saint KS, Arumugam P. Impact of pharmacological stress agent on patient motion during rubidium-82 myocardial perfusion PET/CT. *J Nucl Cardiol.* 2017. ePub ahead of print. doi:10.1007/s12350-016-0767-x.
69. Chow BJ, Ananthasubramaniam K, deKemp RA et al. Comparison of treadmill exercise versus dipyridamole stress with myocardial perfusion imaging using rubidium-82 positron emission tomography. *J Am Coll Cardiol.* 2005;45(8):1227–1234.
70. Chow BJ, Beanlands RS, Lee A et al. Treadmill exercise produces larger perfusion defects than dipyridamole stress N-13 ammonia positron emission tomography. *J Am Coll Cardiol.* 2006;47(2):411–416.
71. Armstrong IA, Memmott MJ, Tonge CM, Arumugam P. The impact of prompt gamma compensation on myocardial blood flow measurements with rubidium-82 dynamic PET. *J Nucl Cardiol.* 2016. EPub ahead of print: doi: 10.1007/s12350-016-0583-3.
72. Armstrong IA, Tonge CM, Arumugam P. Impact of point spread function modelling and time-of-flight on myocardial blood flow and myocardial flow reserve measurements for rubidium-82 cardiac PET. *J Nucl Cardiol.* 2014;21(3):467–474.
73. Johnson NP, Gould L. Regadenoson versus dipyridamole hyperemia for cardiac PET imaging. *JACC Cardiovasc Imaging.* 2015;8(4):438–447.
74. Bateman TM, Dilsizian V, Beanlands RS, DePuey EG, Heller GV, Wolinsky DA. American Society of Nuclear Cardiology and Society of Nuclear Medicine and Molecular Imaging joint position statement on the clinical indications for myocardial perfusion PET. *J Nucl Cardiol.* 2016;23(5):1227–1231.
75. Yu M, Guaraldi MT, Mistry M et al. BMS-747158-02: a novel PET myocardial perfusion imaging agent. *J Nucl Cardiol.* 2007;14(6):789–798.
76. Maddahi J, Czernin J, Lazewatsky J et al. Phase I, first-in-human study of BMS747158, a novel 18F-labeled tracer for myocardial perfusion pet: dosimetry, biodistribution, safety, and imaging characteristics after a single injection at rest. *J Nucl Med.* 2011;52(1):1490–1498
77. Berman D.S., Maddahi J., Tamarappoo B.K. et al. Phase II safety and clinical comparison with single-photon emission computed tomography myocardial perfusion imaging for detection of coronary artery disease. *J Am Coll Cardiol.* 2013;61(4):469–774.
78. Maddahi J, Udelson J, Heller G et al. On behalf of the Flurpiridaz F18 Study 301 Investigators. (2015). Flurpiridaz F 18 MPI: Recent clinical trial data. International Congress on Nuclear Cardiology and Cardiac CT 12 [abstract], Madrid (Spain), May 3–5, 2015;23.

EDITOR'S PERSPECTIVE

Timothy M. Bateman

The evolution of cardiac PET has spanned almost four decades now. The authors of this chapter have chronicled a large evidence base that justifies its prominent place in clinical cardiology today. A few perspectives on its current positioning should be emphasized. First, PET MPI is well-documented to outperform SPECT MPI in those people who require pharmacologic stress testing. Perhaps this should not be surprising: when patients undergo SPECT vasodilator stress, virtually everything about diagnosis and prognosis depends on the static perfusion images. Chest pain and dyspnea are common symptoms even in volunteers. ECG changes are not helpful.[1] The perfusion images most often are not attenuation corrected. The rest and post-stress function images are separated by 30 to 60 minutes so that post-stress stunning is uncommon. Flow quantification is rarely available, so the interpreter would be completely unaware that the vasodilator was ineffective. PET MPI overcomes these shortcomings in several ways. The stress images follow the rest images within just a few minutes, allowing recognition of changes in wall thickening, wall motion, and ejection fraction in response to peak stress imaging. The perfusion images are always attenuation corrected. Flow quantification provides assurances of vasodilator effectiveness, and the amount of flow augmentation improves diagnostic accuracy and prognosis.

Second, rest/stress PET MPI is a much more efficient test than rest/stress SPECT. Most PET MPI protocols, whether performed on legacy dedicated PET cameras or on more state-of-the-art hybrid devices, permit patient scheduling at 30 to 35 minute intervals. The ASNC-recommended protocol for rest/stress SPECT requires several hours. In addition to the long delay between rest and stress, each of the stress and rest images require 15 or more minutes to acquire. Patient fatigue and ensuing body or respiratory motion are a much larger issue than with PET MPI, where the acquisition times are on the order of 5 minutes.

Third, image quality is higher with PET MPI compared to SPECT MPI, when performed in the same patients.[2] A major benefit of PET MPI is that image quality is relatively unaffected by body size or shape, large breasts or breast implants, or whether arms can be lifted or not. Even when SPECT is performed with attenuation correction, PET outperforms in relation to diagnostic accuracy and identification of multivessel CAD.[3-5]Fourth, radiation exposure is much lower with rest/stress PET MPI compared to rest/stress traditional SPECT MPI. The difference is 4-fold lower with PET.[6] Many patients with CAD will undergo multiple radiation-associated imaging sessions over the course of their lives. Clearly, any method that can minimize their total radiation burden is desirable.

In addition, there is the matter of quantification of myocardial blood flow. This is a mature and unique capability of PET MPI, with a strong evidence base for independent and incremental improvement in both diagnostic accuracy and prognostication. Currently, it is the only way to recognize microvascular disease, and to know that vasodilator stress was ineffective.

Despite all these attributes, there is much work to be done. Here are just a few of the questions that need answers.

1. In a patient who can exercise, how would vasodilator PET MPI compare against traditional exercise SPECT MPI with respect to diagnostic accuracy and prognostication?
2. Does PET MPI still maintain superiority when compared against state-of-the-art SPECT, for example, high-resolution CZT SPECT with attenuation correction?
3. Is recently introduced SPECT myocardial blood flow reserve sufficient for most purposes, or do PET-derived absolute blood flow measurements with a superior tracer result in significantly better results?
4. Will F^{18} flurpiridaz, with its better uptake kinetics, improved image quality, and capability of stress first/stress-only imaging change the MPI landscape?

Finally, it needs to be emphasized that there is a major need for a prospective study to show definitively that PET MPI improves outcomes. These may be hard outcomes such as death or myocardial infarction, or other outcomes such as management decisions that improve health status and quality of life.

In summary, much work has already been done, but more is needed. PET has ushered in an entirely new era of accuracy for noninvasive assessment of CAD. It has shown that epicardial disease is only a part of the problem; it might be argued that current excellent therapies for epicardial disease represent a maturity of that portion of the problem. The new challenge is microvascular disease; PET is uniquely positioned to lead the way for both diagnosis and for evaluation of current and potential new therapies.

CHAPTER 2

Coronary Artery Calcium Scanning in Conjunction with Stress/Rest Myocardial Perfusion Imaging: Complementary Uses for Risk Assessment and Clinical Patient Management

Alan Rozanski, Seth Uretsky, and Daniel S. Berman

Stress/rest myocardial perfusion imaging (MPI) is commonly used for the diagnostic assessment of patients with suspected coronary artery disease (CAD) and for aiding clinical management decisions, such as the need for myocardial revascularization versus medical therapy. The latter use is facilitated by the well-documented relationship between the extent and severity of stress-induced myocardial perfusion abnormalities and the risk for subsequent adverse cardiac events. Despite these utilities, stress/rest MPI imaging has an important limitation: while myocardial perfusion abnormalities are useful for assessing the hemodynamic significance of obstructive coronary stenosis, many patients with normal stress/rest MPI studies have a substantial magnitude of subclinical coronary atherosclerosis, which cannot be detected because they are not flow-limiting in magnitude.[1,2] Coronary artery calcium (CAC) scanning is a complementary test that can detect subclinical atherosclerosis.

Over the years, CAC has been primarily used for screening purposes among asymptomatic individuals with risk factors for CAD. However, there is now growing recognition that CAC scanning could also serve as a clinical aid for improving the work-up and management of patients who are candidates for stress/rest MPI.[3,4]

A number of features make CAC scanning make it an appealing test. The presence of CAC is a specific marker of CAD in an individual patient. Even very small amounts of CAC, with scores ranging 1–10, places patients at increased risk compared to patients with normal CAC scans.[5,6] Patho-anatomic studies conducted by Rumberger et al in the 1990s demonstrated a proportional relationship between the amount of CAC and total atherosclerotic burden.[7] Since then, hundreds of outcome studies have consistently demonstrated a strong proportional relationship between the magnitude of CAC abnormality and the frequency of subsequent cardiac events. Most of these studies have been performed in asymptomatic populations. However, more recent studies have also demonstrated a similar proportional relationship between CAC scores and adverse outcomes among patients with chest pain symptoms. For example, in the recent Prospective Multicenter Imaging Study for Evaluation of Chest Pain (PROMISE) trial, a proportional relationship was also noted between the degree of CAC abnormality and the frequency of subsequent clinical events among patients with chest pain symptoms.[8]

For these reasons, there has been growing interest in evaluating the combined use of stress/rest MPI and CAC scanning for diagnostic and prognostic assessment. MPI using positron emission tomography (PET) is particularly well suited for this use because most PET scanners used for cardiac imaging today are hybrid PET/CT scanners, permitting both the anatomic assessment of coronary atherosclerosis and functional assessment of myocardial perfusion in a single study. In addition, hybrid SPECT/CT camera systems are now also increasingly available, although they presently constitute only a small percentage of the SPECT-MPI scanners. At the time of hybrid PET or SPECT imaging, the concomitant low dose non-ECG-gated CT scan is used to perform attenuation correction for the radionuclide images. This permits visual estimation of CAC abnormality, which in one formal study of 492 patients undergoing hybrid PET or SPECT/CT imaging was shown to have favorable agreement to the standard measurement of CAC abnormality during separately acquired ECG-gated calcium scans in the same patient population.[9] Performance of SPECT-MPI with conventional cameras or stand-alone PET systems can also be combined with stand-alone CAC scanning to assess the same functional information that can be derived from hybrid scanners. Accordingly, this chapter reviews potential clinical applications that can be derived from the combined use of stress/rest MPI and CAC scanning. Second, we also examine how CAC scanning can be used as a triage method for optimizing the selection of patients for stress/rest MPI.

USING COMBINED CAC SCANNING AND STRESS/REST MPI FOR DISEASE DETECTION

Studies performed in the early 2000s established a high frequency of atherosclerosis among patients with normal SPECT-MPI. For example, in a study involving 1195 patients that underwent both SPECT-MPI and CAC scanning, we noted that most patients with an abnormal SPECT-MPI study had CAC abnormality, but so too did 78% of 1119 patients with normal SPECT-MPI[2] (Figure 2-1). Among the non-ischemic patients with CAC abnormality, nearly one-third had evidence of CAC scores >400, indicative of extensive subclinical atherosclerosis.

This observation of a high frequency of CAC abnormality among patients with normal SPECT-MPI studies is particularly notable in light of data indicating a declining frequency of abnormal SPECT-MPI studies over time. In our own experience, between 1991 and 2009 the frequency of ischemic SPECT-MPI studies fell from 29.6% to 5.0% among diagnostic

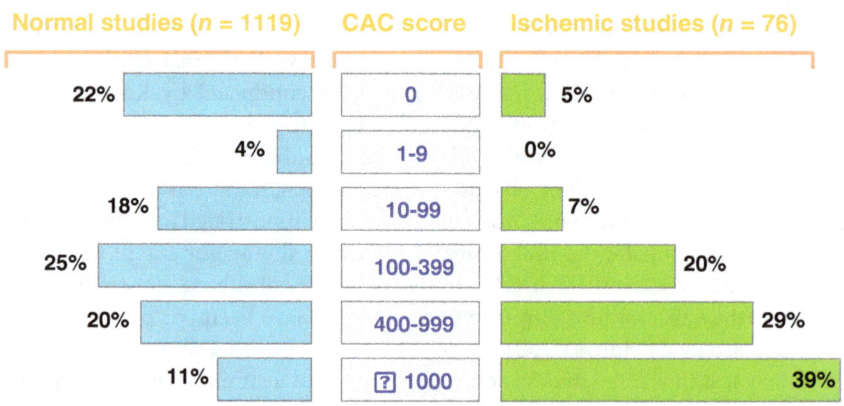

FIGURE 2-1 Distribution of Concomitant Coronary Artery Calcium (CAC) Scores Scores are divided into six categories, among patients with abnormal stress/rest myocardial perfusion SPECT-MPI (right bars) and with normal SPECT-MPI (left bars). (Reproduced with permission from Berman DS, Wong ND, Gransar H, et al. Relationship between stress-induced myocardial ischemia and atherosclerosis measured by coronary calcium tomography, J Am Coll Cardiol. 2004 Aug 18;44(4):923-930)

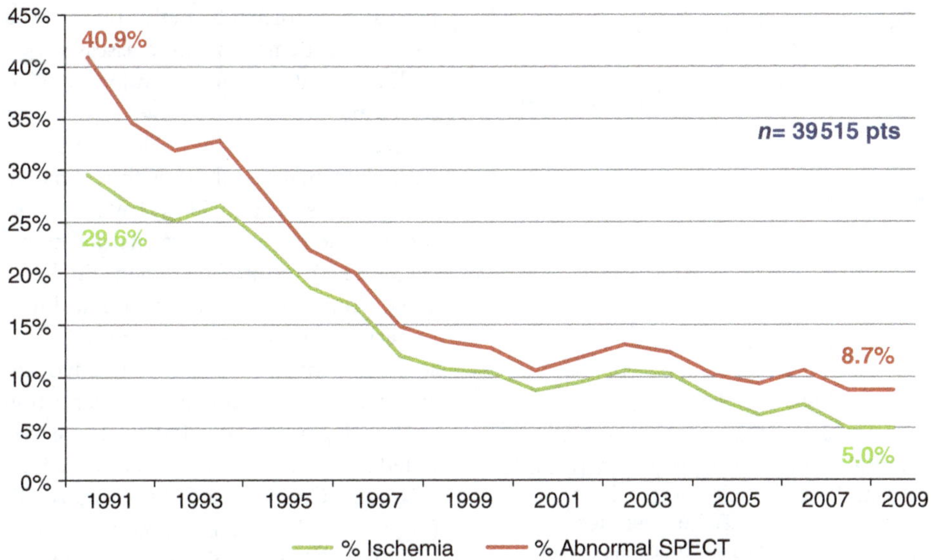

FIGURE 2-2 Marked temporal decline in the frequency of abnormal SPECT-MPI studies and in the frequency of ischemic studies between 1991 and 2009 among 39 515 diagnostic patients referred for testing. (Reproduced with permission from Rozanski A, Gransar H, Hayes SW, et al: Temporal trends in the frequency of inducible myocardial ischemia during cardiac stress testing: 1991 to 2009, J Am Coll Cardiol. 2013 Mar 12;61(10):1054-1065)

patients who were referred for SPECT-MPI at Cedars-Sinai Medical Center[10] (Figure 2-2). The presence of a temporal decline in inducible myocardial ischemia has also been noted in other large patient populations.[11,12] This has implications for patient management, because notwithstanding the important utilities of a normal MPI in guiding acute management decisions, it has generally had limited impact on guiding the intensity of CAD risk factor management. In contrast, concomitant use of CAC scanning with stress/rest MPI allows both improved prognostic risk assessment and opportunities for enhancing patient risk factor management based on the combined test results.

USING COMBINED CAC SCANNING AND MPI FOR RISK ASSESSMENT

For years, the ability of radionuclide stress testing to predict myocardial risk was based on primarily short-term follow-up studies. These studies established that a normal SPECT study was associated with an excellent prognosis. For example, in a meta-analysis of 17 studies, Metz et al found that the annualized event rate associated with a normal exercise SPECT-MPI study was only 0.45% per year.[13] The mean duration of follow-up in the studies constituting this meta-analysis was only 33.8 months. In recent years, however, there has been increasing interest in assessing the long-term outcomes associated with stress/rest MPI, in particular, among patients with normal MPI studies. These studies have demonstrated that long-term outcome among non-ischemic MPI patients is quite heterogeneous, influenced by a variety of clinical factors.

For example, in an extended follow-up of 5762 patients who had a normal stress-rest SPECT-MPI. Supariwala et al found that all-cause mortality increased according to both the number of CAD risk factors and whether stress testing was performed using pharmacologic or exercise stress.[14] The frequency of deaths ranged from 0.8% per year for exercise patients who had no CAD risk factors to 4.2% per year among patients undergoing pharmacologic patients and having >two CAD risk factors, a 5-fold increase in risk (Figure 2-3). Similar findings were noted in another large study.[15]

In similar fashion, the concomitant use of CAC scanning can be used to improve long-term risk prediction among patients undergoing stress/rest MPI. CAC scanning provides complementary prognostic information both among patients with and without a myocardial

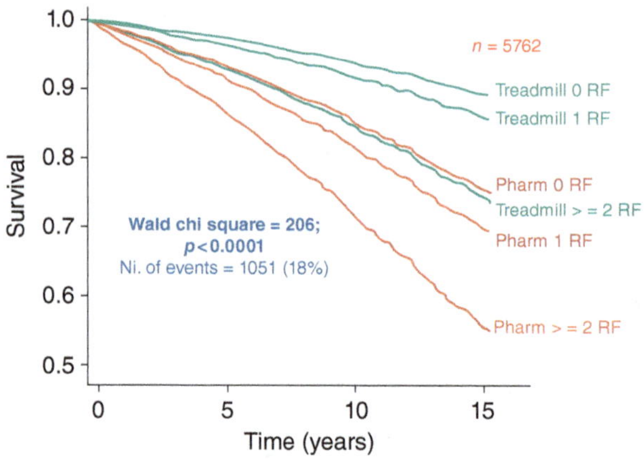

FIGURE 2-3 Kaplan Meier Survival Curves Among 5762 Patients With a Normal SPECT-MPI Study Who Were Followed for All-Cause Mortality Patients are divided according to whether they underwent treadmill exercise or required pharmacologic (Pharm) stress testing and according to the number of CAD risk factors (RF). (Reproduced with permission from Supariwala A, Uretsky S, Depuey EG, et al: Influence of mode of stress and coronary risk factor burden upon long-term mortality following normal stress myocardial perfusion single-photon emission computed tomographic imaging, Am J Cardiol. 2013 Mar 15;111(6):846-850)

perfusion abnormality. In this regard, Chang et al studied 1216 patients who were assessed by both SPECT-MPI and CAC scanning and followed for a median of 6.9 years.[16] There was a progressive increase in adverse clinical events with increasing CAC score in patients with abnormal and those with normal SPECT-MPI. If both CAC scan and SPECT-MPI abnormalities were present, there was a synergistic elevation in patient risk (Figure 2-4). In similar fashion, Engbers et al assessed 4897 symptomatic patients without known CAD who underwent both stress/rest SPECT-MPI with CAC scoring.[17] Adverse events included myocardial infarction, all-cause mortality or late revascularization. The median follow-up period was 940 days. These investigators also noted a stepwise increase in adverse clinical events with increasing CAC score if SPECT abnormality was present (Figure 2-5). Importantly, however, in patients with normal SPECT MPI, while the event rates were lower than in those with abnormal SPECT, there was an increased event rate according to the amount of CAC. A zero CAC scan has also been found to indicate a low likelihood of obstructive CAD when testing patients with a relatively low likelihood of CAD, but this association is

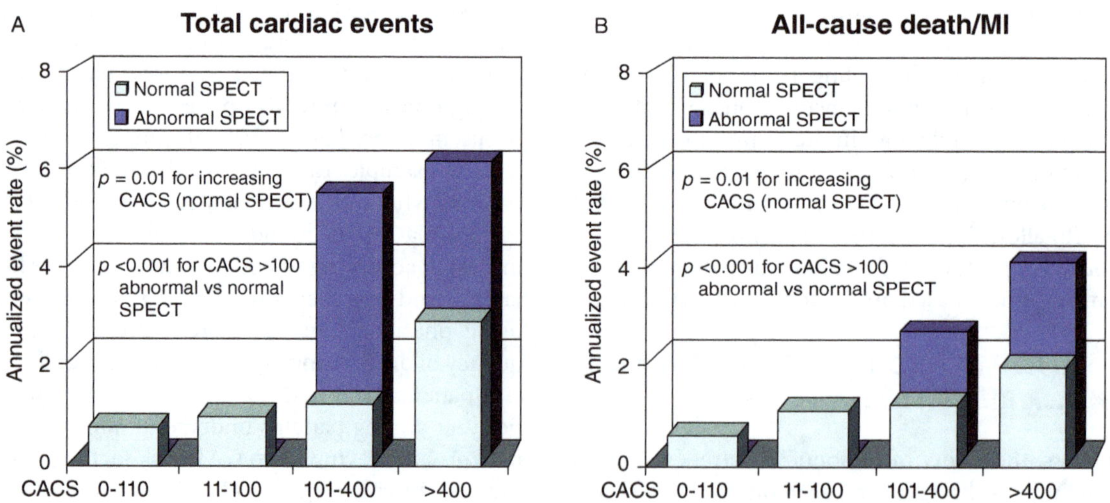

FIGURE 2-4 Annualized event rate for cardiac events (graph A) and all-cause mortality/myocardial infarction (MI) (graph B) among patients undergoing stress/rest SPECT-MPI and concomitant CAC scanning. Patients were subdivided based on both their CAC score and whether their SPECT-MPI was normal (light blue bars) or abnormal (dark blue bars). For both clinical outcomes, event rates increased with increasing CAC scores, and were further increased if inducible myocardial was also present. (Reproduced with permission from Chang SM, Nabi F, Xu J, et al. The coronary artery calcium score and stress myocardial perfusion imaging provide independent and complementary prediction of cardiac risk, J Am Coll Cardiol. 2009 Nov 10;54(20):1872-1882)

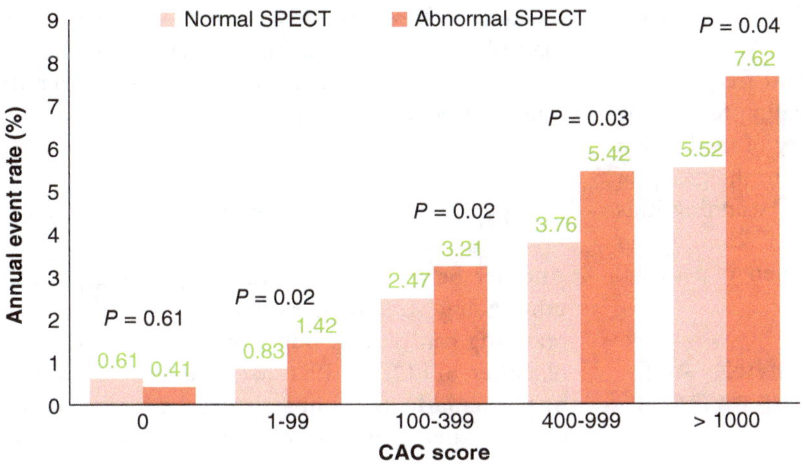

FIGURE 2-5 Frequency of Major Adverse Cardiac Events Among Patients Referred for SPECT-MPI. Patients were stratified based on their CAC score and results of MPI. (Reproduced with permission from Engbers EM, Timmer JR2, Ottervanger JP, et al: Prognostic Value of Coronary Artery Calcium Scoring in Addition to Single-Photon Emission Computed Tomographic Myocardial Perfusion Imaging in Symptomatic Patients, Circ Cardiovasc Imaging. 2016 May;9(5). pii: e003966)

not as reliable when applying CAC scanning to patients with a higher likelihood of CAD.[18,19]

USING COMBINED CAC SCANNING AND STRESS/REST MPI TO IMPROVE PATIENT MANAGEMENT

Among patients referred for stress/rest MPI for clinical reasons, the presence of myocardial ischemia is often a determining factor as to whether myocardial revascularization may be warranted. Further, once ischemia is present, aggressive medical management of CAD risk factors and clinical symptoms becomes warranted in all such patients. Among patients with a normal stress/rest MPI study, the intensity of medical management following testing may be considerably enhanced by considering the results of concomitant CAC scanning. Because any CAC abnormality among patients with a normal MPI puts them at increased long-term clinical risk,[5,6] this finding should signal the physician to intensity their clinical management of patients. The presence and extent of CAC among patients with normal MPI may influence the physician to more closely monitor and aggressively manage other CAD risk factors, such as initiating or increasing the intensity of statin therapy. In addition, knowledge of a high CAC score may be reason for the physician to encourage other lifestyle changes designed to reduce long-term clinical risk and to provide more feedback and/or frequent physician visits to assist patients. Further, for non-ischemic patients with substantial CAC burden, the physician may choose to increase the frequency of follow-up or decrease the threshold for further testing. By contrast, a zero CAC score may be the reason for physicians to increase their threshold for further testing and reduce downstream medical testing.

Whereas, the actual impact of CAC scanning on influencing the behavior of physicians has not yet been studied among patients referred for stress/rest MPI, important insights in this regard can be garnered from the Early Identification of Subclinical Atherosclerosis by Noninvasive Imaging Research (EISNER) trial, a prospective randomized trial that assessed the impact of CAC scanning on subsequent patient management and change in CAD risk factor profiles.[20] For this study, 2137 middle-aged volunteers with CAD risk factors were randomized in a 2:1 fashion into two groups: those receiving CAC scanning at baseline and those who were not scanned. A standard risk-factor counseling session was provided to both groups during an initial clinical visit supervised by a nurse practitioner, but the scan group was also counseled based on the results of CAC scanning. During 4-year follow-up, it became apparent that within the scan group that the intensity of medical risk-factor management, such as statin use and blood pressure medication, paralleled the CAC scores at the start of the study. The higher the CAC score, the greater was the use of these medications. Similarly, the frequency of downstream tests and procedures during follow-up paralleled the baseline magnitude of CAC abnormality. Among patients with a zero CAC score, the intensity of medical management and frequency of downstream medical resource utilization fell during follow-up compared to the frequency of medication or resource utilization that occurred in the group of subjects that were not referred for CAC scanning. This study thus shows that the results of CAC scanning can strongly influence physician management of patients.

USING COMBINED CAC SCANNING AND STRESS/REST MPI TO IMPROVE PATIENT ADHERENCE

Optimizing patient adherence is a continual challenge in patient management. Ideally, patients will adhere to their medications and comply with behavioral suggestions, such as improving their diet, regulating their weight and exercising, but rates of adherence are suboptimal, even for medication use. When physicians talk to their patients about their CAD risk factors or global risk scores, such as the Framingham Risk Score or the ASCVD risk scores, the discussion may often seem theoretical to patients, because the risk represents some future probability of adverse events from data based on observations in patient populations. For example, the physician may frame for the patient their future 10-year risk for developing a cardiac event.[21] By contrast, the CAC scan can be used to provide proof of disease and its associated risk in the individual patient. The finding is not theoretical and thus may be more palpable to patients. This here-and-now quality of CAC scanning may serve to be more motivating to patients.

Various studies suggest that the results of CAC scanning may serve to improve patient adherence to lifestyle changes. For example, in a study of 980 asymptomatic subjects who were followed for 3 years after CAC scanning, dietary changes, exercise, and aspirin use increased with higher baseline CAC scores.[22] Similarly, a 3.6-year follow-up of 505 asymptomatic patients found a progressive increase in statin adherence with increasing CAC scores.[23] Overall, a review of 15 studies found that increasing CAC scores was associated with greater medication adherence in 13 of the studies.[24] To date, however, these findings are not definitive because they have relied on self-reports of behavioral changes rather than objective measurements of behavioral change, such as change in weight, measurement of exercise fitness, or pedometer steps.

IMPROVED TEST INTERPRETATION

Another benefit of CAC scanning among patients undergoing stress/rest MPI is the role that CAC scanning can play in improving the interpretation of either SPECT or PET MPI studies. This might be particularly useful in assisting the interpretation of small perfusion defects for which CAC scanning can be used to resolve diagnostic uncertainty regarding borderline findings. In addition, CAC scanning might be used to help evaluate the results of frankly discordant test results, such as uncertainty in diagnosis among patients having a normal SPECT study but having an abnormal clinical and electrocardiographic response to exercise. A normal CAC scan in such patients may increase the likelihood that the combined stress ECG findings and chest pain represent a false-positive response for ischemia. Presently, there have only been limited studies to assess the impact of CAC scanning on test interpretation. In one study, Mouden et al assessed the interpretation of perfusion images when readers did or did not have concomitant knowledge of patients' CAC scores.[25] The frequency of equivocal SPECT MPI interpretations in this study fell from 21% to 9% when the results of CAC scanning were considered. In a second study, we retrospectively interpreted 162 SPECT-MPI according to the following sequence: (1) assessment of the stress-only images; (2) additional consideration of the patients' clinical data; and (3) additional consideration of patients' CAC data.[26] The end-point of this analysis was to determine how often we felt a patient needed to come back for a rest MPI study to resolve diagnostic uncertainty. Knowledge of the CAC scan data reduced the perceived need for a rest SPECT-MPI in nearly three-quarters of patients with a probably normal test interpretation and in one-half of patients with an equivocal test interpretation. Similarly, CAC scanning is likely to prove beneficial in aiding the interpretation of equivocal defects on PET MPI studies.

Use of CAC Scanning to Assess CAD Likelihood for CAD Prior to Stress/Rest MPI Testing

In addition to using CAC scanning in combination with stress/rest MPI to improve risk stratification and clinical management, CAC scanning can be used as a means for improving the selection of patients for stress/rest MPI in the first place. One utility in this regard may be using CAC scanning to improve the overall estimation of pretest likelihood of obstructive CAD among patients with clinical symptoms. For years, the selection of patients for diagnostic testing with exercise ECG, MPI, and stress echocardiography has been based on the Bayesian analysis of CAD likelihood, as initially proposed by Diamond and Forrester in 1979.[27] This analysis has been based on the assessment of patient age, gender, CAD risk factors, and chest pain symptoms. However, various lines of evidence have now demonstrated that the Diamond-Forrester algorithm no longer accurately predicts CAD likelihood. For example, Cheng et al evaluated 14 048 patients who underwent coronary computed tomography angiography (CTA) because of a suspicion of CAD.[28] According to the Diamond-Forrester algorithm, the mean likelihood of obstructive CAD in this large patient cohort was 51%. However, the actual observed prevalence in this population was only 18%. In particular, the Diamond-Forrester algorithm seriously underestimated the frequency of obstructive disease compared to the observed prevalence among patients with atypical angina (47% vs 15%) and typical angina (71% vs 29%). Similar findings were observed in the PROMISE trial.[29] In this study of 10 003 patients, the calculated mean likelihood of obstructive CAD by the Diamond-Forrester algorithm was 53.3%, but the actual observed prevalence of obstructive CAD was only 10.7%.

This phenomenon is likely a major contributor to the profoundly low prevalence of abnormal stress MPI studies found in recent studies. Thus, there is a need to develop enhanced methods for determining patients' pretest likelihood of obstructive CAD. CAC scanning may be useful in this regard because of a demonstrated strong proportional relationship between the magnitude of CAC abnormality and the frequency of obstructive CAD.[30] As initially suggested by Budoff et al, combining CAC scanning with age, gender, risk factor, and chest pain information is likely to result in a substantially improved estimation of pretest CAD likelihood by Bayesian analysis.[31]

Use of CAC Scanning to Predict the Likelihood of Inducible Ischemia

A more direct way of using CAC scanning to guide the appropriate selection of patients for stress/rest MPI is to consider the relationship between the CAC score and the likelihood of inducing myocardial ischemia during stress testing. This potential was first suggested based on a report by He et al who evaluated the relationship between CAC score categories and frequency of myocardial ischemia during SPECT-MPI in 411 patients.[1] The frequency of ischemia in their study rose progressively with increasing CAC score but remained low for patients with CAC scores <400. Overall, they observed no inducible ischemia among patients with CAC scores <10. The frequency of ischemia was only 2.6% among those with CAC scores of 11 to 100 and rose to 11.3% for those with CAC scores of 100–399. Among those with CAC scores >400, the frequency of ischemia was 46%. In subsequent work we noted a similar progressive relationship between CAC score and inducible myocardial ischemia, but found a lower frequency of inducible ischemia for those patients with CAC scores >400 compared to the results of He et al.[2] More recently, a meta-analysis of 20 studies also found a low frequency of inducible myocardial ischemia among patients with either zero or very low CAC scores in most studies.[32] While the frequency of inducible myocardial ischemia rose with increasing CAC scores, a high variance in the actual frequency of inducible ischemia was noted among studies. A prospective study is thus required to assess the reasons for this variance. Factors to be studied should include the role of risk factors, chest pain symptoms, co-morbid medical conditions, and other factors that affect patient acuity. For instance, in one study, Wong et al found that the presence versus absence of metabolic factors influenced the likelihood of observing inducible myocardial ischemia among patients with intermediate CAC scores.[33] For patients with CAC scores (100–399), the frequency of inducible ischemia was only 4% among patients without diabetes or metabolic syndrome versus 13% for patients who had either diabetes or metabolic syndrome. Other work suggests that the quality of chest pain symptoms can also influence the relationship between CAC score and inducible myocardial ischemia,[34] but more study is required in this regard. In general, however, low CAC scores (<100) are associated with a low frequency of inducible myocardial ischemia among asymptomatic patients and those patients with atypical chest pain.

CASE EXAMPLES OF HYBRID PET/CAC SCANNING FOR DIAGNOSTIC PURPOSES

As we have reviewed, the combined use of stress/rest MPI and CAC scanning differentiates patients with nonischemic MPI studies who are at varying long-term risk for cardiac events. One common group is those patients who have both normal stress/rest MPI images and a lack of CAC abnormality, as exemplified by a patient who underwent hybrid PET/CT imaging in Figures 2-6 and 2-7. Such patients are at quite low risk for subsequent clinical events over a long temporal time span. This combined imaging pattern should thus lead to a higher threshold for initiating aggressive medical management and lower utilization of subsequent medical tests, as occurred in the EISNER study.[20] However, the presence of atherosclerosis is commonly present among patients with a normal stress/rest MPI study,[1,2] as exemplified in another patient who underwent hybrid PET/CT imaging in

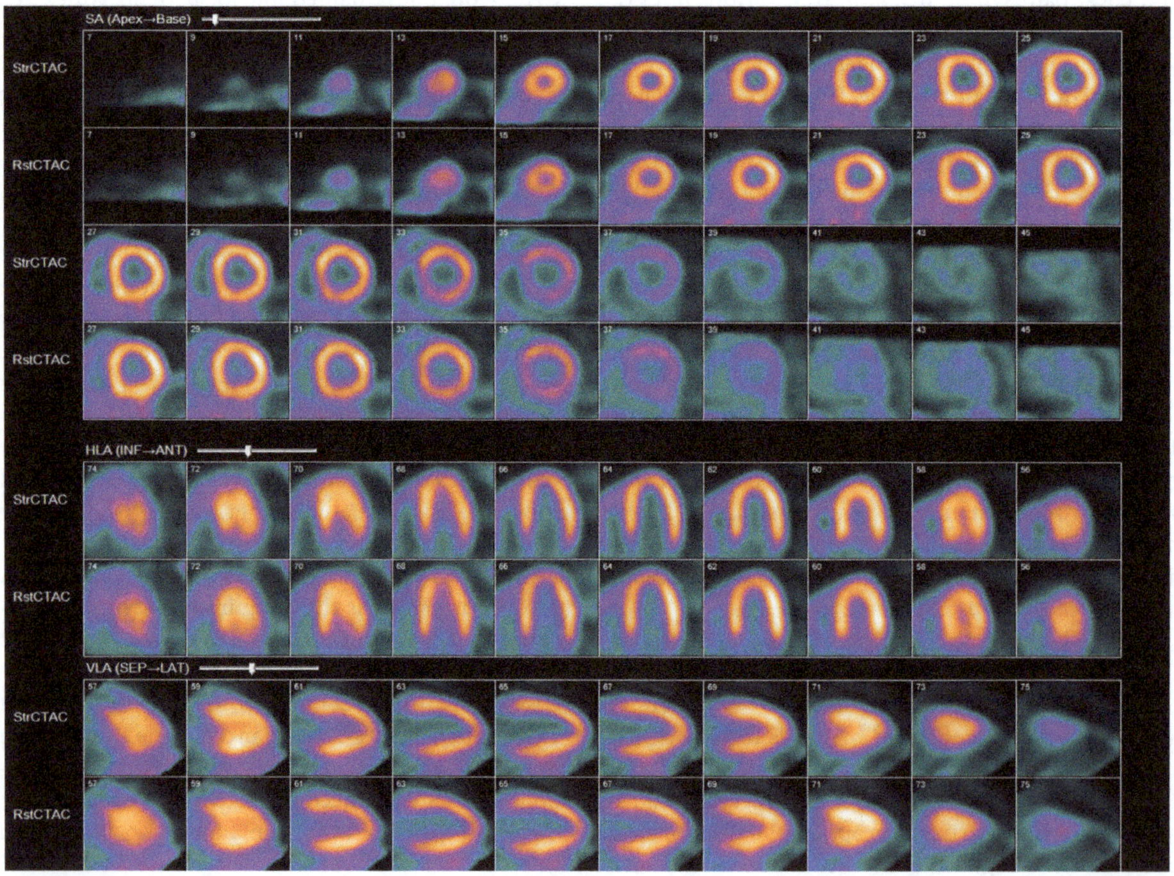

FIGURE 2-6 PET scan in a 40-year-old male with a history of hypertension and obesity referred for testing because of atypical chest pain. The PET scan is normal.

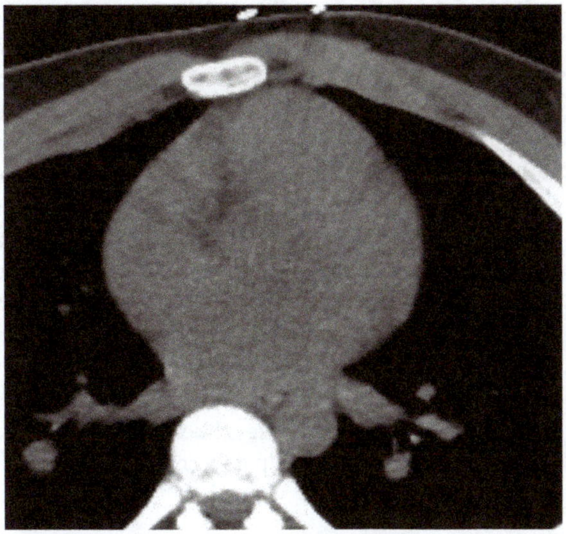

FIGURE 2-7 The corresponding coronary artery calcium scan in the patient in Figure 2-6 is also normal.

Figures 2-8 and 2-9. Even though this patient's PET scan is normal, the patient still deserves aggressive medical management, including strong control of all CAD risk factors, consideration of statin use, and more intensive follow-up. Thus, these two studies illustrate how the addition of CAC scanning can lead to a marked difference in the clinical management of patients with normal SPECT-MPI studies.

Hybrid PET-CAC scanning also permits the assessment of CAC abnormality among patients with ischemic MPI studies. For example, Figure 2-10 shows the PET images for a patient with chest pain who underwent hybrid PET-CT imaging for clinical evaluation. The images illustrate a reversible inferolateral wall defect, indicative of inducible myocardial ischemia within the distribution of the left circumflex

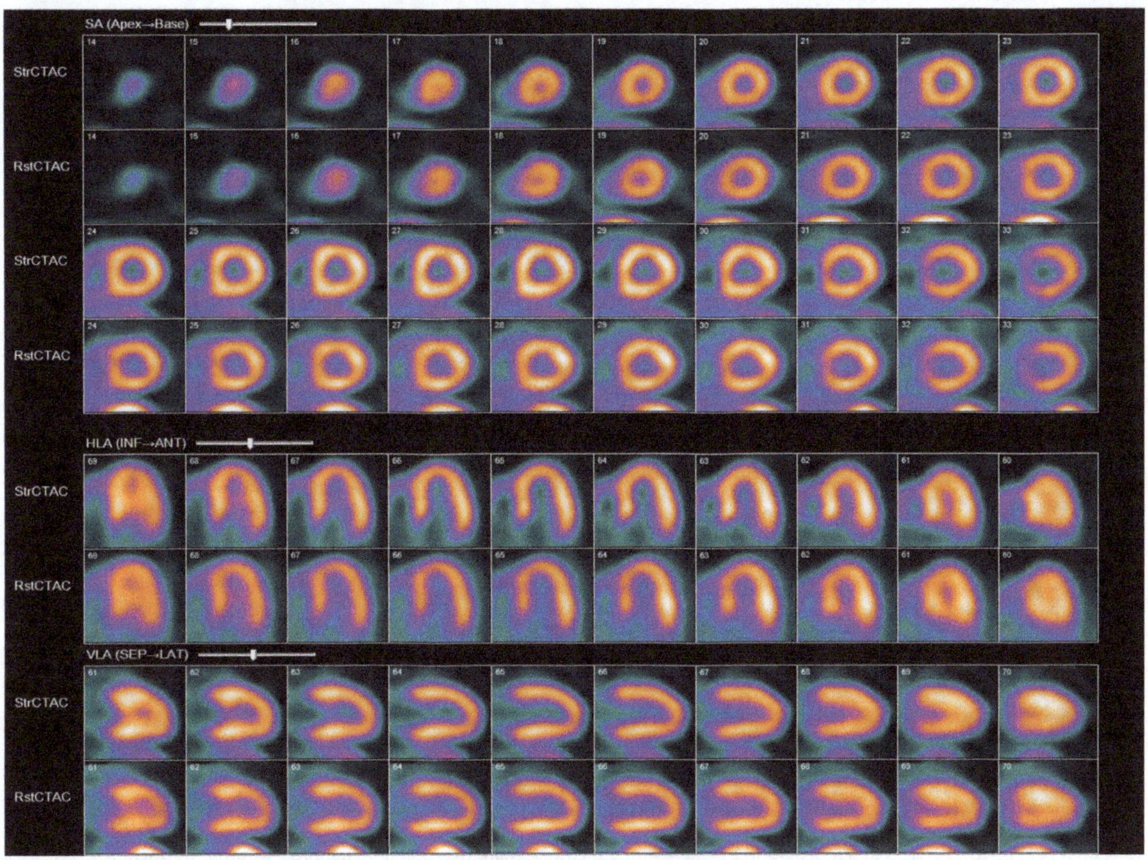

FIGURE 2-8 PET scan in a 62-year-old patient with a history of hypertension, hyperlipidemia, and diabetes referred for testing because of chest pain. The study reveals normal perfusion on the stress and rest perfusion images.

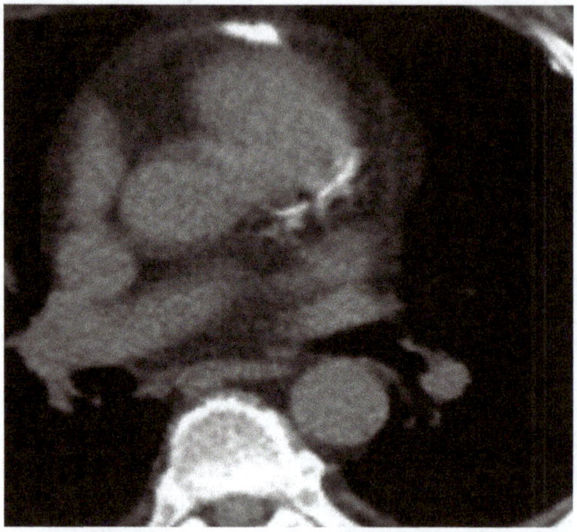

FIGURE 2-9 The corresponding CAC scan in the patient in Figure 2-8 reveals calcium in the left anterior descending coronary artery. The CAC score was 97.

coronary artery. The concomitant CAC scan identifies that this patient also has calcium abnormality in all three coronary arteries (Figure 2-11). Current data suggest that this patient would be at increased risk compared to a patient who has inducible ischemia and little to no CAC abnormality.[16,17] Practically, the use of CAC score data among ischemic MPI patients is most likely to be useful among patients with only a mild stress-induced perfusion abnormality, because the CAC score may shift the assessed clinical risk to higher or lower levels in such patients. By contrast, once severe and/or extensive stress-induced ischemia is present, a high risk for future clinical events is already established and it is less likely that knowledge of the CAC score would help govern patient management in such patients.

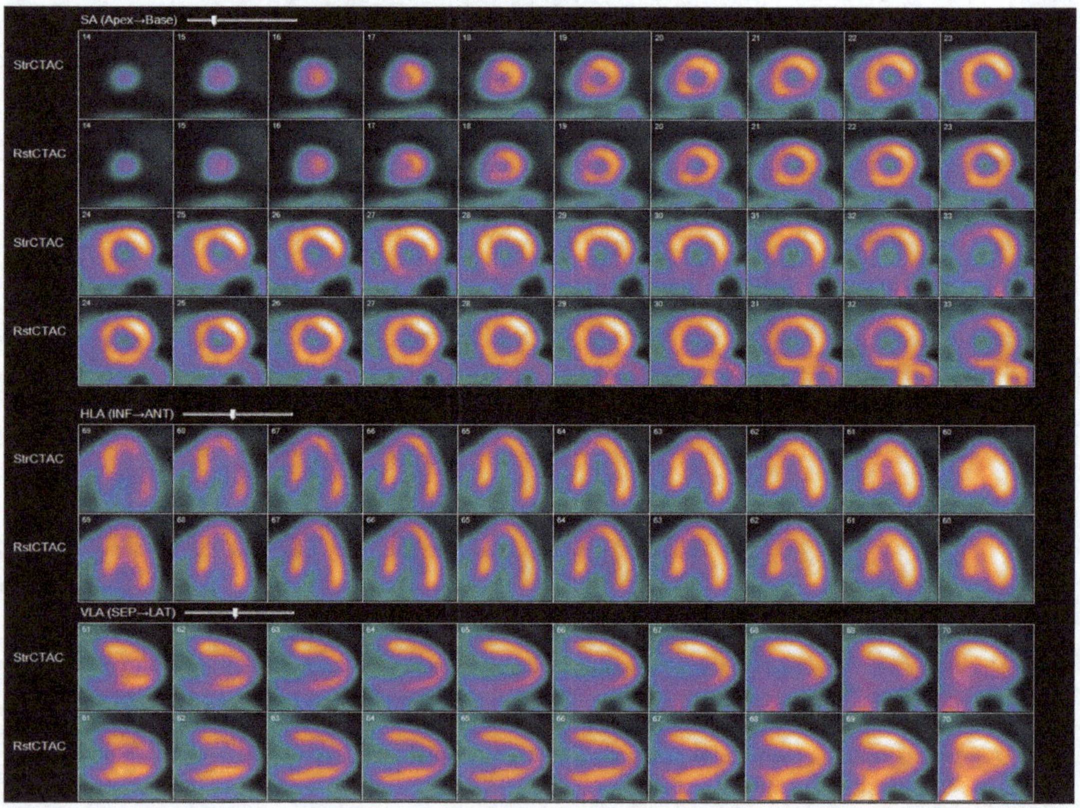

FIGURE 2-10 PET scan in a 62-year-old woman, with a history of hypertension and diabetes, referred for testing because of atypical chest pain. The scan reveals a reversible perfusion defect in the apical and basal portions of the inferolateral wall, indicative of hemodynamically significant disease in the left circumflex coronary artery.

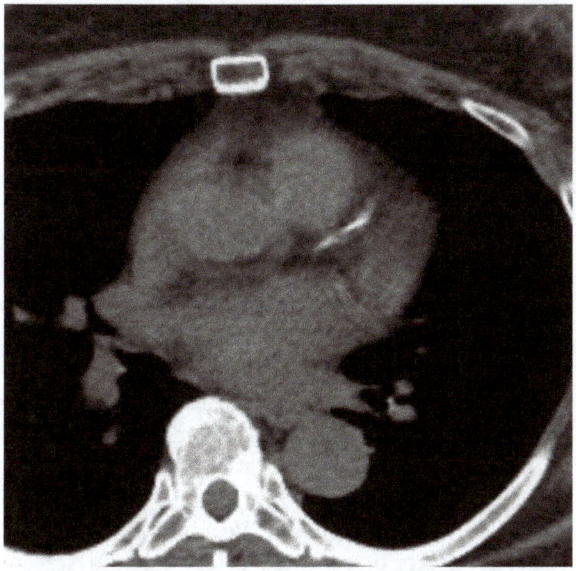

FIGURE 2-11 Coronary artery calcium scan in the same woman as in Figure 2-10, revealing calcium in the left anterior descending artery. She also had calcium in the right and left circumflex coronary arteries (not shown).

CONCLUSIONS

While CAC scanning was initially applied as a standalone screening test for CAD, recent studies suggest that the test may also have broad applications with respect to the clinical management of patients, either as a standalone test or combined with cardiac stress testing, even including exercise electrocardiography.[35] As reviewed in this chapter, combining CAC scanning with stress/rest MPI imaging can be used to improve the detection of CAD, aid in overall patient risk assessment, enhance patient risk factor management, spur improved patient adherence to risk factor modification, and/or improve the interpretation of SPECT or PET images. Accordingly, the routine assessment of CAC scanning should be considered among diagnostic patients who are undergoing stress/rest SPECT or PET MPI because of suspected CAD. In addition, CAC scanning can be used to help triage patients for stress testing by providing enhanced assessment of patients' pretest likelihoods of obstructive CAD and/or their likelihood of manifesting stress-induced myocardial ischemia.

REFERENCES

1. He ZX, Hedrick TD, Pratt CM, et al. Severity of coronary artery calcification by electron beam computed tomography predicts silent myocardial ischemia. *Circulation.* 2000 Jan;101:244–251.
2. Berman DS, Wong ND, Gransar H, et al. Relationship between stress-induced myocardial ischemia and atherosclerosis measured by coronary calcium tomography. *J Am Coll Cardiol.* 2004;44:923–930.
3. Rozanski A, Slomka P, D SB. Extending the use of coronary calcium scanning to clinical rather than just screening populations: ready for prime time? *Circ Cardiovas Imaging.* 2016;9.
4. Berman DS, Rozanski A. Value-based imaging: combining coronary artery calcium with myocardial perfusion imaging. *J Nucl Cardiol.* 2016;23:939–941.
5. Budoff MJ, McClelland RL, Nasir K, et al. Cardiovascular events with absent or minimal coronary calcification: the Multi-Ethnic Study of Atherosclerosis (MESA). *Am Heart J.* 2009;158:554–561.
6. Blaha M, Budoff MJ, Shaw LJ, et al. Absence of coronary artery calcification and all-cause mortality. *JACC Cardiovasc Imaging.* 2009;2:692–700.
7. Rumberger JA, Simons DB, Fitzpatrick LA, Sheedy PF, Schwartz RS. Coronary artery calcium area by electron-beam computed tomography and coronary atherosclerotic plaque area. A histopathologic correlative study. *Circulation.* 1995;92:2157–2162.
8. Budoff MJ, Mayrhofer T, Ferencik M, et al. The prognostic value of coronary artery calcium in the PROMISE study. *Circulation.* 2017 Aug 28;pii:117.030578.
9. Einstein AJ, Johnson LL, Bokhari S, et al. Agreement of visual estimation of coronary artery calcium from low-dose CT attenuation correction scans in hybrid-PET/CT and SPECT/CT with standard Agatston score. *J Am Coll Cardiol* 2010;56:1914–1921.
10. Rozanski A, Gransar H, Hayes SW, et al. Temporal trends in the frequency of inducible myocardial ischemia during cardiac stress testing: 1991 to 2009. *J Am Coll Cardiol.* 2013;61:1054–1065.
11. Chhabra L, Ahlberg AW, Henzlova MJ, Duvall WL. Temporal trends of stress myocardial

perfusion imaging: influence of diabetes, gender and coronary artery disease status. *Int J Cardiol.* 2016;202:922–929.

12. Jouni H, Askew JW, Crusan DJ, Miller TD, Gibbons RJ. Temporal trends of single-photon emission computed tomography myocardial perfusion imaging in patients with coronary artery disease: A 22-year experience from a tertiary academic medical center. *Circ Cardiovasc Imaging.* 2017;10.pii: e005628.
13. Metz LD, Beattie M, Hom R, Redberg RF, Grady D, Fleischmann KE. The prognostic value of normal exercise myocardial perfusion imaging and exercise echocardiography: a meta-analysis. *J Am Coll Cardiol.* 2007;49:227–237.
14. Supariwala A, Uretsky S, Depuey EG, et al. Influence of mode of stress and coronary risk factor burden upon long-term mortality following normal stress myocardial perfusion single-photon emission computed tomographic imaging. *Am J Cardiol.* 2013;111:846–850.
15. Rozanski A, Gransar H, Min JK, et al. Long-term mortality following normal exercise myocardial perfusion SPECT according to coronary disease risk factors. *J Nucl Cardiol.* 2014;21:341–350.
16. Chang SM, Nabi F, Xu J, et al. The coronary artery calcium score and stress myocardial perfusion imaging provide independent and complementary prediction of cardiac risk. *JACC* 2009;54:1872–1882.
17. Engbers E, Timmer JR, Ottervanger JP, et al. Prognostic value of coronary artery calcium scoring in addition to SPECT myocardial perfusion imaging in symptomatic patients. *Circ Cardiovasc Imaging.* 2016;9:pii:e0039966.
18. Mouden M, Timmer JR, Reiffers S, et al. Coronary artery calcium scoring to exclude flow-limiting coronary artery disease in symptomatic stable patients at low or intermediate risk. *Radiology.* 2013;269:77–83.
19. van Werkhoven JM, de Boer SM, Schuijf JD, et al. Impact of clinical presentation and pretest likelihood on the relation between calcium score and computed tomographic coronary angiography. *Am J Cardiol.* 2010;106:1675–1679.
20. Rozanski A, Gransar H, Shaw LJ, et al. Impact of coronary artery calcium scanning on coronary risk factors and downstream testing the EISNER (Early Identification of Subclinical Atherosclerosis by Noninvasive Imaging Research) prospective randomized trial. *J Am Coll Cardiol.* 2001;57:1622–1632.
21. Wilson PW, D'Agostino RB, Levy D, et al. Prediction of coronary heart disease using risk factor categories. *Circulation.* 1998;97:1837–1847.
22. Orakzai RH, Nasir K, Orakzai SH, et al. Effect of patient visualization of coronary calcium by electron beam computed tomography on changes in beneficial lifestyle behaviors. *Am J Cardiol.* 2008;101:999–1002.
23. Kalia NK1, Miller LG, Nasir K, et al. Visualizing coronary calcium is associated with improvements in adherence to statin therapy. *Atherosclerosis.* 2006;185:394–399.
24. Mamudu HM, Paul TK, Veeranki SP, Budoff M. The effects of coronary artery calcium screening on behavioral modification, risk perception, and medication adherence among asymptomatic adults: a systematic review. *Atherosclerosis.* 2014;236:338–350.
25. Mouden M, Ottervanger JP, Timmer JR, et al. The influence of coronary calcium score on the interpretation of myocardial perfusion imaging. *J Nucl Cardiol.* 2014;21:368–374.
26. Uretsky S, Cohen R, Argulian E, et al. Combining stress-only myocardial perfusion imaging with coronary calcium scanning as a new paradigm for initial patient work-up: an exploratory analysis. *J Nucl Cardiol.* 2015;22:89–97.
27. Diamond GA, Forrester JS. Analysis of probability as an aid in the clinical diagnosis of coronary-artery disease. *N Engl J Med.* 1979;300:1350–1358.
28. Cheng VY, Berman DS, Rozanski A, et al. Performance of the traditional age, sex, and angina typically-based approach for estimating pretest probability of angiographically significant coronary artery disease in patients undergoing coronary computed tomographic angiography: results from the multinational coronary CT angiography evaluation for clinical outcomes: an international multicenter registry (CONFIRM). *Circulation.* 2011;124:2423–2432, 1–8.
29. Douglas PS, Hoffmann U. Anatomical versus functional testing for coronary artery disease. *N Engl J Med.* 2015;373:91.

30. Villines TC, Hulten EA, Shaw LJ, et al. Prevalence and severity of coronary artery disease and adverse events among symptomatic patients with coronary artery calcification scores of zero undergoing coronary computed tomography angiography: results from the CONFIRM (Coronary CT Angiography Evaluation for Clinical Outcomes: An International Multicenter) registry. *J Am Coll Cardiol.* 2011;58:2533–2540.
31. Budoff MJ, Diamond GA, Raggi P, et al. Continuous probabalistic prediction of angiographically significant coronary artery disease using electron beam tomography. *Circulation* 2002;105:1791–1796.
32. Bavishi C, Argulian E, Chaterjee S, Rozanski A. Coronary artery calcium score and the frequency of stress-induced myocardial ischemia during myocardial perfusion imaging. J *Am Coll Cardiol Imagining.* 2016.
33. Wong ND, Rozanski A, Gransar H, et al. Metabolic syndrome and diabetes are associated with an increased likelihood of inducible myocardial ischemia among patients with subclinical atherosclerosis. *Diabetes Care.* 2005;28:1445–1450.
34. Rozanski A, Gransar H, Wong ND, et al. Use of coronary calcium scanning for predicting inducible myocardial ischemia: influence of patients' clinical presentation. *J Nucl Cardiol.* 2007;14: 669–679
35. Myers J, Prakash M, Froelicher V, Do D, Partington S, Atwood JE. Exercise capacity and mortality among men referred for exercise testing. *N Engl J Med.* 2002;346:793–801.

EDITOR'S PERSPECTIVE

Timothy M. Bateman

In the 1970s, it became popular in some labs performing planar thallium-201 studies to have patients routinely undergo cardiac fluoroscopy.[1] Fluoroscopy was felt to be useful, because it could detect the presence of coronary artery calcium (CAC), and therefore assist in making a correct diagnosis when combining interpretation of both fluoroscopy and the often equivocal planar scintigrams. With modern technologies, this has now become a reality. In the current era, despite the fact that tomographic single photon and positron images are much more highly resolved and accurate, knowledge of the presence of CAC continues to be an important adjunct to myocardial perfusion data.

The authors of this chapter delineate the strong evidence base in support of routinely measuring or estimating CAC in conjunction with stress/rest MPI tests. As they point out, knowledge of CAC:

- can change a miscommunication about the meaning of a normal scan implying no CAD to a diagnosis of underlying CAD, despite no current flow-limiting lesions;
- carries important independent short- and long-term prognostic information;
- can inform changes in patient management, education about their disease, and frequency and intensity of follow-up.

Fortunately, delineating the presence of CAC is facilitated by the existence of hybrid scanners. Even with non-hybrid devices, the simplicity of the test is such that a CAC score can be gotten in seconds by having the patient undergo this test elsewhere in the facility using a stand-alone CT scanner. This chapter makes the case for such evaluation.

The authors have made the important point that the presence and extent of CAC adds prognostic information regardless of whether the scan is normal or abnormal. In practice, CAC scoring is less useful once a diagnosis of CAD has been made. It has the most value when the MPI has been ordered for a patient with no prior history of CAD.

Readers should also know that with modern scanners the risk in deriving the CAC score is low. In most patients, informed control of tube voltage and current should result in radiation exposures on the order of 1 mSv.[2] Further, inspection of a non-gated low-resolution CT scan acquired for attenuation correction can provide sufficient information to identify the presence of CAC as well as a fairly accurate estimate of its score, at approximately 0.3 mSv.[3]

Report generation, including a statement about the presence and extent of CAC, should be routine for reasons discussed throughout this chapter. However, there remain many questions that hopefully will be answered with further research. Among these are the following:

- In a patient with a very high CAC score but a normal or near-normal MPI performed with vasodilator stress, is there a CAC threshold at which coronary angiography should be considered, regardless of scan appearances, and does myocardial blood flow quantification influence this decision?
- Does a high CAC score carry the same prognostic importance when PET-derived myocardial blood flow is normal, implying healthy coronary physiology despite the presence of CAC?
- Should a normal or low CAC score deter performance of MPI in younger patients with chest pain syndromes?
- Should scan interpreters routinely inspect the non-gated low resolution CT scans for the presence and extent of CAC as well as accuracy of the results, and do these rough estimates result in changes in patient management or in patient outcomes?[3,4]

Based on current understandings, this chapter should serve as an excellent reference in support of the emerging practice of combining an assessment of CAC for all patients with no known CAD history. Careful inspection of the CT scans for other incidental findings such as valvular calcifications, thoracic aorta enlargements, pericardial and pleural effusions, and lung abnormalities is also important.[5,6]

References for Editor's Perspective

1. Bartel AG, Chen JY, Peter RH, Behar VS, Kong Y, Lester RG. The significance of coronary calcification detected by fluoroscopy. A report of 360 patients. *Circulation*. 1974;49:1247-1253.

2. Messenger B, Dong L, Nasir K, Carr JJ, Blankstein R, Budoff MJ. Coronary calcium scans and radiation exposure in the multi-ethnic study of atherosclerosis. *Int J Cardiovasc Img.* 2016;32:525-529.
3. Einstein AJ, Johnson LL, Bokhari S, et al. Agreement of visual estimation of coronary artery calcium from low-dose CT attenuation correction scans in hybrid-PET/CT and SPECT/CT with standard Agatston score. *J Am Coll Cardiol.* 2010;56:1914-1921.
4. Xie X, Zhao Y, de Bock GH, et al. Validation and prognosis of coronary artery calcium scoring in non-triggered thoracic computed tomography: systematic review and meta-analysis. *Circ Cardiovasc Imaging.* 2013;6:514-521.
5. Goetze S, Pannu HK, Wahl RL. Clinically significant abnormal findings on the "nondiagnostic" CT portion of low-amperage-CT attenuation-corrected myocardial perfusion SPECT/CT studies. *J Nucl Med.* 2006;47:1312-1318.
6. Machaalany J, Yam Y, Ruddy TD, et al. Potential clinical and economic consequences of noncardiac incidental findings on cardiac computed tomography. *J Am Coll Cardiol.* 2009;54:1533-1541.

Interpretation of Cardiac PET Myocardial Perfusion Imaging Studies

CHAPTER 3

Dennis A. Calnon

INTRODUCTION

Cardiac positron emission tomographic (PET) myocardial perfusion imaging offers patients and referring health-care providers a superior product with high diagnostic accuracy and risk stratification. As with SPECT, the interpretation of the images is extremely important to the resulting product. Physicians with experience in interpreting single-photon emission computed tomography myocardial perfusion imaging (SPECT MPI) are familiar with the imaging artifacts that reduce confidence in the interpretation of SPECT MPI studies (eg, soft tissue attenuation, gastrointestinal (GI) tracer activity in close proximity to the heart, and patient motion). Interpretation of PET MPI studies requires an understanding of the fundamental differences between PET and SPECT (Table 3-1) and the imaging artifacts unique to PET MPI. As rubidium-82 (^{82}Rb) is the most commonly used radionuclide tracer for PET MPI, the discussion pertains primarily to interpretation of ^{82}Rb PET MPI studies. This chapter examines key aspects to successful interpretation, including differences in interpretation between SPECT and PET, artifacts unique to PET, approaches to interpretation, and, finally, reporting.

As a result of the robust methods for correction for soft tissue attenuation and photon scatter, a normal PET MPI study will generally appear "more normal" than a normal SPECT MPI study. That is, in normal subjects, image quality will typically be good to excellent[1] and myocardial tracer activity will be more homogeneous with PET MPI than SPECT MPI. Unlike SPECT MPI (in which breast attenuation results in variability in normal perfusion patterns for women and men), normal PET MPI perfusion patterns for women and men are similar to one another. Owing to the superior myocardial uptake kinetics of PET MPI tracers and the ability to measure left ventricular systolic function at peak stress, an abnormal PET MPI study will appear "more abnormal" than an abnormal SPECT MPI study. Therefore, interpretative confidence is higher for PET MPI studies than for SPECT MPI studies.[1] However, confident interpretation of PET MPI studies requires that the PET MPI study is performed properly and that study quality is confirmed with automated quality control software. The use of quality control software is mandatory for PET MPI, because it is impossible to exclude artifacts related to patient motion or incorrect attenuation correction (misregistration of transmission and emission datasets) solely by reviewing the reconstructed tomographic slices. Unlike traditional SPECT MPI in which the angular projections are acquired sequentially and the rotating raw planar images are available for review, PET MPI images are acquired simultaneously by circular arrays of detectors. As a result, there are no rotating raw images for visual assessment of study quality with PET MPI.

DIFFERENCES BETWEEN PET AND SPECT INTERPRETATION

There are common normal variants that need to be recognized when interpreting PET MPI studies.

Table 3.1

Fundamental Differences Between Traditional SPECT and ^{82}Rb PET

	Traditional SPECT	^{82}Rb PET
Spatial resolution (mm)	12-15	4-6
Photon energy (keV)	68-167	511
Attenuation correction	Rarely used	Routine and robust
Scatter correction	Rarely used	Routine and robust
GI tracer interference	Common	Minimal
Timing of stress imaging	post-stress	Peak-stress
Acquisition of angular projections	Sequential	Simultaneous

Owing to the partial volume effect and the superior spatial resolution of PET, the apical region will frequently demonstrate a mild reduction in tracer activity on both resting and peak-stress images in normal subjects (Figure 3-1A). The apical defect is a result of the normal anatomic thinning of the apical myocardium relative to the mid- and basilar myocardial regions. This is illustrated in Figure 3-1B. The peak-stress images are displayed directly above the corresponding resting images. There is mildly reduced ^{82}Rb activity in the apical region on both the rest and peak-stress images. There is GI uptake of ^{82}Rb evident on the resting images, but the GI tracer activity does not interfere with image interpretation.

A

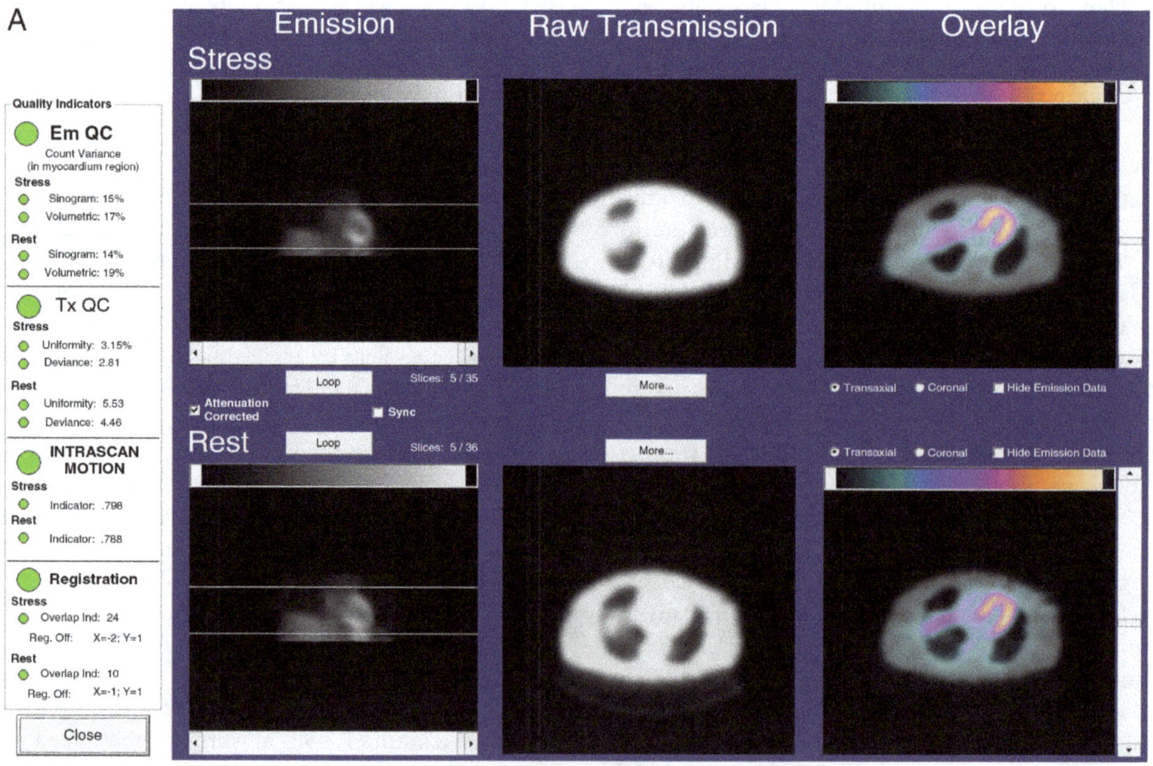

FIGURE 3-1A Normal PET MPI Study With Apical Thinning Variant: Quality Control Display.

B

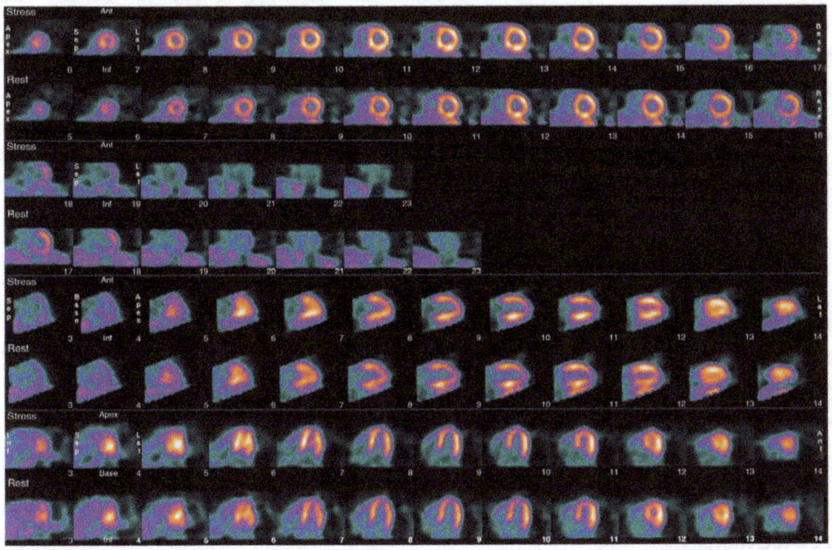

FIGURE 3-1B Tomographic Slices Illustrating Normal Apical Thinning With Rb-82 PET.

C

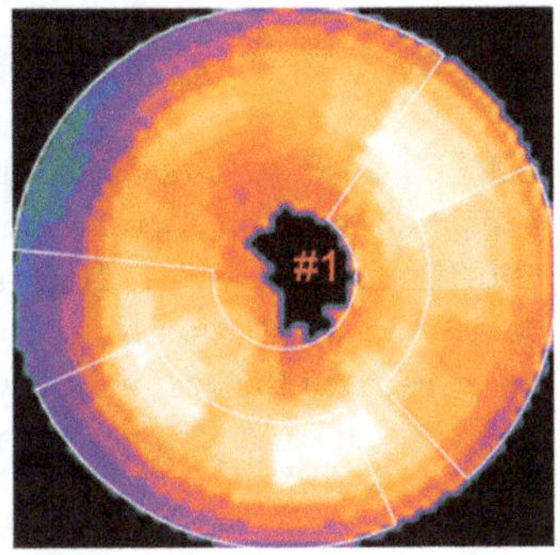

FIGURE 3-1C Polar Map Display of PET Apical Thinning Normal Variant.

Although there are commercially available quantitative PET MPI software programs that include gender-specific normal databases for assessment of regional 82Rb distribution, the software programs can fail to recognize the normal "apical thinning variant" (Figure 3-1C). The mild reduction in apical tracer activity is incorrectly designated as a true perfusion defect by the quantitative perfusion software program. Apical thinning is associated with normal wall motion on peak-stress and resting images. Regional wall thickening is normal in the apical region on both resting and peak-stress confirming the normal apical thinning variant. In this case, the left ventricular ejection fraction (LVEF) increased 5% during stress acquisition, compared to rest. A normal "LVEF reserve" (peak-stress LVEF minus resting LVEF) of 5% is a typical finding in normal subjects.

The apical thinning variant is even more commonly observed during ^{13}N-ammonia imaging because of the higher spatial resolution of ^{13}N-ammonia compared to ^{82}Rb, and fluorine-18 (^{18}F) labeled perfusion tracers (in clinical development) would be expected to demonstrate apical thinning because of the very high spatial resolution of ^{18}F. Another normal variant to recognize is the occasional reduction in lateral wall tracer activity on ^{13}N-ammonia PET images.[2] To date, this defect is unexplained, but may be incorrectly interpreted as being positive for ischemia.

The spatial resolution for PET perfusion tracers varies because of differences in the energy of the positrons emitted from the nucleus during radioactive decay. Positrons with higher energy travel longer average distances before interacting with an electron, resulting in mutual particle annihilation and generation of two 511 keV photons. This distance traveled by the positron from the nucleus to the site of interaction with an electron is referred to as the positron range of the PET radionuclide. Table 3-2 lists the half-lives and positron ranges of PET radionuclides. Perfusion images acquired with radionuclides with a long positron range (eg, ^{82}Rb) demonstrate lower spatial resolution and mild image blurring. Images acquired with radionuclides with a short positron range (eg, ^{18}F) demonstrate higher spatial resolution

Table 3.2

Half-lives and Positron Ranges of PET Radionuclides

Radionuclide	Half-Life (min)	Positron Range (mm)
Fluorine-18	110	0.23
N-13 ammonia	9.8	0.57
O-15 water	2	1.02
Rubidium-82	1.27	2.60

and sharper delineation of the left ventricular cavity and endocardial surface. Despite these apparent limitations, it is clear that the overall image quality of any PET tracer is superior to the lower-energy technetium (SPECT) tracers.

PET IMAGING ARTIFACTS

All PET MPI studies are routinely processed using robust attenuation correction, either with a radionuclide line source or CT. Thus, the routine artifacts of soft tissue attenuation from body habitus are no longer present in the vast majority of patients. The three primary causes of artifact with PET are discussed in the next sections.

Patient Motion During Image Acquisition

Similar to SPECT MPI, patient motion during image acquisition produces motion artifacts on PET MPI studies (Figures 3-2, 3-3, and 3-4). Patient motion is a more significant problem for PET MPI than for SPECT MPI, primarily because PET motion cannot be "corrected"[3] owing to the continuous acquisition of the PET data, which means that one cannot isolate where the motion occurred. Thus, recognition of this artifact with PET, particularly if it affects the stress study alone, is important in reducing false-positive interpretations.

Table 3-3 outlines the factors influencing the impact of patient motion on PET and SPECT MPI. As mentioned previously, PET MPI images are acquired simultaneously by circular arrays of detectors, and, because of the continuous acquisition of data on each detector, visual identification of patient motion during image acquisition cannot be identified by reviewing rotating images. Therefore, patient motion is harder to detect on PET MPI studies, although some software programs can alert the reader to its presence. Positive identification of patient motion is left to evaluation of the processed images. Thus, being able to recognize the presence of motion on PET images is very important. Visually, the image appears distorted and blurred, similar to an extreme example of motion artifact during SPECT. Two examples of patient motion during cardiac PET MPI with rubidium-82 are shown in Figures 3-2, 3-3, and 3-4.

Figure 3-2 is an example of substantial motion artifact on the peak-stress data. This is characterized by a distortion of the entire image, with elongation of the ventricle on the short axis images. There are both anterior and inferior abnormalities, which cannot be mistaken for CAD but are consistent with motion artifact. This defect is so severe that the study should be repeated, rather than assuming that the study is normal (with motion artifact) or abnormal. A second example of less severe patient motion artifact is shown in Figure 3-3. This, too, affects only the peak-stress data. There are "contralateral" defects in the anterior and inferior regions, with distortion of the entire image. The patient motion produces a "slit-like" appearance, which does not appear typical for CAD. This can be interpreted as "probably normal" if the reporting physician were comfortable with this. Also note that the TID ratio may be spuriously abnormal (TID >1.13) because of the patient motion affecting the measured cavity volumes. A third example of motion is shown in Figure 3-4. In this case, patient motion is present on both peak-stress and resting images. In both "cool" and gray-scale, the left ventricle appears square rather than round on short axis projections. There are slit-like deformities in the septal, lateral, and inferior segments that do not have the typical appearance of CAD, with similar characteristics on peak-stress and resting images. This study can be considered "probably normal" or the study can be repeated.

Quality-control software is capable of detecting and quantifying patient motion, but robust methods for motion correction are not yet available for PET MPI and are difficult because of the continuous acquisition of data, such that individual datasets cannot be corrected. On account of the short 75-second half-life of ^{82}Rb, the presence of severe patient motion requires repeat image acquisition, which can be accomplished easily on the rest image, but more difficult on stress image due to the short-lived hyperemic phase. Therefore, prevention of patient motion is much more important for PET MPI than for SPECT MPI. The shorter scan times for emission image acquisition for PET (5–7 minutes) compared to traditional SPECT (12–14 minutes) reduces the likelihood of patient motion during imaging. However, unlike traditional SPECT in which the patient leaves the imaging table between rest and poststress

Table 3.3

Factors Influencing the Impact of Motion Artifact on SPECT and PET

	Traditional SPECT	Rubidium-82 PET
Acquisition of angular projections	Sequential	Simultaneous
Review of cine images for motion	Yes	No
Time per image acquisition (min)	12-15	5-6
Continuous time under camera (min)	12-15	30-40
Motion detection software	Yes	Yes
Motion correction software	Yes	No
Able to repeat image for motion	Yes	No

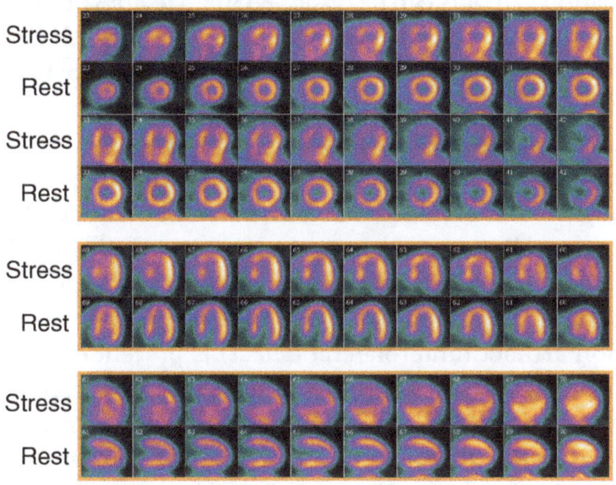

FIGURE 3-2 Example of Motion Artifact During Stress Acquisition. There is distortion of the image, which could be interpreted as CAD.

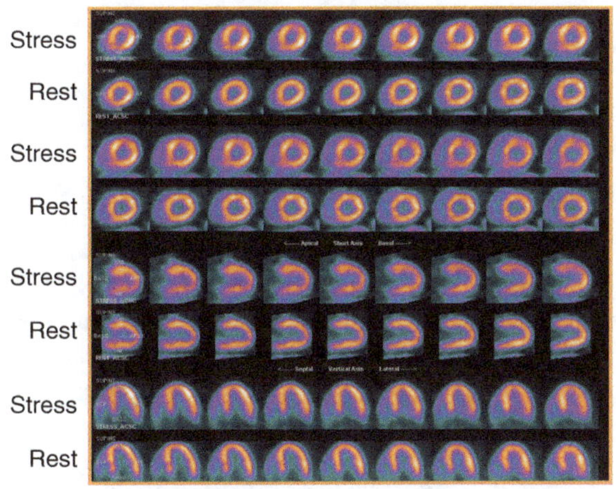

FIGURE 3-3 Example of Less Severe Motion During Stress Contralateral defects in the anterior and inferior segments are consistent with motion artifact.

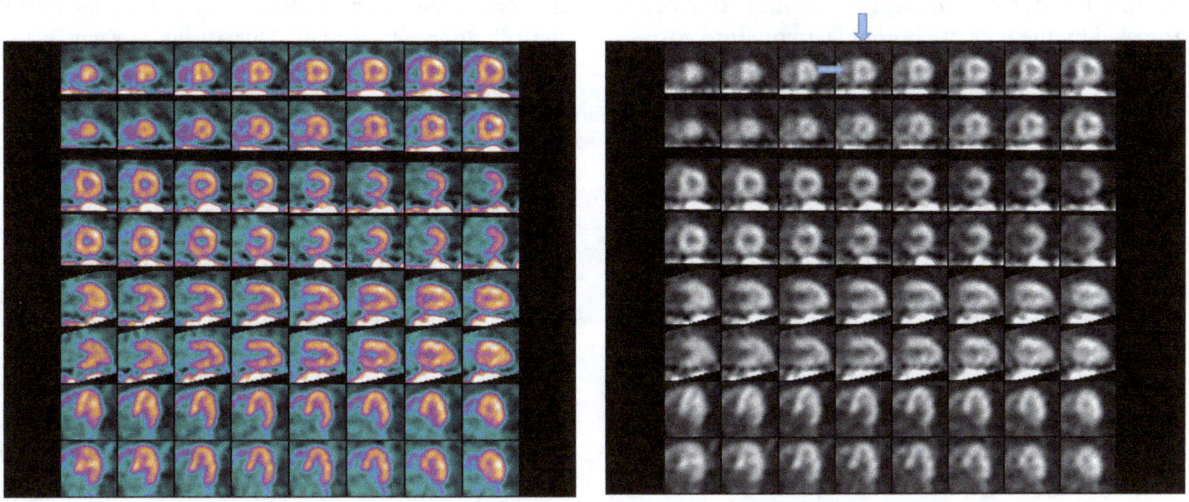

FIGURE 3-4 Example of Motion Artifact During Both Stress and Rest Images are in "cool" color as well as gray scale. Arrows point to slit-like defects consistent with motion. The images are abnormal but do not have the appearance of CAD.

image acquisitions, the patient remains continuously in the PET scanner for the full 30–40 minute duration of a standard rest-stress ^{82}Rb PET MPI protocol. Therefore, patient comfort and patient cooperation are critically important for PET MPI. It is particularly important for the technologists to coach the patient to not move specifically during the short acquisition phases of rest and stress PET. One approach to addressing the problem of patient motion is to acquire dynamic sequential images rather than a single static image. In this way, the frames degraded by patient motion can be rejected and the remaining frames that are free of patient motion can be used for image reconstruction.[4]

Misregistration of the Emission and Transmission Images

It is a common misconception that because of the high 511 keV energy of the photons produced by PET radionuclides, soft tissue attenuation is less problematic for PET MPI than for SPECT MPI. In fact, the opposite is true. Accurate assessment of the anatomic distribution of a PET radionuclide requires nearly simultaneous (coincidence) detection of a pair of photons by detectors on opposite sides of the patient. Therefore, each pair of photons must traverse the entire diameter of the patient's thorax. If either of the two photons fails to reach the detector, the positron annihilation event will not be registered. For this reason (and the combined distance traveled by the pair of photons), attenuation correction is mandatory for high-quality PET MPI. This is accomplished successfully with all PET systems, and robust attenuation correction is a routine part of every PET study.

Transmission scans are used to define the soft tissue attenuation characteristics of the patient. The transmission scans can be obtained with either dedicated line source in the form of the radionuclide germanium or with CT sources. In both cases, data are collected separately from the perfusion (emission) data. In processing, the two images are superimposed. If the emission and transmission datasets are not properly aligned, misregistration artifacts will occur. The typical perfusion defect produced by misregistration is an anterolateral wall defect caused by portions of the anterolateral wall of the left ventricle extending into the left lung field; however, septal and inferior abnormalities can also be the result of nonalignment. The affected myocardial region (eg, the anterolateral region) is then incorrectly assigned a very low attenuation value (consistent with lung tissue) and the attenuation correction algorithm produces a perfusion defect in the anterolateral region. If the misregistration artifact is not recognized, this perfusion pattern might be mistaken for the presence of left main or left circumflex coronary artery disease. False-positives can occur in other affected areas, such as inferior and septal regions as well. Studies have noted that clinically relevant misregistration artifacts can be observed in up to 40% of PET/CT studies.[5] Misregistration is less likely with line source attenuation correction because the patient does not move within the camera. It is important to inspect the quality control overlay of the emission and transmission datasets to confirm proper alignment. If needed, the datasets can be shifted into proper alignment, using misregistration software. If misregistration is apparent on review of the quality control display and a typical appearing misregistration artifact (anterolateral defect) is present on perfusion images, the misregistration must be corrected and the properly aligned images be reconstructed and reviewed. An example of anterior misregistration is shown in Figure 3-5. In this example, the upper images show an anterolateral defect that has the appearance of CAD. However, the axial images demonstrate that the emission (PET data) are out of the CT attenuation map. This study, as seen in the second set of images, was registration corrected with available software, and is now normal.

Gastrointestinal (GI) Tracer Activity With Cardiac PET

Intense GI tracer activity in close proximity to the heart is a very common source of imaging artifact on SPECT MPI studies, especially those obtained at rest or following pharmacologic stress. As a result of the superior spatial resolution of PET, the robust scatter/attenuation correction, and the slightly lower intrinsic GI uptake of ^{82}Rb compared to the ^{99m}Tc-labeled SPECT tracers, GI tracer interference is substantially less problematic with ^{82}Rb PET MPI (Figure 3-1B). In a clinical comparison of SPECT and PET patients,

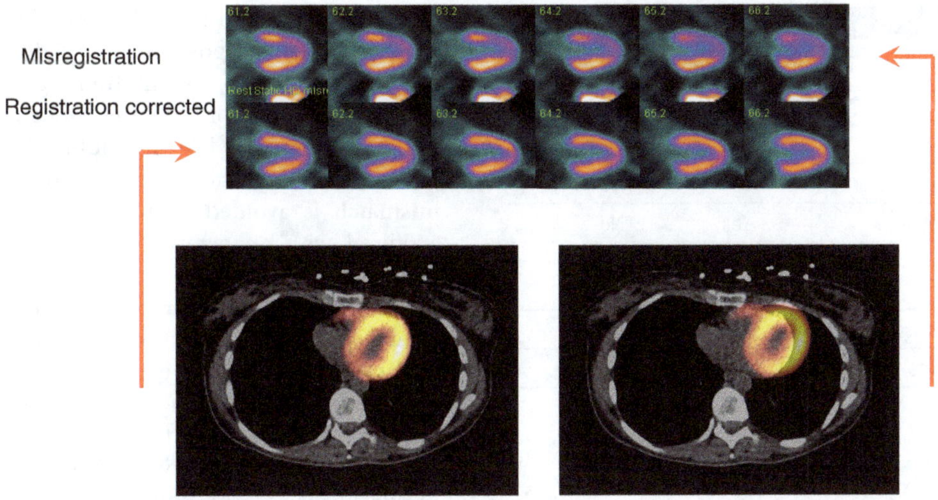

FIGURE 3-5 Misregistration on Rest Image With Software Correction. The corrected image is shown below. Axial images demonstrate misregistration.

Bateman et al reported significantly fewer patients with PET who had gut and liver interference (1). Even when present, gut and/or liver activity rarely affects diagnostic performance (1).

Low Tracer Counts During PET

Owing to the 75-second half-life of ^{82}Rb, approximately 95% of the useful counts are obtained in the first 5 minutes of imaging. Optimal timing of the ^{82}Rb image acquisition is critically important to ensure adequate counts. For patients with normal left ventricular function, imaging is typically initiated 70–90 seconds after completion of the ^{82}Rb infusion to avoid blood pooling, which interferes with interpretation (the ^{82}Rb infusion should be accomplished in < 30 seconds).[4] However, the myocardial uptake and blood pool clearance of ^{82}Rb is delayed in patients with reduced left ventricular systolic function, severe pulmonary hypertension, hemodynamically significant left to right shunts, or severe valvular regurgitation. In these situations, emission images are typically initiated 110–130 seconds after completion of the ^{82}Rb infusion. If imaging is begun too early after ^{82}Rb infusion, residual left ventricular blood pool tracer activity will scatter into the myocardial counts, degrading image quality and interfering with accurate assessment of perfusion defect size and severity.

ARTIFACTS UNIQUE TO PET/CT

Attenuation correction can be accomplished by transmission scans acquired using computed tomography (CT) or an external radioactive line source (Table 3-4). PET/CT imaging allows for detailed anatomic localization of tracer activity for clinical applications, such as assessment of cardiovascular device infections and cardiac sarcoid assessment. PET/CT also permits coronary artery calcium scoring, which can refine long-term cardiac risk stratification for patients with normal PET perfusion studies.[6] The value of calcium scoring during PET/CT is discussed in Chapter 3. CT-based transmission scans can be acquired rapidly during a single breath hold. The required breath hold duration will vary from <10 seconds (for a CT scanner with 16 or more slices) to >20 seconds (for CT scanners with only 2 to 4 slices).[3] In contrast, dedicated PET scanners using radioactive line sources require 60 to 180 seconds to acquire a transmission scan.

There are two important disadvantages of the use of CT for attenuation correction: respiratory mismatch and metal artifacts (Table 3-4). Respiratory mismatch occurs because the CT transmission images are acquired during a rapid breath hold, while the emission images are acquired over 5 minutes during free breathing. The breath hold CT transmission images might therefore fail to accurately represent the attenuation

Table 3.4

Comparison of CT vs line-source (dedicated PET) for attenuation correction

	CT	Line Source
CTA and calcium score	Yes	No
Anatomic detail	Yes	No
Transmission scan time (sec)	10-25	60-180
Respiratory mismatch	Common	No
Metal artifacts	Yes	No

pattern of the patient's chest during emission image acquisition. Examples of respiratory motion are demonstrated in Figure 3-6.[3] In Figure 3-6, the patient on the left took a deep breath in the middle of the scan resulting in the liver being imaged in two different locations. The patient on the right took a smaller breath, resulting in a choppy boundary between the mediastinum and the lung. The artifacts present in these transmission images might produce perfusion artifacts when the attenuation coefficients are applied to the emission dataset.

Several approaches have been proposed to address this potential source for artifacts. CT images can be acquired multiple times during free breathing, then averaged to obtain a CT transmission scan reflecting the average diaphragm position during free breathing. The disadvantages of this method include potentially higher radiation exposure and degradation of the spatial resolution of the CT images. The other approach is to acquire the CT during an end-expiratory breath hold. Because the diaphragm spends most of the time in light expiratory phase during a normal breathing cycle, the end-expiratory breath hold more closely approximates the average position of the diaphragm during free breathing. Patient training is mandatory prior to transmission imaging, since most patients find end-expiratory breath holding to be less natural than end-inspiratory breath holding. Respiratory mismatch is avoided by using transmission scans acquired with an external radioactive line source during free breathing.

Metal artifacts occur because of the high efficiency of metals to absorb x-rays and because of differences in attenuation effects between x-rays and photons generated though positron-electron annihilation. Metal objects attenuate x-rays primarily via the photoelectric effect, while Compton scatter primarily affects 511 keV photons and the photoelectric effect is relatively small.[3] The CT-derived attenuation values, therefore, do not accurately reflect the attenuation of the 511 keV photons. Metallic objects can also produce streak artifacts and beam-hardening artifacts, which further corrupt the transmission images and can produce (or mask) perfusion defects. It has been estimated that 50% of patients with metal objects near the heart can be subject to metal artifacts.[7] Metal artifacts are avoided by using an external radioactive line source for attenuation correction.

APPROACH TO THE INTERPRETATION OF CARDIAC PET MPI STUDIES

As with SPECT, the interpretation of a cardiac PET MPI study is dependent on the quality of the study presented to the interpreting physician. Thus, assessment of the quality of the collected and processed data is an important aspect before providing an interpretation. Quality evaluation and interpretation and

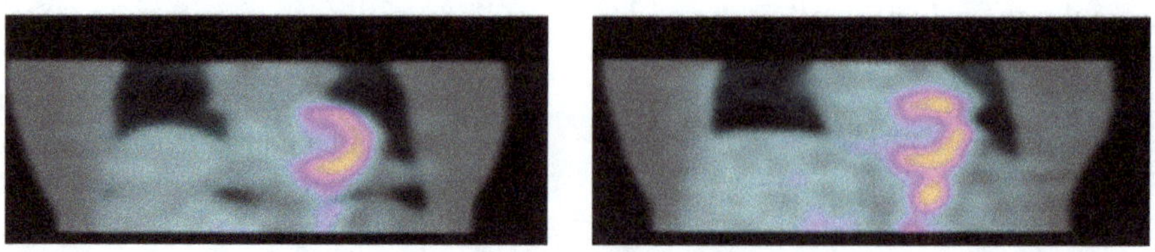

FIGURE 3-6 Breathing Artifacts During a Free Breathing CT Transmission Scanning Protocol. (Reproduced with permission from Case JA, Bateman TM: Taking the perfect nuclear image: Quality control, acquisition, and processing techniques for cardiac SPECT, PET, and hybrid imaging, J Nucl Cardiol. 2013 Oct;20(5):891-907)

reporting of cardiac PET MPI is discussed in the next section.

Quality Control Evaluation Prior to Interpretation

The quality control software display should be carefully inspected, with close attention to the overlay representation of the emission and transmission scan to confirm proper alignment. This can be observed in the coronal and axial views to determine proper overlay. If there is overlap, the study should be reprocessed before interpretation. In addition, evaluation of the data collection by way of rotating (raw) images should also be examined. Although one cannot observe motion as in SPECT because of the continuous acquisition of data, the position of the patient in the camera field as well as extraneous structures can be evaluated. There are several software displays for quality control, one of which is illustrated in Figure 3-1. The quality indicators on the left are displayed in a color format, with green, yellow, or red lights representing good, moderate, or poor quality for each individual parameter. Quality parameters include emission scan quality, transmissions scan quality, motion, and registration of the emission and transmission scans with one another. The emission scans can be viewed in a simulated rotating format, both as attenuation corrected and uncorrected images. Transmission scans (in this case obtained using a germanium line source) can be viewed alone (center panel) or as an overlay of the emission and transmission images (right panel).

If the heart is positioned too close to the upper or lower aspect of the camera head, artifact in the anterior or inferior walls could result. An example of the patient being out of the field affecting the inferior wall of the perfusion image is shown in Figure 3-7A, B, and C. As seen in the still image of the stress rotating images (blue arrow), during the stress data collection the inferior wall is below the camera field (Figure 3-7A). This results in the inferior wall of the processed data being absent on peak-stress, but not on resting images (Figure 3-7B), which could be interpreted as a reversible inferior perfusion abnormality consistent with ischemia. The patient returned for a repeat stress imaging at a later time, as shown in Figure 3-7C. The study now shows a fixed inferior defect.

SEQUENTIAL INTERPRETATION OF A CARDIAC PET STUDY

Once the quality control data are examined and thought to be satisfactory, the perfusion images are reviewed as tomographic slices in a manner identical to the review of SPECT MPI images. As with SPECT, it is recommended that the PET MPI perfusion images should be interpreted initially without clinical information in order to minimize bias.[4] Relevant clinical information should be subsequently reviewed. There are subtle differences in the interpretation between SPECT and PET. First, the slice thickness of both rubidium-82 and ammonia-13 are one-half that of SPECT, thus there are approximately 2-fold more slices for the same size heart. This should be taken into account when determining the size of a given perfusion abnormality. Second, because of robust scatter and attenuation correction, tracer distribution on PET images should appear homogeneous, since the impact of attenuation artifact is virtually eliminated. Therefore, any perfusion abnormality, particularly if reversible, should be considered consistent with CAD. In general, PET is read for sensitivity while SPECT is read for specificity owing to the number of attenuation artifacts. Gut and liver activity are less frequent with the two PET tracers, but are not uncommonly still present. A primary difference between SPECT and PET is that with the latter it is rare that gut/liver tracer activity interferes with interpretation, again owing to higher spatial resolution, scatter, and attenuation correction.

While these characteristics lend toward a higher diagnostic accuracy, including specificity, both rubidium and ammonia have artifacts that reduce accuracy. This is most likely related to their unfavorable positron range, which leads to apparent perfusion abnormalities that are not associated with CAD. In the case of ammonia, the unexplained lateral defects need to be recognized, while rubidium is associated with small reversible inferior wall perfusion abnormalities.

The ratio of peak-stress to resting left ventricular cavity volume (transient ischemic dilation or TID)

A

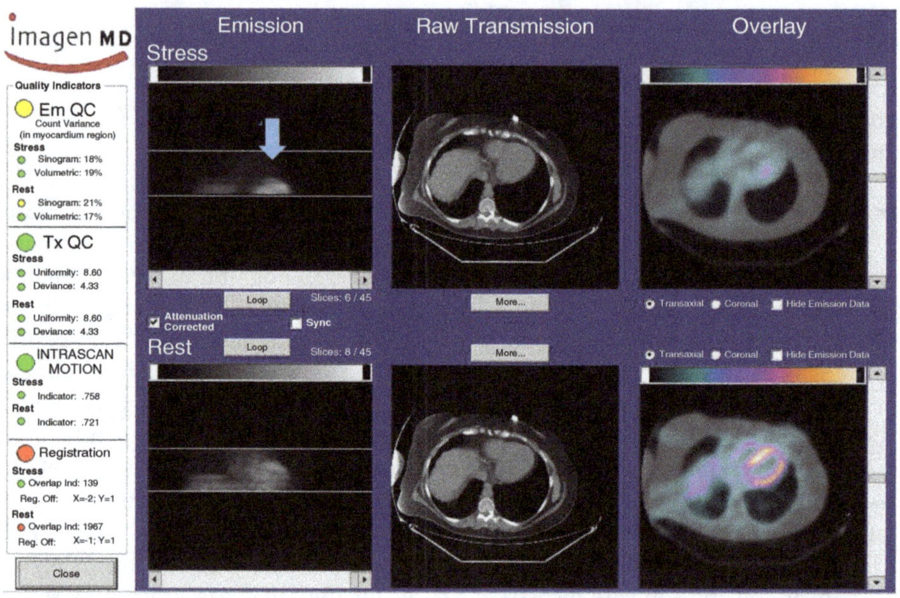

FIGURE 3-7 A Quality Control Page Demonstrating Stress Emission Study Partially. Below Camera Edge (Blue Arrow)

B

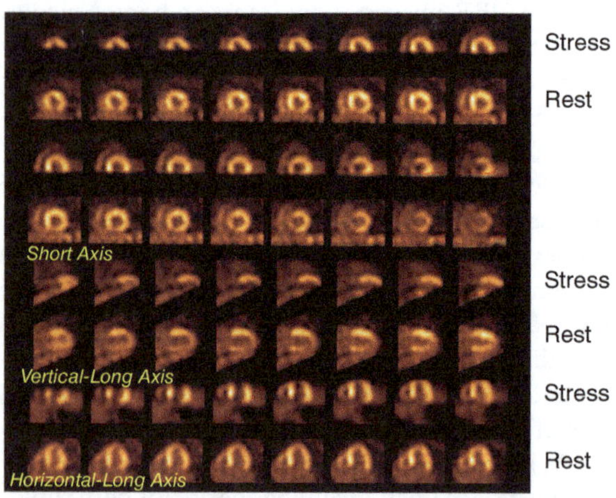

FIGURE 3-7B Rest/Stress PET Study With Inferior Wall Out of Camera Field. This creates a reversible defect.

C

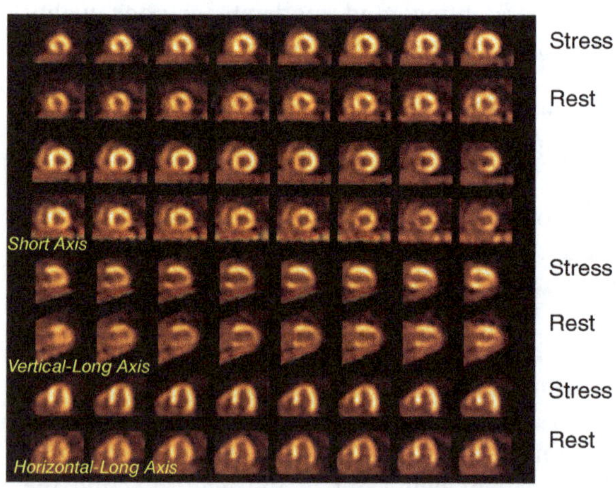

FIGURE 3-7C Repeat Stress Study With Image Collected Within the Camera Field. The study now shows a fixed inferior defect.

can be assessed subjectively and quantitatively. Because PET MPI images are acquired at peak-stress (rather than 30–60 minutes poststress as for SPECT MPI), TID is observed relatively commonly on PET MPI studies in the presence of ischemia. The threshold for elevated TID for ^{82}Rb has been reported to be 1.13 (based on a mean of 0.98 ± 0.06 in normal subjects; 0.98 + 2.5 SDs = 1.13) with a second study reporting similar results.[8,9] However, these studies were small and the TID threshold may vary depending on the patient population, the imaging protocol, and the specific quantitative software used. There are fewer studies evaluating TID in PET, but TID is a relatively common occurrence in both single vessel and multivessel CAD, and presence of TID on PET MPI studies does not always indicate extensive (multivessel) disease at catheterization, in contrast to SPECT.

Similar to SPECT MPI, subjective assessment of TID is most reliably accomplished by comparison of the peak-stress and resting images on vertical and horizontal long-axis projections. Inadvertent misalignment of the short-axis images can produce the appearance of TID because the apparent cavity dilation on peak-stress images will be evident on all slices from the apex to the base of the left ventricle. For this reason, the appearance of TID on short-axis slices should always be confirmed by reviewing the long-axis slices. Relative myocardial perfusion (assessment of regional tracer activity relative to the most normal myocardial region) can be assessed using semiquantitative methods (17 segment model and summed stress, summed rest, and summed difference scores) and by using quantitative polar perfusion maps derived from ^{82}Rb imaging in subjects with a low-likelihood of coronary artery disease, available on most software packages that display PET images.

LVEF and regional wall motion can be assessed on gated PET MPI imaging at rest and peak-stress, and the LVEF reserve is defined as the peak-stress LVEF minus the resting LVEF.[9] As described by Dorbala et al (9), in patients with normal myocardial perfusion, the LVEF typically rises during vasodilator stress (the LVEF reserve is positive) and the left ventricular end-systolic volume declines (Figure 3-8A).[9] As the extent and severity of coronary artery disease increases, the LVEF reserve declines and becomes negative in the presence of multivessel or left main disease (Figure 3-8B).[9] Because the gated PET MPI images are acquired during peak-stress (in contrast to gated SPECT MPI images that are acquired 30–60 minutes poststress), reduced regional left ventricular wall thickening is more commonly observed on peak-stress gated PET images and may represent acute myocardial ischemia rather than postischemic myocardial stunning.

A reversible wall motion abnormality (in the same area as a reversible perfusion defect) is observed more frequently with PET than SPECT because of the data collection in close proximity to peak hyperemic pharmacologic stress. It can be observed in conjunction with a drop in ejection fraction, or independent of that finding. As with SPECT, it assists in assuring that the reversible perfusion abnormality is consistent with CAD and usually associated with high-grade stenosis (>80%) at cardiac catheterization.

Because of the higher spatial resolution of PET MPI, the right ventricle is frequently well delineated. Right ventricular dilation or increased right ventricular tracer activity relative to the left ventricle can be seen in the presence of pulmonary hypertension. Some PET software programs are able to provide a right ventricular ejection fraction, although the validity of such data have not yet been defined. If a relative increase in right ventricular activity is only apparent on the peak-stress images, the reader should consider the possibility of balanced left ventricular ischemia as a result of left main disease.[10]

Increased lung tracer activity can be observed on the quality control display in patients with elevated left ventricular filling pressure, infiltrative lung disease, or active tobacco use.[4] Lung tracer activity is typically reported qualitatively.

Extra-cardiac tracer uptake can be seen in the presence of malignancy or localized inflammation. PET/CT systems provide more precise anatomic localization of the site of increased tracer activity, but important extra-cardiac findings can also be identified using dedicated PET systems. Figure 3-9A-C shows examples of findings on transmission images acquired using an external germanium line source. Figure 3-9A shows (arrows) left arm noted on the side of the patient in both the overlay and transmission images. Figure 3-9B illustrates a patient with a breast implant observed on the transmission data. The left breast implant (center and right panels, white arrows) is positioned more anteriorly than the native right breast, which falls laterally to the patient's right side while in the supine position on the imaging table. The position and density of the left breast implant is reflected by the transmission images and the emission images are corrected for the specific pattern of photon attenuation. Figure 3-9C shows an example of localized ^{82}Rb uptake in the left breast in a patient with breast cancer. The left breast uptake is evident on the simulated rotating emission images (left panel, red arrows) and in the overlay of the transmission and emission images (right panel, white arrows). The images were acquired with the left arm down in the field of view, which can be seen on the raw transmission images

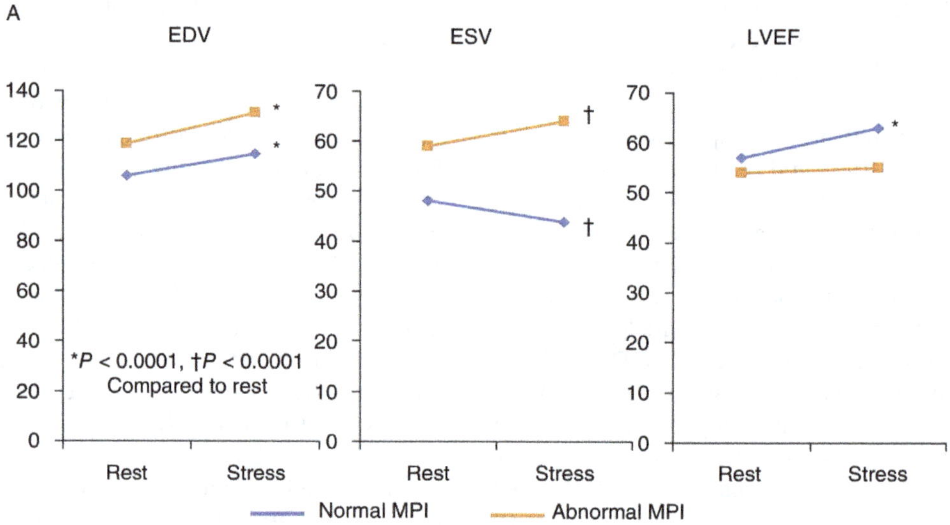

FIGURE 3-8A Left Ventricular Volumes and Ejection Fraction by Gated PET at Rest and During Regadenoson Stress. ("Reproduced with permission from Hsiao E, Ali B, Blankstein R, et al: Detection of obstructive coronary artery disease using regadenoson stress and 82Rb PET/CT myocardial perfusion imaging. J Nucl Med. 2013 Oct;54(10):1748-1754")

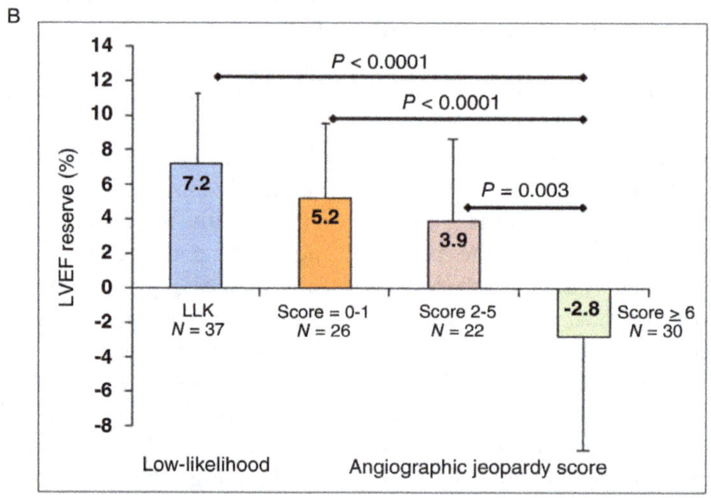

FIGURE 3-8B LVEF Reserve as a Function of the Extent and Severity of Coronary Artery Disease. (Reproduced with permission from Hsiao E, Ali B, Blankstein R, et al: Detection of obstructive coronary artery disease using regadenoson stress and 82Rb PET/CT myocardial perfusion imaging. J Nucl Med. 2013 Oct;54(10):1748-1754)

(center panel) and the overlay of the emission and transmission images (right panel).

PET/CT systems allow for quantification of coronary artery calcium, which can provide important incremental information regarding long-term cardiac risk for patients with normal PET perfusion studies.[6]

Interpretation of the absolute myocardial blood flow data requires careful review of the quality control parameters and a thorough understanding of the clinical factors that impact myocardial flow reserve.[3,4] These topics are covered in detail in Chapters 4 and 5.

A

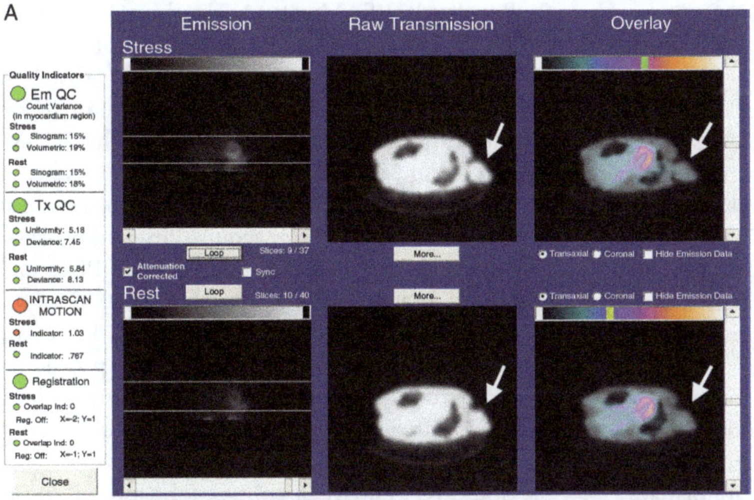

FIGURE 3-9A Left Arm at Side of Patient Noted on Quality Control Page

B

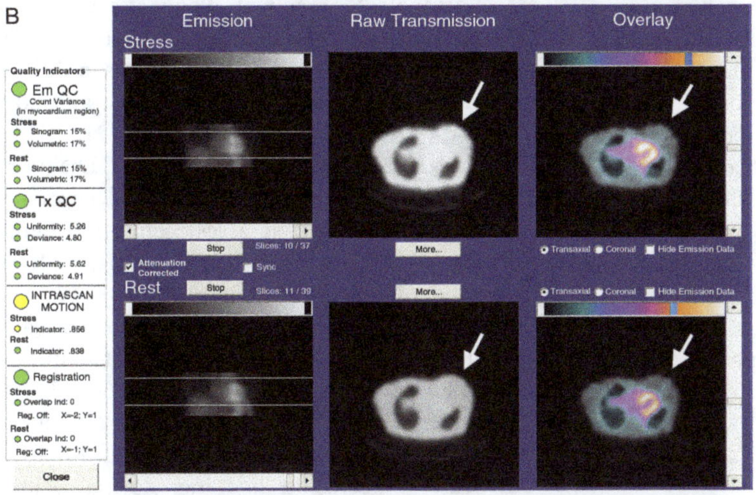

FIGURE 3-9B Left Mastectomy and Breast Implant Seen on Quality Control Page

C

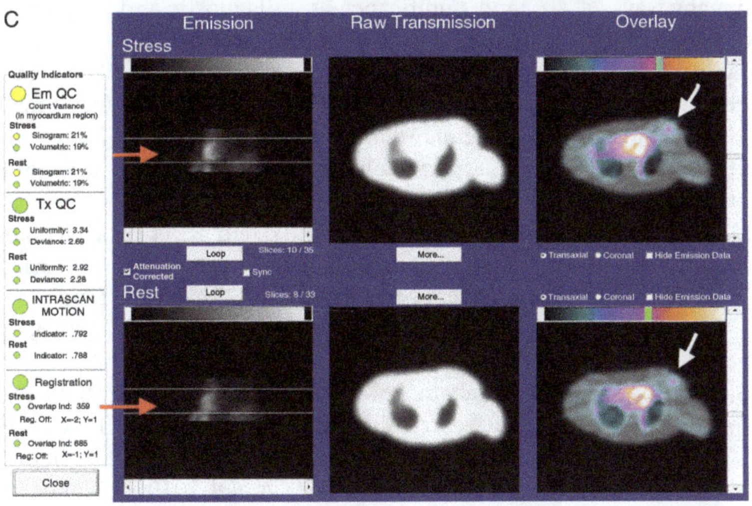

FIGURE 3-9C Female Patient With Left Breast Cancer on Quality Control Page

REPORTING OF CARDIAC PET MPI STUDIES

The general approach to reporting of PET MPI studies is similar to reporting of SPECT MPI studies.[4] The ECG response to pharmacologic stress should be reported, as well as the hemodynamic response and presence or absence of symptoms. If the patient has no prior history of coronary artery disease and if the study was acquired using a PET/CT system, the calcium score can be included in the report. As with SPECT, the TID ratio during PET should be reported, as well as image quality if it is an issue for interpretation. Rest and stress perfusion data should be reported with regard to size, severity, and location. The degree of reversibility of a perfusion abnormality should be reported. Global and regional wall motion should be reported at both peak-stress and rest, and the change in ejection fraction (LVEF reserve) should be reported. As mentioned previously, a rise in LVEF of approximately 5% from rest to peak-stress is anticipated in a normal study. The absolute myocardial blood flow and myocardial blood flow reserve (MBFR) results should be included in the report if the interpreting physician is confident in the accuracy of the data (based on a careful review of the quality control parameters) and if the MBFR results add incremental diagnostic or prognostic information.[4] This important topic is discussed in Chapters 5 and 6.

CONCLUSIONS

Interpretation of cardiac PET studies is in many ways similar to that of SPECT, and the transition from SPECT to PET can be accomplished as long as there is an appreciation for the differences. This chapter covers the important aspects of cardiac PET MPI, including how artifacts differ between PET and SPECT as well as unique aspects of quality evaluation, interpretation, and reporting of PET MPI studies.

REFERENCES

1. Bateman TM, Heller GV, McGhie AI, et al. Diagnostic accuracy of rest/stress ECG-gated Rb-82 myocardial perfusion PET: comparison with ECG-gated Tc-99m sestamibi SPECT. *J Nucl Cardiol.* 2006;13:24–33.
2. Beanlands RS, Muzik O, Hutchins GD, Wolfe ER Jr, Schwaiger M. Heterogeneity of regional nitrogen 13-labeled ammonia tracer distribution in the normal human heart: comparison with rubidium-82 and copper 62-labeled PTSM. *J Nucl Cardiol.* 1994;1:225–235.
3. Case JA, Bateman TM. Taking the perfect nuclear image: quality control, acquisition, and processing techniques for cardiac SPECT, PET, and hybrid imaging. *J Nucl Cardiol.* 2013;20:891–907.
4. Dilsizian V, Bacharach SL, Beanlands RS, et al.. ASNC imaging guidelines/SNMMI procedure standard for positron emission tomography (PET) nuclear cardiology procedures. *J Nucl Cardiol.* 2016;23:1187–1226.
5. Gould KL, Pan T, Loghin C, Johnson NP, Guha A, Sdringola S. Frequent diagnostic errors in cardiac PET/CT due to misregistration of CT attenuation and emission PET images: a definitive analysis of causes, consequences, and corrections. *J Nucl Med.* 2007;48:1112–1121.
6. Bybee KA, Lee J, Markiewicz R, et al. Diagnostic and clinical benefit of combined coronary calcium and perfusion assessment in patients undergoing PET/CT myocardial perfusion stress imaging. *J Nucl Cardiol.* 2010;17(2):188–196.
7. DiFilippo FP, Brunken RC. Do pacemaker leads and ICD leads cause metal-related artifact in cardiac PET/CT? *J Nucl Med.* 2005;46:436–443.
8. Rischpler C, Higuchi T, Fukushima K, et al. Transient ischemic dilation ratio in ^{82}Rb PET myocardial perfusion imaging: normal values and significance as a diagnostic and prognostic marker. *J Nucl Med.* 2012;53:723–730.
9. Shi H, Santana CA, Rivero A, et al. Normal values and prospective validation of transient ischemic dilation index in 82 Rb PET myocardial perfusion imaging. *Nucl Med Commun.* 2007;28(11):859–863.
10. Hsiao E, Ali B, Blankstein R, et al. Detection of obstructive coronary artery disease using regadenoson stress and 82Rb PET/CT myocardial perfusion imaging. *J Nucl Med.* 2013;54:1748–1754.
11. Abraham A, Kass M, Ruddy TD, et al. Right and left ventricular uptake with Rb-82 PET myocardial perfusion imaging: markers of left main or 3 vessel disease. *J Nucl Cardiol.* 2010;17:52–60.

EDITOR'S PERSPECTIVE

Parthiban Arumugam and Gary V. Heller

The growth of cardiac PET MPI in many countries has been impressive, most likely due to an increased awareness of its high clinical value. As one moves from SPECT to PET, it is important to understand the differences in interpretation of these two modalities in order to maximize the value of PET. For those who wish to start or have recently begun a cardiac PET program, this well-written chapter on cardiac PET interpretation is very useful in elucidating those differences. The chapter is supported by excellent examples, provides a clear and concise guide to systematic image interpretation, and affords an appreciation of important differences between PET and SPECT perfusion images, including artifacts unique to PET.

From the start, a reader new to PET will notice the consistently high image quality, regardless of which PET tracer is used or patient body characteristics. With the rigorous attenuation correction, attenuation artifact is a thing of the past. Gut and liver activity can be seen in some patients, but due to better image quality, scatter compensation, and spatial resolution, it is rarely a problem for interpretation. Overall, the incidence in comparison to pharmacologic SPECT is substantially less. TID will be more frequent and helpful for confirming extensive ischemia. The use of ECG gating for wall motion at rest and peak hyperemic stress will provide more information on ischemia and severity of stenosis. The presence of reversible wall motion abnormalities as well as fall in or lack of augmentation of EF at stress provides additional diagnostic and prognostic value. With the rapid acquisition of rubidium data during hyperemia, the wall motion changes are somewhat analogous to a dobutamine stress echo.

A word of caution: with cardiac PET MPI come new challenges. While attenuation artifact for the most part is eliminated, other technical issues arise. This is primarily in the form of mis-registration and breathing and motion artifact. Both mis-registration and movement artifact need to be recognized by the interpreting physician and this chapter provides information on recognizing and dealing with them. Mis-registration can be corrected with appropriate software. Motion artifact cannot be corrected due to the continuous acquisition aspect of PET.

In a well-performing laboratory the presence of mis-registration and motion artifact should be minimized. It follows that the removal of the vast majority of artifact from PET images leaves the reader with a different mind-set. For most SPECT readers, the skill set is to appreciate attenuation artifact and try to minimize its effect for false positive studies. Thus, the reader inadvertently interprets for specificity. In contrast, since artifact for PET is generally removed, an abnormality with this modality should be considered consistent with CAD. Therefore the PET interpreter reads more for sensitivity.

In summary, the successful transition from SPECT to PET interpretation, as elucidated in this chapter, is in the recognition of new types of artifact as well as an understanding that attenuation artifact is no longer an important issue. Thus abnormal is abnormal. Once accomplished, interpretation of cardiac PET studies is a pleasure!

SECTION

3

QUANTITATIVE MYOCARDIAL BLOOD FLOW ASSESSMENT

Assessing Myocardial Blood Flow with Cardiac PET: Acquisition, Processing, and Quality Control

CHAPTER 4

James A. Case

INTRODUCTION

The introduction of routine absolute myocardial blood flow assessments for cardiac PET adds unique information that is difficult, if not impossible, to acquire using other noninvasive modalities. Specifically, the assessment of absolute myocardial blood flow with cardiac PET improves the determination of normalcy,[1,2] detection of multivessel disease,[3] detection of balanced flow reduction,[4] detection of microvascular disease,[5] and risk stratification.[6–8] These benefits can only be obtained if the quantitative values are accurate.[9]

The assessment of myocardial blood flow with PET uses the measurement of the transport of tracer from the blood pool into the myocardium[10–13] to calculate the blood flow in the coronary arteries. First, this requires an accurate dynamic scan across a wide range of count rates. In many systems, the count rate can be 10 times the activity of a conventional perfusion scan, with the entire, undecayed bolus in the field of view at once. In the case of ^{82}Rb, that activity will decay to near background levels during the course of the study. This complex, quantitative study must be accomplished without adding to significantly the radiation dose or compromising the quality of the clinical study.[14,15]

The choice of the radiotracer used to measure blood flow, in principle, should not have an impact on the blood flow. However, protocols and flow models for measuring blood flow are typically specific to the radiotracer used and have challenges particular to that agent.[10–13] In addition, quality control and data processing steps depend heavily on the choice of radiotracer. Clinicians must carefully assess data quality for patient motion,[16] accuracy of the placement of the blood pool region of interest (ROI),[17,18] and the accuracy of myocardial boundaries. Quality control in the assessment of myocardial blood flow carries a greater importance than in visual analysis of perfusion data because quantitative flow can correctly contradict visual assessment.

Ultimately, the assessment of myocardial blood flow with cardiac PET can greatly increase the diagnostic information available to the cardiologist; however, this information may complement, complicate, or even contradict the visual assessment of the study. Because of this, the utility of absolute blood flow assessment requires an understanding of the entire acquisition, processing, and quality control procedures by both the technologist and the interpreting nuclear cardiologist. This chapter describes the scientific foundation of myocardial blood flow assessment, methods for optimizing myocardial blood flow measurements, and strategies for assessing the quality of myocardial blood flow PET studies.

ACQUISITION AND PROCESSING

Acquisition

The assessment of myocardial blood flow with PET is made possible because of two characteristics of PET imaging: (1) all PET studies are attenuation and scatter corrected, and (2) PET studies are always acquiring a full 360 degrees of data. This constant collection of tomographic data allows for the creation of high-quality dynamic data at very short time intervals. It is this dynamic measurement of the kinetics of the uptake and washout of the tracer from the myocardium that allow for the quantitative assessment of the blood flow. The dynamic acquisition used for the assessment of myocardial blood flow uses a series of short tomographic images over the duration of the study to measure the transport of the tracer out of the blood pool into the myocardium. There are two primary means of acquiring blood flow data. The most common technique for acquiring the dynamic data is using a list-mode acquisition, illustrated in Figure 4-1. These acquisitions record each true coincidence event in a file so that multiple virtual "acquisitions" can be performed post-acquisition over the entire acquisition. This type of acquisition allows for rebinning of the gated, perfusion, and dynamic datasets from the single list-mode acquisition (Figure 4-1).

A second approach uses a short dynamic framed acquisition at the beginning of the study. This technique then is followed by a longer perfusion and gated study (Figure 4-2). Both techniques have been validated and can produce accurate results; however, different flow models must be employed depending on the type of acquisition used.[19,20] This method has the advantage of being less susceptible to the effects of tracer washout and patient motion, and it can be implemented on list-mode and non-list-mode PET systems.

The dynamic PET study is a set of short, continuous tomographic acquisitions starting prior to the start of the infusion (or injection) of the radiotracer and concluding in a final frame representing the cumulative uptake and washout of tracer. This dynamic study can be produced in real time as a series of sinograms or from a virtual rebinning of list-mode data. The dynamic scan typically uses shorter acquisition times near the peak of the blood pool bolus activity and then longer acquisition times during the uptake phase of the study.[9–11] For accurate calculation of the myocardial blood flow, it is necessary to measure the entire uptake process of the tracer into the myocardium; from prior to the start of the infusion to the final uptake frame. Technologists should allow for sufficient time between the start of the acquisition and start of the injection of the radiotracer to establish that no part of the blood pool activity is missed.

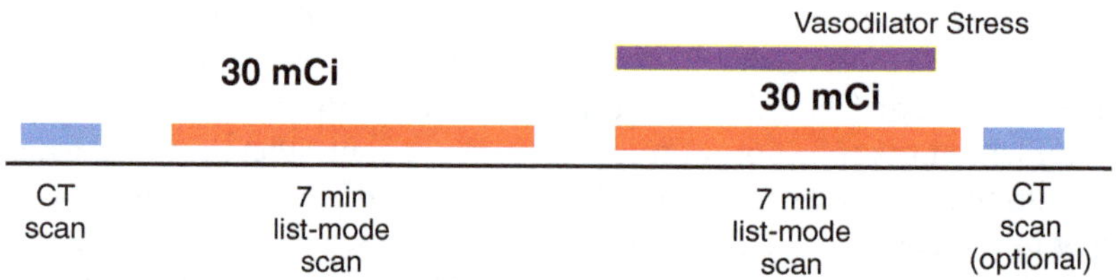

FIGURE 4-1 Dynamic study can be created from a replay of list-mode PET study. These protocols allow the list-mode dataset to be parsed into the three main studies: perfusion, gating and dynamic. The resulting frames are then reconstructed into tomographic volumes.

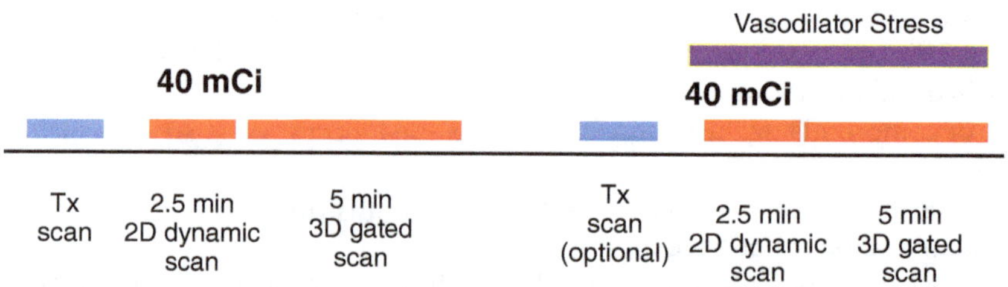

FIGURE 4-2 Framed Mode Acquisition Begins With a Short Dynamic Study Followed by a Longer ECG-Gated Perfusion Study. These acquisition times collect the dynamic data during the blood pool clearance phase of the study and do not require a second injection of tracer.

During the dynamic acquisition, technologists should ensure that the patient avoids motion. Patient motion, either position movement or respiratory, can lead to inaccurate flow values that can be difficult to detect.[16,21] For some flow models, it is recommended that patient motion be corrected prior to evaluating myocardial blood flow. This motion correction differs from misregistration correction and artifact-producing patient motion. Motion correction of the dynamic study must be performed to ensure that the blood pool region of interest tracks is correctly registered over the myocardium and not the blood pool or outside the cardiac region.

The processing of myocardial blood flow PET studies is similar to the processing of conventional myocardial perfusion PET studies. It requires that the sinogram data be corrected for misregistration of transmission and emission datasets, and using an appropriate iterative algorithm. It is important that in the processing myocardial blood flow PET studies to use image-filtering parameters as are required by the specific quantitative software. Altering these values can change the quantitative accuracy of blood flow estimates. Once the dynamic volumes are created by reconstruction software, the myocardial blood flow study must be reoriented onto conventional cardiac oblique angles and the myocardial boundary and blood pool region of interest (ROI) identified.[17]

Last, it is essential that sufficient counts are obtained throughout the dynamic series. Technologists and clinicians should inspect entire dynamic series to ensure the myocardium and blood pool images are of sufficient quality to obtain accurate measurements.

Quantitative Models

Calculating myocardial blood flow from measurements of tracer uptake and blood pool concentration requires a model for transport of tracer activity into the myocytes. The most common model for tracer transport is a multicompartment model. Each compartment of the model represents a location the tracer can be in during the acquisition. In the simplest model, the tracer begins in the blood (compartment one) and then is transported into the cell (compartment two). More complicated models include parameters for washout from the cell, compartments for the interstitial layer, metabolism of the tracer, and different subcomponents within the cell.

The choice of a compartmental model for calculating myocardial blood flow is based on an understanding of the underlying kinetics of the tracer and the parameters of the acquisition. In addition, consideration should be given common imaging artifacts, such as image noise, patient motion, and noncardiac uptake. These practical considerations become essential as the complexity of the model increases.

The general form of a three compartment model is[12]:

$$C_3 = \frac{K_1 k_2}{k_2 + k_3} e^{-(k_2 + k_3)t} \otimes C_a(t) + \frac{K_1 k_3}{k_2 + k_3} \int_0^t C_a(\tau) d\tau$$

where C_m is the myocardial uptake, K_1 is the uptake into the first tissue compartment, k_2 is the washout from the first compartment, k_3 is the uptake into the second tissue compartment, ^{t} is the timepoint the uptake is measured and $C_m(t)$ is the arterial concentration at timepoint ^{t}. This model is also often referred to as a two-tissue compartment model (2TCM) where one compartment represents the blood and the two-tissue compartments represent the cell.

To calculate the myocardial blood flow from the compartmental model, a model for the tracer extraction is needed. The extraction of activity from the blood is often modeled using the Renkin-Crone formula[22,23]:

$$K_1 = \text{MBF} \cdot (1 - a \times exp(^{-b}/_{MFB}))$$

where MBF is the myocardial blood flow and a and b are fit parameters. A list of common a and b parameters is given in Table 4-1.[11,23–28]

Early studies of the 2TCM for ^{13}N-ammonia demonstrated a high degree of accuracy compared to microspheres. Choi et al in 1999 examined the quantitative myocardial blood flow of ^{13}N-ammonia using four different quantitative models.[24] In that study, the 2TCM was demonstrated to have low dispersion (0.15) and correlated well with microspheres results. The authors also noted the importance of the correction of washed out metabolite. In a separate study comparing blood flow models using ^{13}N-ammonia, it was demonstrated that the single-tissue compartment

Table 4-1

Common Parameters for the Multicompartmental Model for Perfusion Tracers

	A	*B*	k_2 (Rest/Stress)	k_3 (Rest/Stress)
Rb-82 (10)	0.77	0.63	0.12/0.21	NA
N-13 ammonia (10)	0.607	1.25	0.23/0.89	0.14/0.13
C-11 acetate (23)	0.64	1.20	3.0	1.0
F-18 flurpiridaz (20,27)	0.06	0.0	NA	NA
O-15 water (25)	0	0	Freely diffusible	NA
Tc-99m sestamibi (19)	0.86	0.267	NA	NA

a and *b* are the fit parameters for the Renkin-Crone model, k_2 is the washout rate at rest and stress from the first tissue compartment and k_3 is the uptake into the second compartment.

model did not accurately represent the myocardial blood flow as well as the two-tissue compartment model.

^{82}Rb is a potassium analog and thus is not metabolized by the myocytes. Because of this ^{82}Rb can be modeled using a single-tissue compartment model (1TCM). Lortie et al in 2007 presented a simplified single-tissue compartment model for calculating the myocardial blood flow using ^{82}Rb.[11] This model uses a nonlinear fit to a series of dynamic measurements of uptake arterial blood pool to estimate the K_1 (uptake), k_2 (washout), and partial volume corrections (f).

The 1TCM can be derived by setting $k_3 = 0$:[10]

$$C_m = K_1 e^{-k_2 t} \otimes C_a(t)$$

1TCM has been shown to accurately represent the estimate of myocardial blood flow for ^{82}Rb myocardial blood flow[11] and is highly repeatable.[29]

This model can be further simplified by setting $k_2 = 0$. This model is referred to as the net retention model.[9] Comparison of the net retention model with the full 1TCM demonstrates a high degree of correlation between blood flow calculations in the first 2 minutes of a study. Following the first 2 minutes, the influence of the washout reduces the accuracy of this model. One of the advantages of this simple model is that it can be performed on non-list-mode, frame-mode PET systems. Another advantage of this technique is that the myocardial uptake is calculated from a single late frame, making it less susceptible to motion artifacts. One of the limitations of this technique is that the partial volume correction cannot be determined from the data and must be supplied as a parameter.

A major concern of clinicians is the robustness and interchangeability of myocardial blood flow measurements. In a large study comparing myocardial blood flow calculation techniques in ^{82}Rb, net retention, 1TCM and 2TCM models produced similar results for the mean rest and stress values for flow; however, there were differences observed on a patient-by-patient basis depending on the kinetic model that was used[19] (Table 4-2). These results confirm the overall robustness of these methods and demonstrates their interchangeability.[30] In addition, software packages using the same compartmental modeling algorithm produced interchangeable results. This further validates the consistency of these software packages, despite varying implementation strategies. The key limitation of this study is that no gold standard was available and, therefore, the overall accuracy of particular techniques cannot be assessed relative to true myocardial blood flow.

BLOOD FLOW CHARACTERISTICS OF PET TRACERS

In principle, with an accurate model of a PET tracer's extraction and retention properties, and a high-quality dynamic acquisition, all PET tracers can produce identical results. However, variations in each tracers uptake and retention properties can create both systematic and random errors in the measurement

Table 4-2

Comparison of Differences in the 15 Software Packages Compared in the Ruby 10 Study

	Rest (mL/g/min)	Stress (mL/g/min)	MFR
Min	0.97	1.85	1.58
Max	1.69	3.57	2.42
Average	1.19	2.41	2.13
Stdev	0.18	0.38	0.20

Though there were differences between the software packages on a patient-by-patient basis, the means and standard deviations over all patients were very similar. Though the software packages are not completely interchangeable (differing primarily based on the kinetic model employed), the average performance across all patients was similar. This would imply that limits of normal for rest, stress and myocardial blood flow reserve are similar across the packages examined.

of myocardial blood flow. In addition, some PET tracers present particular challenges for accurate acquisition of the dynamic data. An illustration of *K1* versus MBF is given in Figure 4-3. The most highly extracted of the PET tracers is ^{15}O water, followed by ^{18}F flurpiridaz, ^{13}N-ammonia, and ^{82}Rb. In terms of the visual appearance of images, the more highly extracted the tracer, the greater contrast perfusion defects product. In quantitative terms, more highly extracted tracers can more precisely estimate quantitative blood flow.

O-15 Water

The gold standard for the estimation of myocardial blood flow is O-15 water. This tracer has particularly favorable characteristics with freely diffusing across the cell boundary. This property gives O-15 water a linear, 1-1 relationship between K_1 and blood flow. The challenge with O-15 water is the very short half-life of oxygen 15 (122 seconds). This makes chemistry and delivery of the radiotracer very difficult. In addition, O-15 water is not retained in the myocytes. Because of this, there is very little contrast between the blood pool and the myocardium parameters making traditional assessment of wall motion thickening and visual interpretation challenging if not impossible.[31] O-15 water is best imaged parametrically, to assess absolute blood flow without the conventional visual and functional assessments.

^{82}Rb Rubidium

^{82}Rb rubidium is the most common PET perfusion agent used in the United States. It is most commonly

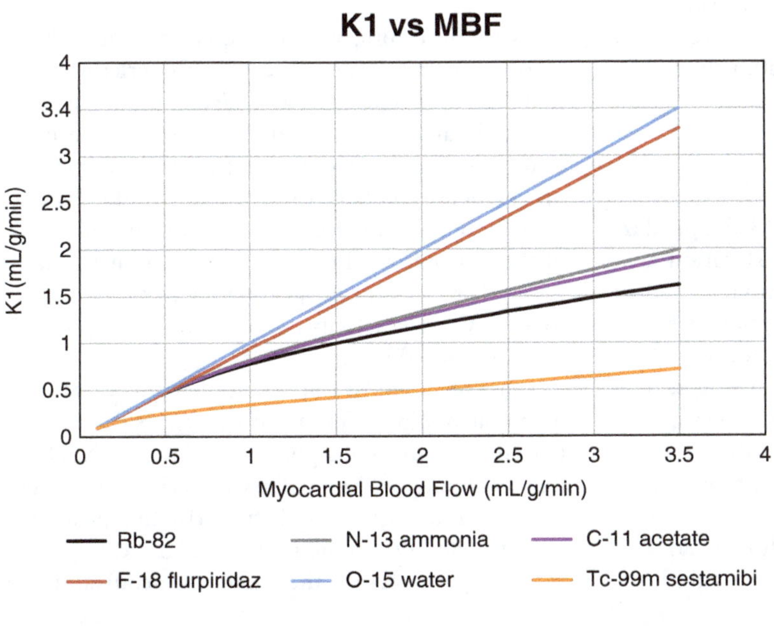

FIGURE 4-3 As Myocardial Blood Flow Increases, Fraction of Extracted Tracer Is Reduced Tracers with a lower extraction fraction at higher blood flow rates will produce smaller visual defects that more highly extracted agents. Furthermore, low extraction fraction can reduce the quantitative accuracy of blood flow estimates.

delivered using an infusion system as rubidium chloride solution. As a potassium analog, rubidium is taken up by the potassium pump into the cell. Once inside the cell, the rubidium is not bound and will slowly wash out ($k_2 \approx 0.14$/min at rest). ^{82}Rb properties are similar to thallium chloride.

Because of the efficient uptake slow washout, ^{82}Rb can be modeled well with a net retention, single-tissue compartment model, or two-tissue compartment model. For the net retention model, a short (<3 minutes) dynamic acquisition is necessary to avoid errors due to tracer washout.[10] For longer acquisitions either the single-tissue compartment model or two-tissue compartment model is recommended.[11,30]

^{13}N-ammonia

^{13}N-ammonia is a cyclotron-produced tracer with a 9.93 minute half-life. This radiotracer has excellent first-pass extraction and with a longer half-life produces high-quality perfusion and functional images. Quantitative measurements of myocardial blood flow are complicated by the fact that ^{13}N-ammonia is only partially retained in the cell. Upon first extraction from the blood pool a portion of the ammonia is converted to glutamine and retained in the cell. A smaller fraction is then converted into a ^{13}N-metabolite and washes out into the blood pool. This metabolite cannot be re-extracted from the blood pool and can artifactually increase the estimate of the arterial input function. For accurate measurement of myocardial blood flow with ammonia a 2TCM that includes corrections for the metabolite must be used.[12]

F-18 Flurpiridaz

A new ^{18}F-labeled cardiac tracer, F-18 flurpiridaz, is currently under FDA Phase 3 investigation as a myocardial perfusion agent. Preliminary studies of this agent demonstrate a high signal to background, high extraction fraction, and excellent resolution properties.[32] In addition, this agent has the advantage of unit dose delivery opening up the opportunity for laboratories to utilize cardiac PET without the challenge of owning a generator or cyclotron. More recently, quantitative blood flow modeling has indicated that F-18 flurpiridaz has more superior flow characteristics than rubidium and ^{13}N-ammonia[26] with a high extraction fraction (0.94) that is constant up to flows of 5.06 mL/g/sec[33] and is well retained.

QUALITY ASSESSMENT OF MYOCARDIAL BLOOD FLOW STUDIES

Overview

Quality control of myocardial blood flow requires an understanding of the hardware and software that is being used to Despite vendor-specific differences, there are some common quality control steps that can be used. Quality control myocardial blood flow studies begin by assessing:

1. Accurate location of the blood pool ROI
2. Accurate location of the myocardial ROI
3. Acquiring entire arterial input function
4. Using dosage below deadtime limitations of the system for all dynamic frames
5. Adequate dose for blood pool calculation, perfusion, and gating

Table 4-3 is a summary of common quality control problems associated with myocardial blood flow calculations.

Locating the Blood Pool ROI

To assess the timing of the input, a technologist should inspect the first frame of the dynamic series to ensure that no counts are present. Second, the dynamic series should be inspected to verify that the blood pool images are well defined prior to the myocardial uptake phases. Finally, the last frame of the dynamic series should be inspected to verify sufficient uptake of the tracer from the blood pool into myocardium. A simple process for inspecting the dynamic series is to display a time activity curve for the blood pool ROI and myocardial ROI.

One of the most important quality control steps, quantitative blood flow measurement is the accurate placement of the blood pool ROI (Figure 4-4). A high-quality blood pool ROI will have nearly zero counts at the beginning of the acquisition, rise to a peak, then clear to equilibrium value that is significantly lower than the peak value at the end of the acquisition. For

Table 4-3

Summary of Common Quality Control Problems Associated with Myocardial Blood Flow Calculations

QC Issue	Cause and Prevention	Effect on MBF Calculation	Assessment
Misplacement of blood pool ROI	User selects an inappropriate location for blood pool ROI.	Inaccurate MBF and reserve calculations.	Visually inspect blood pool location for accuracy and review all frames to ensure ROI stays over blood pool for entire dynamic sequence.
Misplacement of myocardial ROI	Automatic boundary detection fails to identify myocardial ROI. Noncardiac uptake, poor user selections for ROI and patient motion.	Inaccurate MBF and reserve calculations.	Inspect the myocardial ROI in all frames used for determining flow to insure ROI is over the myocardium.
Missing portion of arterial input function	Starting dynamic imaging after the infusion or injection. Always start camera prior to injecting or infusing patient.	Increases MBF calculation by underestimating blood pool counts	Visually inspect first dynamic first to ensure no counts are present. For ^{13}N-ammonia, residual activity can be present in first frame; however, it must be subtracted from all dynamic frames.
Deadtime limits exceeded for camera	Activity delivered to patient exceed deadtime limits of system. These limits are particularly strict for 3D acquisition protocols.	Increases MBF calculation by underestimating blood pool counts and possibly introducing dark bands in early dynamic image.	Visually inspect dynamic reconstructions to ensure there is no streaking. Inspect blood pool curve to ensure peak activity is not blunted.
Adequate counts	Use of inappropriately low dosage. Increase dose to appropriate level without exceeding deadtime limitations. If this cannot be achieved blood flow measurement should not be attempted.	Inaccurate regional flow and reserve calculations. Counts should also be sufficient to acquire a high-quality gated and tomographic perfusion study without the need to apply a second dose of radiotracer to the patient.	Review of the dynamic images show reveal clearly a defined myocardium in the later frames and clearly defined blood pool in the early frames.

Careful inspection of dynamic data must be made to insure blood flow calculations are reliable.

constant activity delivery systems, the peak in activity will be less pronounced, and continue at approximately the same level until the end of infusion. If the blood pool ROI includes too much myocardial or extra cardiac activity, the arterial input function can be overestimated thereby reducing the overall measurement of myocardial blood flow (Figure 4-5). If the blood pool ROI is placed offset the blood pool, the arterial input function can be underestimated thereby overestimating myocardial blood flow. Different software packages require specific locations for the blood pool ROI and technologists should consult with their vendor on proper placement.

Location of Myocardial ROI

The assessment of the myocardial boundary can be performed by inspecting and overlay of the boundary on the dynamic volume series. Technologists should ensure that the myocardial boundary accurately represents the position of the myocardium at all phases of the dynamic study. Patient motion during the dynamic series can introduce inaccuracies in the measurement of myocardial blood flow when the single tissue compartment model is used.[16] The net retention model is less susceptible to motion artifacts because it only relies on

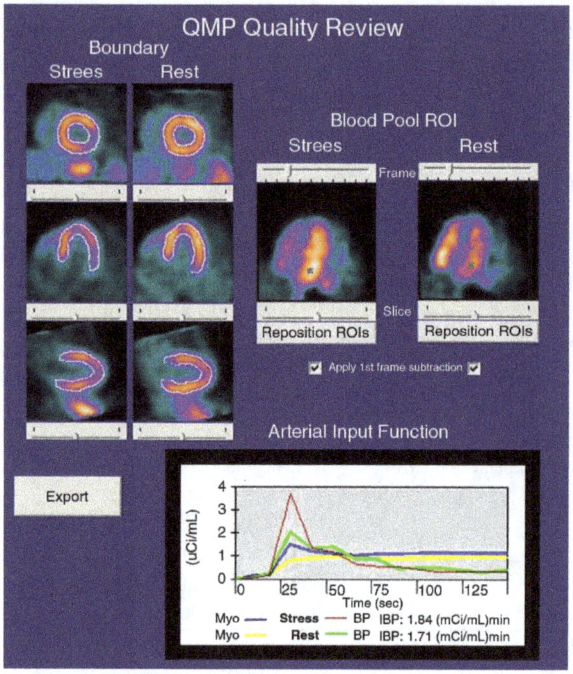

FIGURE 4-4 Proper identification of the blood pool is the most important step in accurate quantification of blood flow. For the net retention models, a left atrial ROI is recommended. For the 1TCM, a left ventricular cavity ROI is recommended.

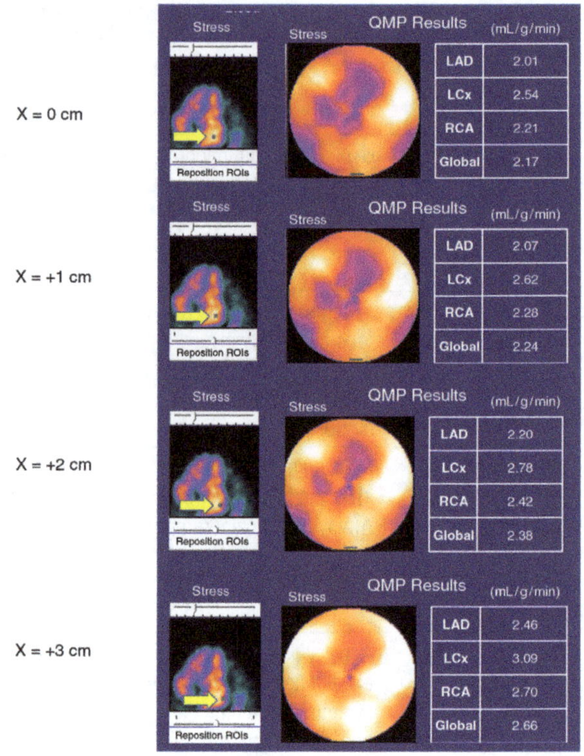

FIGURE 4-5 Accurate placement of the blood pool ROI is essential for accurately estimating the myocardial blood flow. In this example, the blood pool is shifted from its optimal location in 1 cm increments to the left (displayed vertically above). Within the blood pool, small shifts have little impact on the calculation of myocardial blood flow. As the blood pool ROI nears the edge of the left atrium, the estimate of the arterial input function decreases, thereby overestimating the blood flow.

the uptake present in the final frame of the acquisition. Regardless of kinetic model used, the myocardial boundary should also be inspected to ensure proper placement the base of the heart and that no noncardiac structures have been included in the boundary.

Acquiring Entire Arterial Input Function

To accurately estimate the myocardial blood flow, it is necessary to acquire the entire transit of the activity from the blood into the myocardium. For this, a dynamic acquisition is needed, beginning *prior* to the injection or infusion of the radiotracer. If the scanner is started after the start of infusion, the estimate of myocardial blood flow will be inaccurate and should not be used. The dynamic acquisition should continue until the activity has cleared the blood pool (Figure 4-6). This can be measured in terms of the peak blood pool-to-plateau blood pool counts (the equilibrium count level). Alternatively, they can be measured in terms of the blood pool to myocardium ratio.

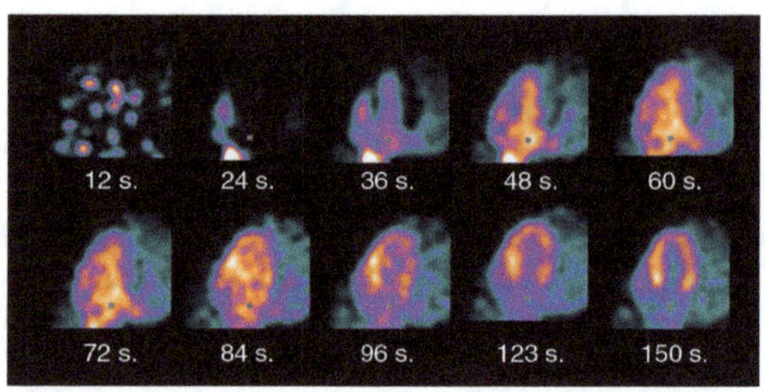

FIGURE 4-6 Dynamic series used in blood flow assessment requires higher sampling of the time activity curve when the initial bolus passes through the ventricle As the tracer is taken up into the ventricle, time bins can be extended to allow for better uptake assessment.

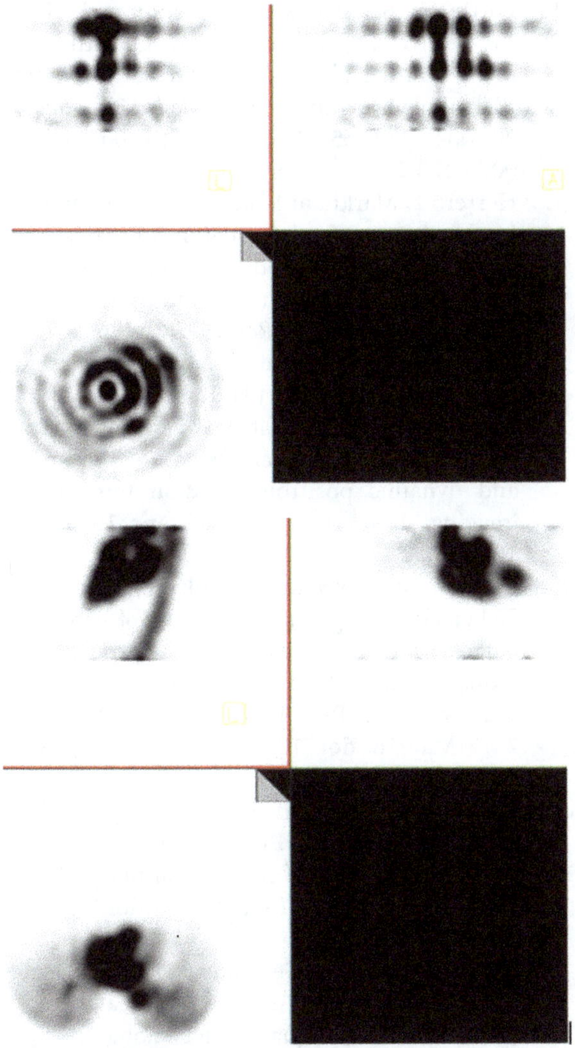

FIGURE 4-7 High doses of activity can saturate the detector crystals producing extreme artifacts in the blood pool images and reducing the accuracy of myocardial blood flow measurements. (A) An image of the blood pool at its maximum count level form a 50 mCi infusion of ^{82}Rb. (B)The same patient's blood pool image using a 29 mCi infusion. The threshold for introducing the artifacts is dependent on the electronics of the PET system and varies between systems. Images displayed are from a Siemens 64-slice PET/CT system.

Using Appropriate Dosages: Deadtime and Image Quality Considerations

Accurate determination of the myocardial blood flow and blood flow requires not exceeding the count rate limitations of the imaging system. For most applications, the initial input count rate can be 10-fold higher than the equilibrium count rate. For many systems, this high count rate can exceed the operational range of the system and can create artifacts (see Figure 4-7). Nuclear laboratories must verify that the dosage prescribed does not exceed the count rate capabilities of the imaging system.

For systems acquiring in 3D list-mode, this can be particularly challenging. Early activity rates can be 70% deadtime or higher. Reducing injected doses below recommended dosages for the perfusion and gated study is not justified for the purpose of obtaining accurate blood flow measurements.

For systems that cannot acquire accurate 3D blood pool measurements at high enough doses to acquire a quality perfusion and gated study, and alternative is to acquire the blood pool input function in 2D and the perfusion and gating in either 2D or 3D. These measurements can be applied to most systems with a minimal increase of acquisition time and provide myocardial blood flow and blood flow reserve measurements that are comparable to modern PET/CT measurements.[34]

SUMMARY

Accurate assessment of absolute myocardial blood flow and blood flow reserve is revolutionizing nuclear cardiology by improving the diagnosis, risk stratification, and management of patients. Furthermore, the models for the assessment of myocardial blood flow and flow reserve have been well validated for a wide variety of radiotracers, imaging systems, and blood flow quantification software packages. Successful quantification of myocardial blood flow requires an understanding of the correct acquisition and processing of dynamic PET studies and the application of appropriate quality control steps. When these steps are applied, myocardial blood flow number should be reliable and provide essential information in assessing cardiac patients.

REFERENCES

1. Bateman TM, Dilsizian V, Beanlands RS, DePuey EG, Heller GV, Wolinsky DA. American Society of Nuclear Cardiology and Society of Nuclear Medicine and Molecular Imaging joint position

statement on the clinical indications for myocardial perfusion PET. *J Nucl Cardiol.* 2016. Epub ahead of print.

2. Yoshinaga K, Katoh C, Manabe O, et al. Incremental diagnostic value of regional myocardial blood flow quantification over relative perfusion imaging with generator-produced rubidium-82 PET. *Circ J.* 2011;75:2628–2634.
3. Kajander S, Joutsiniemi E, Saraste M, et al. Cardiac positron emission tomography/computed tomography imaging accurately detects anatomically and functionally significant coronary artery disease. *Circulation.* 2010;122(6):603–613.
4. Ziadi MC, Dekemp RA, Williams K, et al. Does quantification of myocardial flow reserve using rubidium-82 positron emission tomography facilitate detection of multivessel coronary artery disease? *J Nucl Cardiol.* 2012;19(4):670–680.
5. Schindler TH, Schelbert HR, Quercioli A, Dilsizian V. Cardiac PET imaging for the detection and monitoring of coronary artery disease and microvascular health. *JACC Cardiovasc Imaging.* 2010;3:623–640.
6. Herzog BA, Husmann L, Valenta I, et al. Long-term prognostic value of 13N-ammonia myocardial perfusion positron emission tomography added value of coronary flow reserve. *J Am Coll Cardiol.* 2009;54(2):150–156.
7. Murthy VL, Naya M, Foster CR, et al. Improved cardiac risk assessment with noninvasive measures of coronary flow reserve. *Circulation.* 2011;124(20):2215–2224.
8. Taqueti VR, Hachamovitch R, Murthy VL, et al. Global coronary flow reserve is associated with adverse cardiovascular events independently of luminal angiographic severity and modifies the effect of early revascularization. *Circulation.* 2015;131(1):19–27.
9. Moody JB, Lee BC, Corbett JR, Ficaro EP, Murthy VL. Precision and accuracy of clinical quantification of myocardial blood flow by dynamic PET: a technical perspective. *J Nucl Cardiol.* Apr 2015. doi:10.1007/s12350-015-0100-0.
10. Yoshida K, Mullani N, Gould KL. Coronary flow and flow reserve by PET simplified for clinical applications using rubidium-82 or nitrogen-13-ammonia. *J Nucl Med.* 1996;37(10):1701–1712.
11. Lortie M, Beanlands RSB, Yoshinaga K, Klein R, Dasilva JN, DeKemp RA. Quantification of myocardial blood flow with 82Rb dynamic PET imaging. *Eur J Nucl Med Mol Imaging.* 2007;34(11):1765–1774. doi:10.1007/s00259-007-0478-2.
12. Herrero P, Markham J, Shelton M, Bergmann S. Implementation and evaluation of a two-compartment model for quantification of myocardial perfusion with rubidium-82 and positron emission tomography. *Circ Res.* 1992;70:496–507.
13. Hutchins GD, Schwaiger M, Rosenspire KC, Krivokapich J, Schelbert H, Kuhl DE. Noninvasive quantification of regional blood flow in the human heart using N-13 ammonia and dynamic positron emission tomographic imaging. *J Am Coll Cardiol.* Apr 1990;15(5):1032–1042.
14. Case JA, deKemp RA, Slomka PJ, Smith MF, Heller GV, Cerqueira MD. Status of cardiovascular PET radiation exposure and strategies for reduction: an information statement from the Cardiovascular PET Task Force. *J Nucl Cardiol.* 2017 May 16. doi: 10.1007/s12350-017-0897-9. Epub ahead of print.
15. deKemp RA, Yoshinaga K, Beanlands RSB. Will 3-dimensional PET-CT enable the routine quantification of myocardial blood flow? *J Nucl Cardiol.* 2007;14(3):380–397. doi:10.1016/j.nuclcard.2007
16. Otaki Y, Betancur J, Germano G, Dey D, Berman D, Slomka P. Patient motion significantly affect measurements of quantitative global regional myocardial blood flow assessment by Dynamic PET. *JACC*, Mar 2017, 69(11). Supplement, doi:1.1016/S0735-1097(17)35000-3.
17. Case JA, Bateman TM. Taking the perfect nuclear image: quality control, acquisition, and processing techniques for cardiac SPECT, PET, and hybrid imaging. *J Nucl Cardio.* 2013;20(5):891–907.
18. Chareonthaitawee P, Christenson SD, Anderson JL, et al. Reproducibility of measurements of regional myocardial blood flow in a model of coronary artery disease: comparison of $H_2{}^{15}O$ and $^{13}NH_3$ PET techniques. *J Nucl Med.* Jul 2006;47(7):1193–1201.
19. Nesterov SV, Deshayes E, Sciagra R, et al. Quantification of myocardial blood flow in

absolute terms using Rb-82 PET imaging: results of RUBY-10 study. *J Am Coll Cardiol Imaging.* 2014;7:1119–1127.

20. Bateman TM, Case JA. Variability in normal myocardial blood flow measurements: physiologic, methodologic, or protocol related? *J Nucl Cardio.* Feb 2015;22(1):85–88.
21. Hunter CRRN, Klein R, Beanlands RS, deKemp RA. Patient motion effects on the quantification of regional myocardial blood flow with dynamic PET imaging. *Med Phys.* 2016;43(4):1829. doi:10.1118/1.4943565.
22. Renkin EM. Transport of potassium-42 from blood tissue in isolated mammalian skeletal muscles, *Am J Physiol.* 1959;197:1205–1210.
23. Crone C. The permeability of brain capillaries to non-electrolytes. *Acta Physiol Scand.* 1965;64:407–417.
24. Choi Y, Huang S-C, Hawkins RA et al. Quantification of myocardial blood flow using 13n-ammonia and PET: comparison of tracer models. *J Nucl Med.* 1999;40:1045–1055.
25. Hsu B, Hu LH, Yang B et al. SPECT myocardial blood flow quantitation toward clinical use: a comparative study with 13N-ammonia PET myocardial blood flow quantitation. *Eur J Nucl Med Mol Imaging.* Jan 2017;44(1):117–128. Epub Sep 1, 2016.
26. Sherif HM, Nekolla SG, Saraste A, et al. Simplified quantification of myocardial flow reserve with flurpiridaz F18: validation with microspheres in a pig model. *J Nucl Med.* 2011;52(4):617–624.
27. Van den Hoff J, Borner AR, Fricke F, et al. ^{11}C acetate as a quantitative perfusion tracer in myocardial PET. *J Nucl Med.* 2001;42(8, Aug 1): 1174–1182.
28. Van den Hoff J, Burchert W, Wolper HG, Meyer GJ, Hundeshagen H. A kinetic model for cardiac PET with [1-Carbon-11]-Acetate. *J Nucl Med.*1996;37:521–529.
29. Klein R, Ocneanu A, Renaud JM, Ziadi MC, Beanlands RSB, deKemp RA. Consistent tracer administration profile improves test-retest repeatability of myocardial blood flow quantification with (82)Rb dynamic PET imaging. *J Nucl Cardiol.* Nov 2016:1–13.
30. Nesterov SV, Deshayes E, Sciagrà R, et al. Quantification of myocardial blood flow in absolute terms using (82)Rb PET imaging: results of RUBY-10 study. *JACC Cardiov Imaging.* Oct 2014. doi:10.1016/j.jcmg.2014.08.003.
31. Bergmann SR, Herrero P, Markham J, Weinheimer CJ, Walsh MN. Noninvasive quantitation of myocardial blood flow in human subjects with oxygen-15-labeled water and positron emission tomography. *J Am Coll Cardiol.* 1989;14(3):639–652.
32. Berman DS, Maddahi J, Tamarappoo BK, et al. Phase II safety and clinical comparison with single-photon emission computed tomography myocardial perfusion imaging for detection of coronary artery disease: flurpiridaz F 18 positron emission tomography. *J Am Coll Cardiol.* Jan 29 2013;61(4):469–477.
33. Maddahi J, Packard RS. Cardiac PET perfusion tracers: current status and trends. *Semin Nucl Med.* Sep 2014;44(5):333–343.
34. Case JA, VanVickle S, Courter SA, Burgett EV, Bateman TM. A rapid acquisition protocol for measuring perfusion, gating and absolute blood flow using dedicated frame-mode 3D PET scanners. *J Nucl Cardiol.* 21:768, 2014.

EDITOR'S PERSPECTIVE

Timothy M. Bateman

I vividly recall reading a document in 1979 on how a scintillation camera could produce valid images of myocardial perfusion. And then re-reading it several times. It seemed like my one year of college-level physics was simply inadequate to permit me to understand how all this worked, at least when the process was described by a physicist. It took me many years to finally "get it," and I appreciated the efforts of several clinical experts to simplify the concepts so that a clinical cardiologist could understand how the technology worked. We are confronting a similar challenge today with myocardial blood flow (MBF) quantification during rest/stress myocardial perfusion PET studies.

Clinicians are taught right from the start to look for patterns in making diagnoses—the commonality. Most disease processes can be identified by the convergence of several patterns, so we look for as many identifiers as possible that point in the same direction. We also look suspiciously on outlier data points. We want verification. Sometimes this is through repeat blood work. Sometimes, by personally inspecting an image with the image specialist. In the case of rest/stress PET myocardial perfusion imaging, clinicians are learning that there are many verifiable data points: image appearance; semi-quantified population-based image analysis; presence or absence of transient ventricular dilation (TID); changes in ejection fraction, wall motion, or wall thickening between rest and peak hyperemia; and either a quantification or an estimate of coronary artery calcium. All of these parameters can be verified by visual assessment of the image data. The clinician gains great confidence by personally being shown these data, thereby convincing him or her of the veracity in the ensuing management decision.

Unfortunately, one of the most powerful attributes of rest/stress PET MPI, the ability to quantify myocardial blood flow (MBF) and MBF reserve (MBFR), is not visually verifiable. These are numerical descriptors that can improve diagnostic accuracy, inform about short- and long-term outcomes, and affect patient management.

This chapter simplifies the concepts that underlay accurate MBF quantification. It is not easy for a physicist to translate complex concepts into terms that a clinician can understand. Without handholding, a clinician cannot grasp the veracity of a net retention, one compartment or two compartment model for quantifying MBF. Further, the basic pre-conditions that must be in place need to be spelled out and shown to clinicians as quality control essentials, in order for the clinician to comfortably incorporate MBF measurements into management decisions.

This chapter is an important effort aimed at educating clinicians in the critical factors that underlay the accuracy of MBF measurements. It attempts to explain to clinicians the complex concepts that underlay MBF measurements, and to provide confidence in the outputs. The most important take-home message is that clinicians need to understand the software they are using to quantify MBF, to explicitly follow its directions, and to critically analyze its outputs before incorporating these into patient management decisions.

Quantitative Myocardial Blood Flow: Practical Clinical Perspective with Case Examples

CHAPTER 5

Timothy M. Bateman

INTRODUCTION

Measurement of blood flow to the myocardium represents a quantum leap forward for the field of nuclear cardiology. Quantification of myocardial blood flow as a routine part of rest/stress myocardial perfusion imaging is a unique attribute of cardiac PET. Although the quantification is actually measured in mL/min/g of myocardium, it is usually expressed as a ratio between peak hyperemia and rest. This ratio is termed myocardial blood flow reserve (MBFR) or coronary flow reserve (CFR). In this chapter we use the term MBFR to be in agreement with a recently published joint position paper of the American Society of Nuclear Cardiology (ASNC) and the Society of Nuclear Medicine and Molecular Imaging (SNMMI).[1] MBFR can be measured on a pixel-by-pixel basis if there are sufficient counts, but for clinical applications MBFR is reported globally (an average for the entire myocardium), segmentally, or by coronary territory. Some patients have high resting flows that can artifactually lower MBFR; therefore, it is important to also consider peak hyperemic myocardial blood flow (MBF) in some cases, especially in patients with low MBFR and high resting MBF. There has not been a consensus as to whether peak hyperemic MBF or MBFR is superior for assessing epicardial and microvascular health.[2,3] A recent study examined cardiovascular mortality in more than 4000 consecutive patients, and found that MBFR was a stronger predictor of outcomes than peak flow.[4] In keeping with many studies in the literature, in this chapter we focus primarily on MBFR.

Why is myocardial perfusion PET and the ability to quantify MBFR such an important advance for nuclear cardiology? One of the important attributes of SPECT myocardial perfusion imaging is its ability to risk-stratify populations based on the size and severity of perfusion defects.[5,6] Those whose findings suggest moderate to high risk are often referred to coronary angiography with the expectation of revascularization.[7] Unfortunately, clinicians and interventionists have recognized the shortfalls of traditional spatially relative interpretations of myocardial perfusion studies. When in the catheterization laboratory with an individual patient, decisions need to be made when the coronary angiography appearances deviate from those anticipated from the MPI reports. Publications from the nuclear cardiology community acknowledge the deficiencies of spatially relative interpretation, in which image appearances may suggest limited CAD in patients found to have multivessel CAD at angiography.[8,9] Other publications emphasize the false-positive potential of MPI due primarily to attenuation artifacts.[10,11] Hence, the issues with strong population-based evidence and yet management challenges with application of this population-based evidence to a significant number of individual patients. Cardiac PET MPI has several attributes that can address these problems. First, every study is attenuation corrected. Second, with ^{82}Rb, the gated stress images are acquired under peak hyperemia conditions, such that regional changes in wall thickening or motion indicate ischemia and hence highly narrowed coronaries. Under conditions of increased myocardial blood flow, global increases in function such as LVEF are anticipated; drops in LVEF correlate with extensive CAD independent of the spatially relative MPI appearances.[12,13] Finally, PET studies permit a segment-centric as opposed to a spatially relative assessment of changes in myocardial blood flow, by virtue of its ability to quantify changes in blood flow between resting and peak hyperemic conditions. Numerous studies have shown the independent and incremental value of this information for both diagnosis and prognosis after consideration of all other clinical and imaging data.[14–24] This chapter examines many aspects of myocardial blood flow with cardiac PET, including acquisition of flow data, patient selection, evaluation of validity of flow data, assessing the importance of the findings, and reporting of the findings.

ACQUISITION OF FLOW DATA

Most commonly a patient is positioned in the PET camera, and vital signs and a rest ECG are acquired, followed by an infusion of ^{82}Rb , the most common PET tracer used in the United States. Acquisition begins at the start of the ^{82}Rb infusion, so that the infusion can be tracked as it travels through the heart chambers. Then the patient is "stressed" with an arteriolar vasodilator, such as dipyridamole, adenosine, or regadenoson, or a beta-adrenergic agonist, such as dobutamine, followed by the ^{82}Rb infusion with the same acquisition sequence. After completion of image acquisition, the data are transferred to work stations for processing. This involves two different operations: one for preparation of the images, and one for measurement of blood flow. Prior chapters have described the technical details of these steps.

If the PET tracer used is NH_3-ammonia, the rest study is completed and then this longer-lived tracer (9.8 minutes vs 75 seconds for ^{82}Rb) is given time to decay prior to starting the stress component of the test. Therefore, usually the patient is removed from the camera after the rest acquisition and returns later for the stress study. Otherwise, the study is similar to a ^{82}Rb PET MPI.

Regardless of tracer used, it is important to appreciate that acquiring the data to permit flow quantification can be done routinely as part of a rest/stress PET MPI study. It does not prolong image acquisition and does not expose the patient to any additional radiation. What it contributes is a full interrogation of the integrity of the delivery system to the myocardium, including the epicardial coronary arteries and the microvasculature, and adequacy of the stressor agent.

IMPORTANT CONSIDERATIONS WHEN EVALUATING FLOW DATA

From the clinical perspective, there are several important considerations when the interpreter is presented with the MBF measurements. These include an assessment of whether the measurements would have any useful clinical value for a particular patient, an evaluation for quality and face-validity, a conceptual framework for understanding the meaning of the measurements, and finally a useful way of reporting the information as a guide to next steps in patient management.

Patient Selection for MBFR Reporting: Appropriate and Inappropriate Patients

Many labs acquire flow data as part of the routine performance of a rest/stress myocardial perfusion PET study. However, there are several circumstances where the flow data is likely to be inaccurate. Some examples include patients with moderate to severe valvular regurgitation or large shunts, such as with VSDs or ASDs, and patients who cannot lie still such that precise registration for attenuation correction is not possible. Recent guidelines also caution against the routine reporting of flow values in cases where the information may not add diagnostic value and could be misleading to a referring physician.[25] The guidelines specifically mention patients with severe cardiomyopathies, large prior infarctions, advanced kidney disease, and those post-CABG. These are all examples where flows will usually be abnormal and in patients already known to be high-risk (Table 5-1). Obviously, some of these patients would benefit from reporting of flows, especially if there was found to be no flow augmentation (suggesting the likelihood that the vasodilator stress was ineffective). However, interpreters should always carefully consider the individual patient before incorporating a flow value

Table 5-1

Some Situations Where Flow Measurements May Be Less Useful and, Depending on the Circumstances, Might Best Be Not Reported

1. When technical errors are suspected (eg, patient motion, misregistration, acquisitions starting too late, detector saturation).
2. When patients are already known to be at high risk, and in whom flow measurements may mislead or confuse referring physicians and lead to erroneous management decisions.
   a. Long-standing severe kidney disease, often associated with advanced epicardial and microvascular disease
   b. Post-CABG patients, in whom flow is often abnormal because of extensive CAD despite patent grafts
   c. Patients who have had large transmural infarcts, in whom flow reserve may appear normal despite small increases over rest, but only because resting flows are severely reduced
   d. Patients with advanced cardiomyopathies in whom flow reserve is likely to be reduced on basis of myocardial fibrosis, damaged microvasculature, or high intramyocardial pressure

(Data from Dilsizian V, Bacharach SL, Beanlands RS, et al: ASNC imaging guidelines/SNMMI procedure standard for positron emission tomography (PET) nuclear cardiology procedures, J Nucl Cardiol. 2016 Oct;23(5):1187-1226)

because the flow information can sometimes lead to confusion or wrongful patient management.

Most other patients will have potential benefit of combining the image appearances with flow quantification. The guidelines specifically focus on patients with no known CAD but with symptoms suggestive of CAD, patients with known CAD in whom more definitive information about physiologic significance is desired, posttransplant patients, those in whom multivessel CAD is a concern, and in symptomatic patients with normal coronaries when microvascular disease is a possibility (Table 5-2).

A unique, relatively small but important group of patients are those who have no change in MBF in response to vasodilator stress.[25] Patients whose stress MBF is not changed from baseline may not have responded to the vasodilator applied. In essence, then, there was no real stress. This may reflect the inhibiting effects of caffeine or excess adrenergic tone. Only the flow measurements will be helpful in these situations, because changes in neither blood pressure nor heart rate carry certainty about changes in MBF.[26] The mechanisms that augment myocardial blood flow are different from those that affect symptoms, heart rate, or blood pressure. Patients who have no augmentation in MBF with a vasodilator need consideration for either repeat vasodilator testing after a confirmed 24-72–hour abstinence from caffeine or testing with dobutamine. This situation arises most frequently with emergency department patients who have arrived unprepped for an MPI; it is this same group of patients who are at high risk for acute myocardial infarctions if discharged on the basis of a normal-appearing MPI but who in reality did not have a valid rest/stress MPI. Figure 5-1 shows such

Table 5-2

Examples of Clinical Situations Where Reporting of Flows Is Likely to have Value for Diagnosis and Prognosis

1. Patients with no prior history of CAD
2. Ruling in or out presence of multivessel CAD
3. When physiologic assessment of angiographic CAD is needed
4. In cardiac transplant patients where diffuse CAD is common, such that balanced flow reduction may be more difficult to identify
5. Symptomatic patients with apparently normal coronary arteries by CTA or invasive coronary angiography, if microvascular disease is suspected
6. When rest and stress flows are nearly the same; in such cases the test may need to be repeated after a longer caffeine-free period or using dobutamine instead of a vasodilator for stress

(Data from Dilsizian V, Bacharach SL, Beanlands RS, et al: ASNC imaging guidelines/SNMMI procedure standard for positron emission tomography (PET) nuclear cardiology procedures, J Nucl Cardiol. 2016 Oct;23(5):1187-1226)

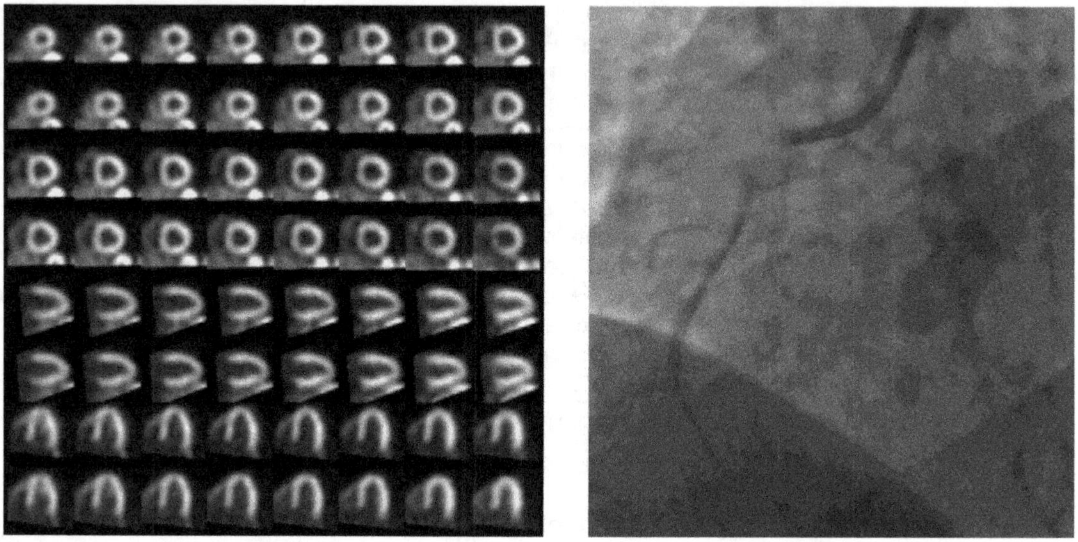

FIGURE 5-1 37-Year-Old Male Presenting to the Emergency Department. He had 20 minutes of chest pain, relieved en route with2 SL NTG. Serum TnI was normal. The scan was normal. However, the CACS was 250 and the MBFR was only 1.1. The patient was dismissed from the ED but returned 24 hours later with a STEMI caused by an occluded right coronary artery. This is an example of a non-stressed MPI. The essentially absent MBFR was the only indicator that the vasodilator stress was ineffective.

an example. One of the major benefits of flow quantification is assuredness that the vasodilator actually "worked." It is essential that the report include language about the test being nondiagnostic when there is no difference in flows at rest and following injection of the vasodilator.

Confidence in the Measurement—An Evaluation for Quality and Face-Validity

The reading physician needs some guidance in order to be confident in the robustness of the MBF measurement. Just as with other forms of cardiac imaging, there needs to be careful attention to detail or the flow measurements can be erroneous. The reading physician expects cases where the flow data will be concordant with other clinical information, such as perfusion appearances, regional and global function at rest and at peak stress, and clinical parameters. However, flow information is often the only clue warranting a change or modification in diagnosis and prognosis. For example, abnormal flow with normal perfusion and function nonetheless places a patient at higher risk for events[20] and in many cases will identify otherwise unsuspected multivessel CAD.[24] Most patients with globally low-flow reserve will need further testing with either coronary CTA or invasive coronary angiography to rule in or out multivessel CAD. Multivessel CAD will be present in less than 50% according to one study, [24] while moderate diffuse CAD with or without microvascular disease is also a common cause (Figure 5-2). On the contrary, globally normal flow in a patient with a perfusion defect can serve to rule out multivessel CAD[23] and establish a relatively low likelihood for mortality.[20,22] Numerous studies have shown the independent and incremental information about both the diagnosis and prognosis of patients based on flow measurements acquired as part of PET MPI, independent of whether the images appear normal or contain perfusion defects.[14–24]

There are a number of common factors that can easily lead to an erroneous flow measurement. Some of these include beginning the acquisition too late; interruption of the radionuclide travel by line kinking, anatomic causes of slowing, or extravasation;

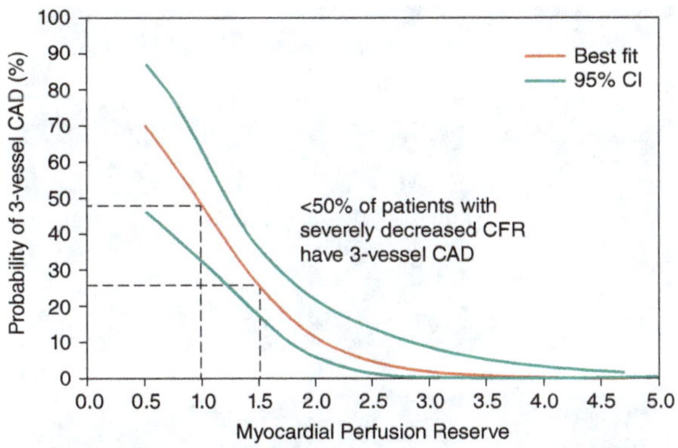

FIGURE 5-2 While probability of multivessel CAD increases as MBFR decreases, there are other causes of reduced MBFR so that down-stream testing is positive for multivessel CAD in <50% of patients. (Reproduced with permission from Ziadi MC, Williams K, Guo A, et al: Does quantification of myocardial flow reserve using rubidium-82 positron emission tomography facilitate detection of multivessel coronary artery disease? J Nucl Cardiol. 2012 Aug;19(4):670-680)

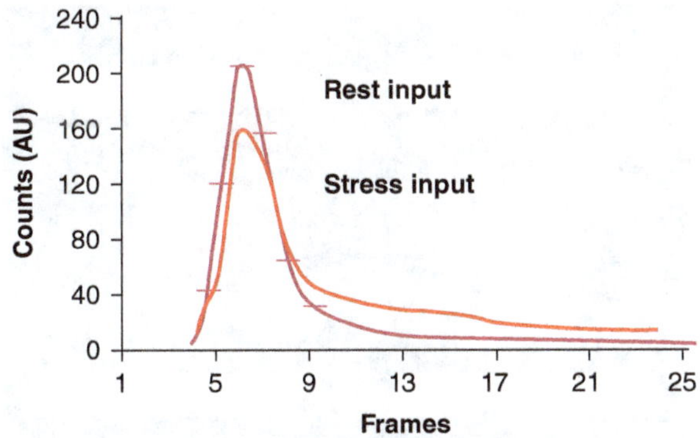

FIGURE 5-3 Example of Good Rest and Stress Time-Activity Curves. Note that the acquisition started prior to the tracer arriving at the blood pool region of interest. The rate of rise of the time-activity curves is relatively steep and the curves are relatively narrow. The stress peak is usually lower than the rest peak. The downward portion of the curves is smooth. Given sufficient time, the curves will approach zero.

scanner count saturation; patient motion; improper placement of the blood pool region of interest; or poor delineation of the myocardial uptake. These can be investigated by the interpreting physician by careful inspection of the blood pool and myocardial uptake curves, and visual inspection of the blood pool region of interest and the myocardial uptake contours. Figures 5-3 through 5-6 show some examples of adequate and inadequate time-activity curves, correct and incorrect blood pool regions of interest, and proper identification of the myocardium. Further information is available from several other sources.[1,27–32] This topic is also discussed in Chapter 4.

Another important quality control step is a critical look at the flow numbers for "face validity." As indicated in Chapter 4, there are some difficult to recognize problems, such as imprecision in the placement of the blood pool region of interest throughout the passage of the radionuclide, and respiratory motion such that attenuation correction is unable to be applied in an exact manner. Here are a few additional helpful tips:

1. **Resting global flow should track with the rate-pressure product.**[1,33,34] It is well known that the two major determinants of myocardial oxygen consumption are heart rate and systolic blood pressure. Therefore, MBF will be higher when the rate-pressure product (systolic blood pressure × heart rate) is higher, and will be lower when the RPP is lower. The correlation describing the relationship has been studied in normal volunteers with both NH3-ammonia PET and with ^{82}Rb

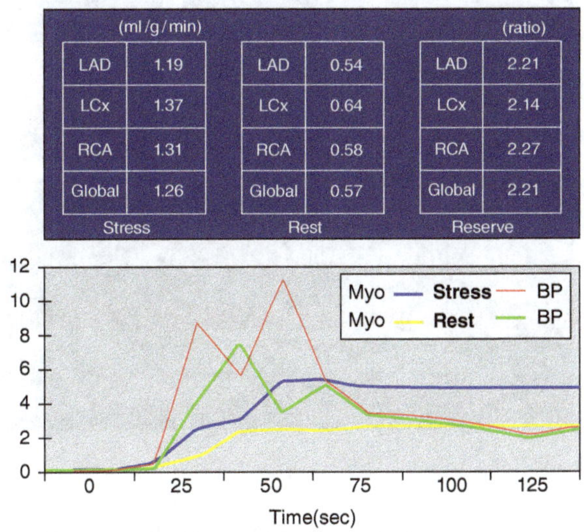

FIGURE 5-4 Example of major technical problems identified by inspection of time-activity input and myocardial curves. Note that the flow measurements by themselves provide no clues that there has been a technical problem likely making the flow measurements highly erroneous. Only by inspecting the curves would an interpreting physician be aware that the flow measurements are likely inaccurate. In this case, the likely problem is a combination of kinking of the intravenous line as well as patient motion.

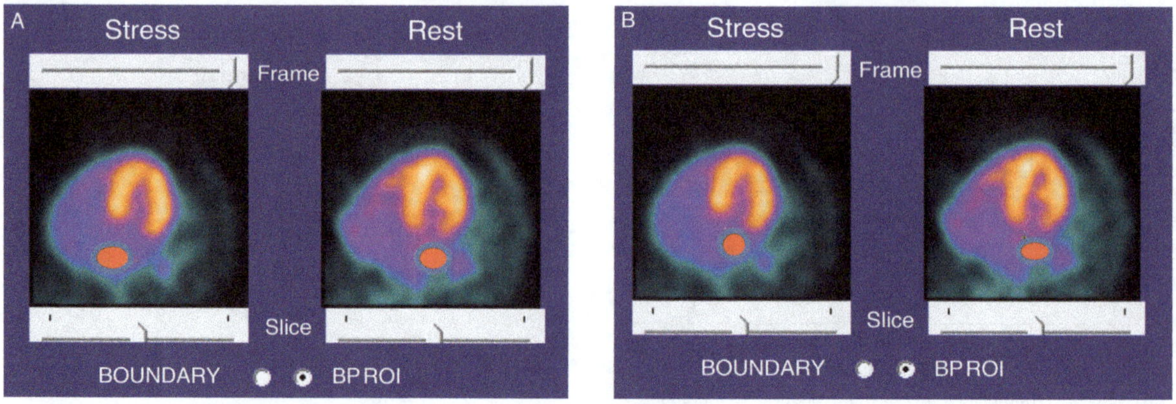

FIGURES 5-5 Input Regions of Interest for MBF Program Utilized Were Intended to Be in the Left. Atrium Note that the placement in (A) is different at stress compared to rest. Note also the global MBFR measurement for (A) showed under the image and compare this with the measurement shown in (B), when the regions of interest are properly positioned.

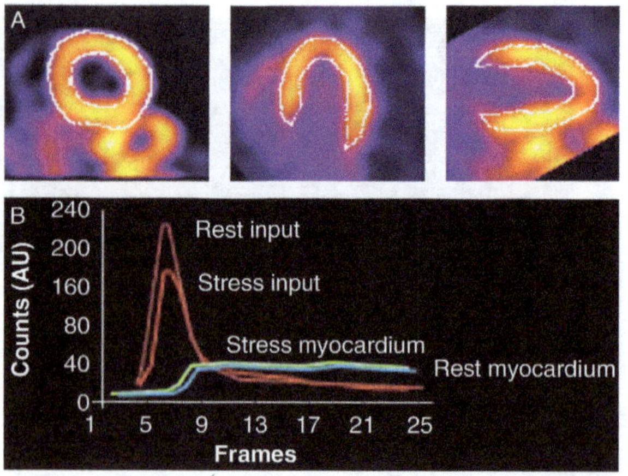

FIGURE 5-6 (A) shows an example of good myocardial boundary definition despite intense subdiaphragmatic tracer uptake immediately adjacent to the myocardium. The myocardial boundaries closely track visual myocardial appearances, and exclude adjacent structures that may be taking up tracer (such as liver or lung or hiatal hernias). (B) shows normal myocardial uptake curves added to the normal input curves displayed in Figure 5-3.

PET.[1,33,34] More recently, Omer et al[35] reexamined this relationship with ^{82}Rb PET in typical patients being referred for PET MPI. They found that the rate-pressure product/9700 was closely predictive of resting MBF. As such, an interpreting physician might as a first step for accepting a baseline flow as accurate, roughly calculate anticipated resting flow by dividing double product by ~10,000; if the resting flow is not within +/- 20%, the resting flow measurements may be misleading, and, therefore, may also be the MBF and MBFR (Figures 5-7A and 5-7B).

2. **If the rest images are normal, large differences in regional rest flow should not be expected.** In general, if the rest perfusion images appear normal, there should be relative homogeneity of regional rest flow. If there are differences of more than 20%, there needs to be concern about patient or cardiac motion and hence misregistration. Severe aortic stenosis may be an exception, where resting flows in the RCA territory may be higher owing to lower-pressure run-off into the right ventricle; variants of asymmetric ventricular hypertrophy may also result in regional differences in resting flow.

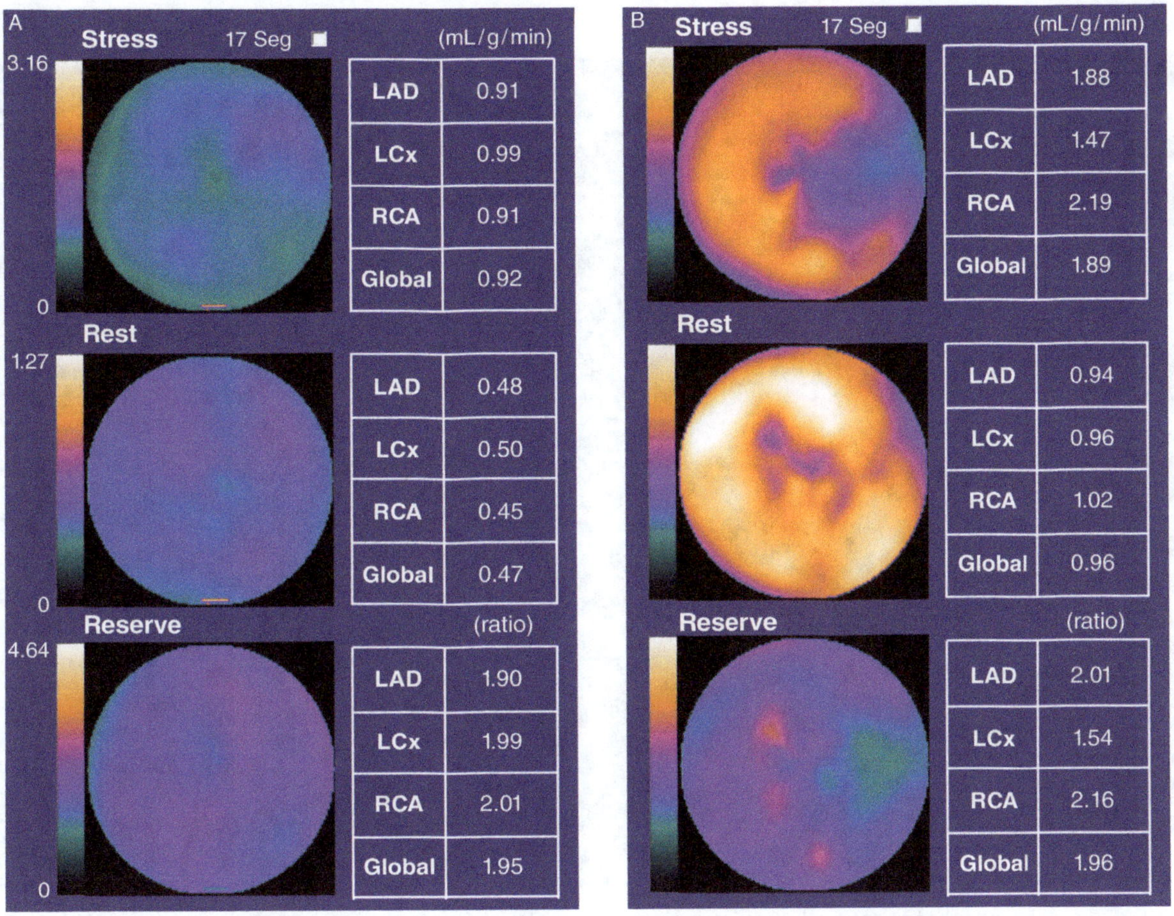

FIGURE 5-7 Note the low resting global flow measurement of 0.47 mL/g/min in patient 7A whose resting heart rate was 50 and resting systolic blood pressure was 97 mmHg (double product 4850). Contrast this with the resting global flow measurement of 0.96 in patient 7B with resting heart rate of 76 and resting systolic blood pressure of 135 mmHg (double product 10260).

3. **Obvious perfusion defects at rest should correlate with corresponding low flows.** Most often, perfusion defects at rest indicate regions of myocardial infarction (scar) or hibernation. Resting flow into such regions are lower compared to areas without perfusion defects. Figure 5-8 shows an example of a partially fixed inferior wall perfusion defect and the low resting flows in the infarct region. The inferior wall was nearly akinetic.
4. **Obvious perfusion defects at stress should correlate with relatively reduced peak flows and MBFR** (Figure 5-9). Regional perfusion defects and regional reductions in MBFR are indicators of epicardial coronary disease. Global and balanced reductions of flow are consistent with moderate diffuse epicardial disease and/or microvascular disease, or, in the case of minimal or no change in MBF between rest and stress, a nonresponder to vasodilator stress.

A CONCEPTUAL FRAMEWORK TO UNDERSTAND THE MEANING OF MBFR AND ITS RELATIONSHIP TO FFR

As outlined earlier, MBFR as measured by PET evaluates the entirety of the delivery system to the myocardium: flow through the epicardial coronaries

A

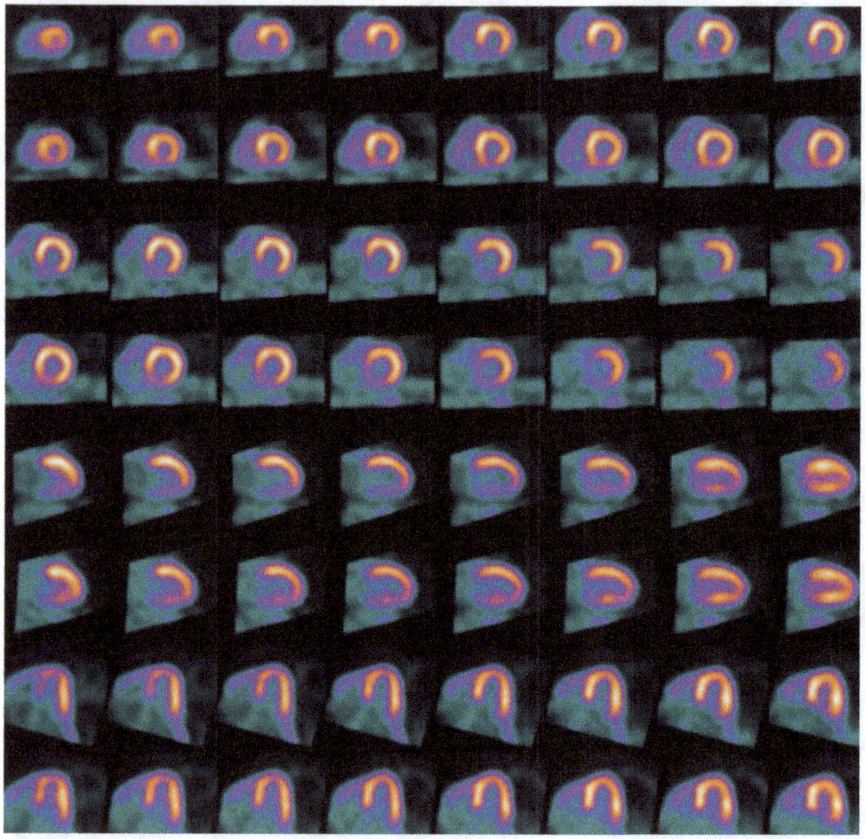

B

LAD	0.67
LCx	0.68
RCA	0.44
Global	0.60

(mL/g/min)

LAD	0.51
LCx	0.51
RCA	0.39
Global	0.48

(ratio)

LAD	1.31
LCx	1.33
RCA	1.13
Global	1.26

FIGURE 5-8 This patient had a transmural infarction involving portions of the inferior wall; note the partially reversible perfusion defect shown in (A). Note in (B) the very low rest flows in the infarct area.

and the microvasculature. Abnormalities affecting flow can occur in either the epicardial coronaries or the microvasculature, or in both. Therefore, a simplistic but clinically useful way to conceptualize the information provided by flow quantification, is to consider the four possibilities. The coronaries and the microvasculature are both normal or both are abnormal; or the coronaries are diseased with a normal microvasculature; or the coronaries are normal in the presence of microvascular disease. When both the coronaries and the microvasculature are healthy, MBFR will be normal (>2) globally and within each of the three coronary artery distributions. Global MBFR <1.5–1.6 (depending on software used) correlates with poor outcomes and can indicate diffuse epicardial disease, microvascular disease, or both. This pattern frequently is followed by further testing with either coronary CTA or invasive coronary angiography. Regional abnormalities of MBFR are strongly suggestive of epicardial coronary disease. The following sections go into greater detail about how flow measurements can be used to enhance patient management.

1. ***Diagnosis of epicardial coronary disease warranting referral to angiography:*** Spatially relative perfusion interpretation often suffices to identify regional abnormalities of flow. However, there are several situations where flow (see Figure 5-9 as an example) quantification will dramatically change the diagnosis and patient management.
    a. **Normal-appearing perfusion images with global abnormality of MBFR.** The concern here is presence of multivessel CAD. Further

A

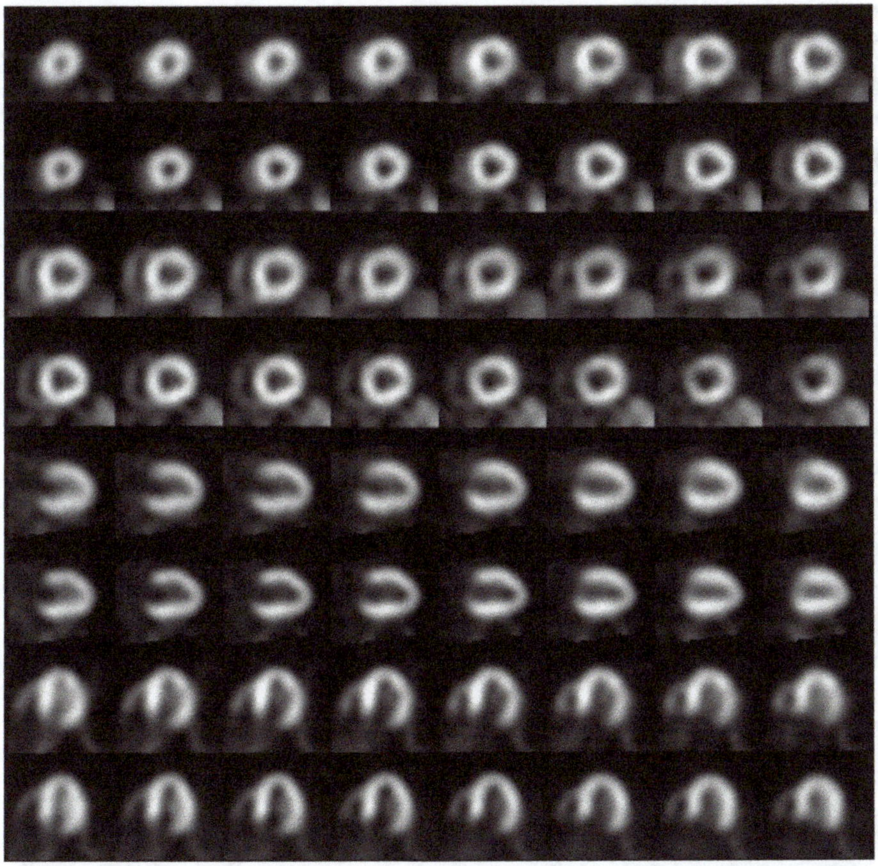

B

LAD	2.32
LCx	1.87
RCA	2.73
Global	2.35

(mL/g/min)

LAD	0.91
LCx	1.09
RCA	1.12
Global	1.01

(ratio)

LAD	2.55
LCx	1.72
RCA	2.44
Global	2.35

FIGURE 5-9 Lateral wall reversible perfusion defect is evident in the perfusion images note the relatively low MBFR for the affected area.

workup is usually recommended to determine if there is balanced epicardial disease requiring revascularization. In the presence of normal coronaries, the reduced MBFR indicates microvascular disease and/or diffuse moderate coronary disease. Studies show that the addition of flow quantification improves sensitivity for detection of coronary disease, but the specificity is affected by the presence of moderate diffuse coronary disease and/or microvascular disease. Figure 5-10 shows normal-appearing images in a patient with globally low MBFR. The PET MPI was followed by coronary angiography that showed multivessel CAD requiring CABG. More often, however, the coronary arteries are found to be normal or to have moderate diffuse disease (see as an example, Figure 12). Therefore, clinical judgment must determine which patients with apparently normal perfusion and low MBFR should undergo an anatomic assessment of their coronary arteries.

b. **Stress-induced perfusion defect.** Because of the spatially relative appearances, scans that show a defect in a single region can misguide the interpreter to believe that there is only single-vessel disease. In other words, the regions that appear better than the easily identified abnormality may also be abnormal. Figures 5-11A and 5-11B show examples of how flow quantification affects diagnosis and management. Both

A

B

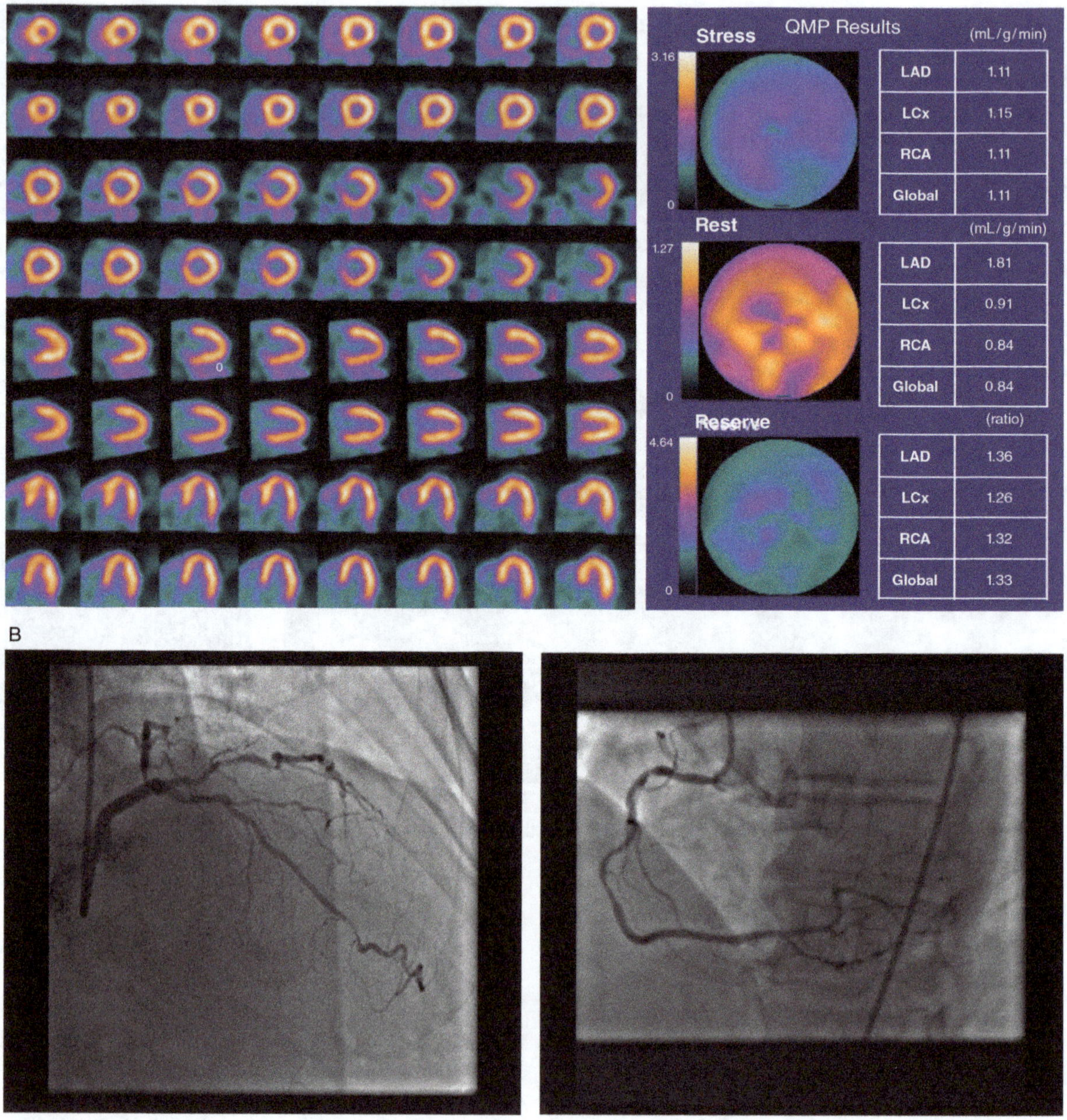

FIGURE 5-10 (A) Normal-appearing perfusion images with globally and regionally low MBFR. The patient underwent coronary angiography revealing severe and diffuse coronary disease as shown above in B, followed by CABG.

scans are similar, showing a single territory of severe reversible perfusion defect. The remainder of the perfusion pattern appears normal, so that the presumption is single-vessel CAD. In one case, however, the MBFR is very low in the remaining two coronary territories, signaling the likelihood of multivessel CAD. In contrast, the other example provides confidence that there is a single likely chronic total occlusion of the right coronary artery, while the other

A

LAD	0.67
LCx	0.68
RCA	0.44
Global	0.60

(mL/g/min)

LAD	0.51
LCx	0.51
RCA	0.39
Global	0.48

(ratio)

LAD	1.31
LCx	1.33
RCA	1.13
Global	1.26

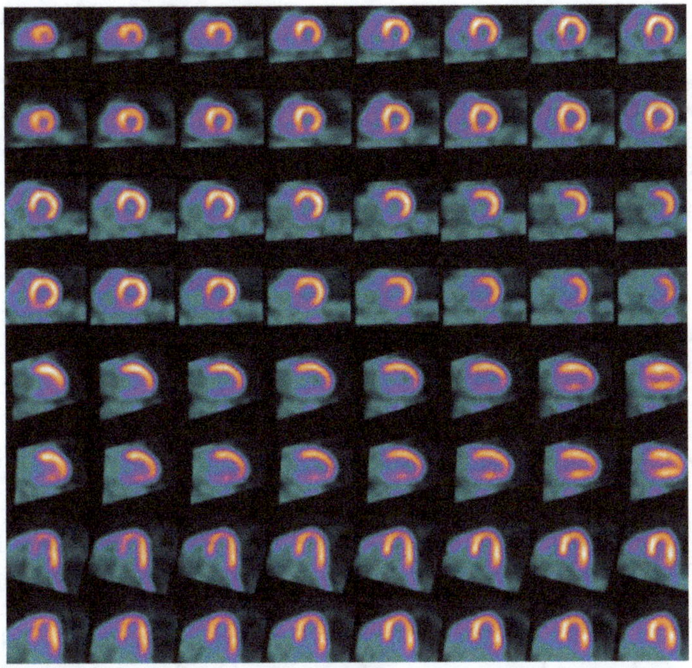

B

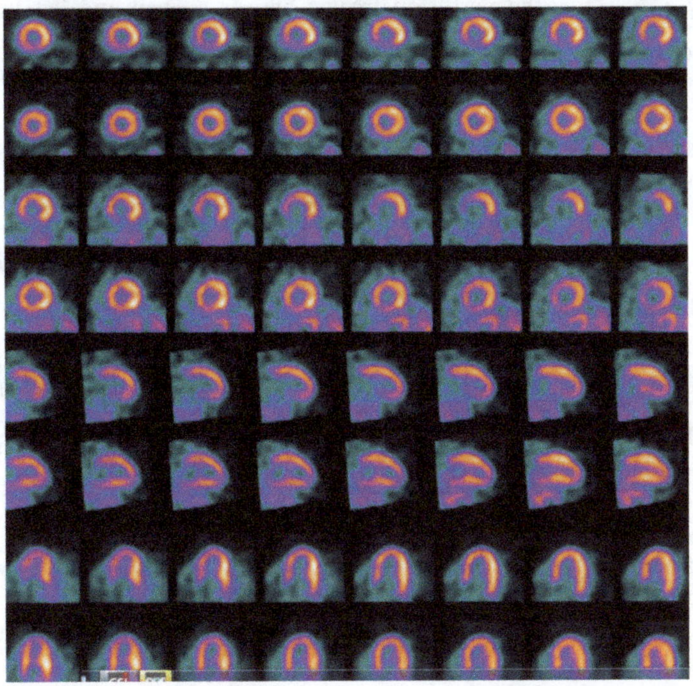

LAD	1.64
LCx	2.32
RCA	0.98
Global	1.58

(mL/g/min)

LAD	0.63
LCx	0.83
RCA	0.69
Global	0.69

(ratio)

LAD	2.60
LCx	2.80
RCA	1.42
Global	2.29

FIGURE 5-11 (A) Perfusion images from a patient with known chronic total occlusion of the RCA. MBFR is very low in the RCA territory, but also is low in both the LAD and LCx regions. Coronary angiography revealed severe 3-vessel CAD, and the patient underwent CABG. (B) shows a localized reversible perfusion defect of the inferior wall, with concomitant reduced MBFR in that region. Note, however, that global MBFR is normal, and is normal for the LAD and RCA regions. The patient was managed medically without referral to coronary angiography.

coronaries are widely patent as evidence by normal MBFR.

   c. **Normal perfusion images and globally and regionally normal MBFR.** The combination of normal perfusion, normal function, and normal MBFR places patients at very low likelihood for significant coronary artery disease. While the positive predictive value for significant CAD of abnormal flows is reduced owing to microvascular disease and mild to moderate diffuse epicardial CAD, the negative predictive value of normal MBFR (>2) for left main or multivessel CAD is high and is very high when MBFR is >2.5.

2. ***Diagnosis of microvascular disease:*** Microvascular disease is a particular concern in diabetics, advanced renal failure, postcardiac transplant, and in women. Although it can in some instances be difficult to distinguish pure microvascular disease from the effects of diffuse epicardial coronary disease, the important point is that MBFR is reduced to a level capable of causing symptoms and increasing the likelihood for type 2 infarctions when the affected person is put into circumstances where myocardial oxygen demand exceeds the delivery capability. Figure 5-12 shows an example.
3. ***Prognosis in relation to MBFR:*** Independent of image appearances, prognosis varies in relation to both hyperemic MBF and MBFR. Events are uncommon when MBFR exceeds 2, and increases in proportion to lower MBFR measures. A significant proportion of patients with normal or near-normal scans are reclassified as high or low risk based on MBFR quantification (Figure 5-13).
4. ***Correlation with FFR***: Data has shown, and physiologic understanding would predict, that there would not be a 1:1 relation between the two. FFR is designed to measure the physiologic significance of a stenosis in a coronary artery. MBFR is designed to measure the physiology of the entire coronary vasculature. If there is no microvascular disease, there will be a concordance between FFR and MBFR. Studies suggest this to be the case in about 60% of cases. However, many symptomatic patients have flow limitations not because of a singular stenosis, but rather to diffuse coronary disease with or without microvascular disease. In these cases, MBFR may be abnormal while FFR is within normal limits. Less often, MBFR is normal but FFR is abnormal. Presumably, this indicates an FFR measurement that is below a population-based threshold, but nonetheless is not creating ischemia in this particular patient. Intervention would unlikely be of benefit. Figure 5-14 provides a diagrammatic depiction of the different interactions between MBFR and FFR.

REPORTING OF MYOCARDIAL BLOOD FLOWS

Often, flow measurements are confirmatory of suspicion based on the imaging data. This does not mean the MBFR should not be reported. On the contrary, astute clinicians have learned the limitations of MPI based on imperfect sensitivity and specificity. Therefore, this measurement that is independently derived versus the images can be an important source of confidence that a study is truly normal or abnormal.

Consider, for instance, an MPI study in which the perfusion images appear normal and left ventricular function is also normal. Because virtually all MPI PET studies today are performed with pharmacologic means of stress, there is rarely any clinical information of value from the stress test itself. The normal appearing images and LVEF are consistent with a completely healthy delivery system (both the epicardial coronary arteries and the microvasculature), balanced flow reduction, moderate diffuse epicardial disease, diffuse microvascular disease, an ineffective vasodilation, low risk for future events, or even high risk for future events. Therefore, reporting that MBFR is completely normal (between 2 and 4 times baseline) provides confidence that the study is indeed normal, that there is no physiologic impairment to blood flow to the myocardium, and that the prognosis is excellent. We conclude our MPI reports in a numerically ordered sequence as follows:

1. No ischemia and no regions of infarction
2. Normal ventricular function segmentally and globally with LVEF (sic) 60%
3. Normal increase in LVEF to 65% in response to vasodilation stress
4. Normal myocardial blood flow reserve, averaging (sic) 2.6 times baseline flows, and within normal limits for all three coronary territories

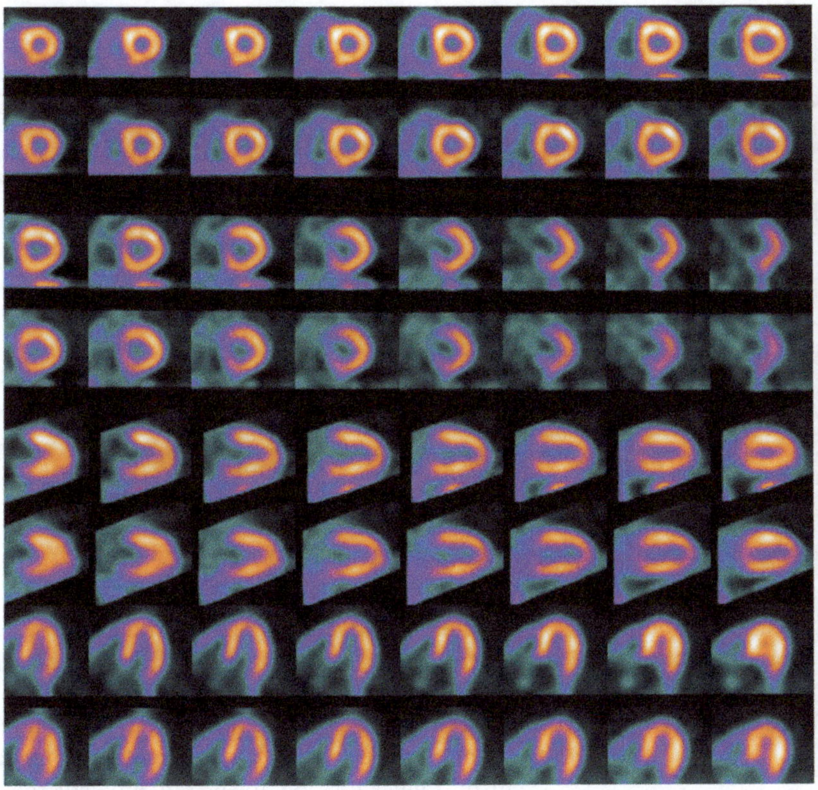

LAD	1.18
LCx	1.08
RCA	1.02
Global	1.11

(mL/g/min)

LAD	0.68
LCx	0.65
RCA	0.62
Global	0.66

(ratio)

LAD	1.73
LCx	1.66
RCA	1.64
Global	1.69

FIGURE 5-12 A 77-Year-Old Man Has Exertional Dyspnea. His MPI images are normal, but he has low MBFR. He sustained a type2 MI while hiking at 10,000 feet in Colorado. His coronary angiogram was near normal.

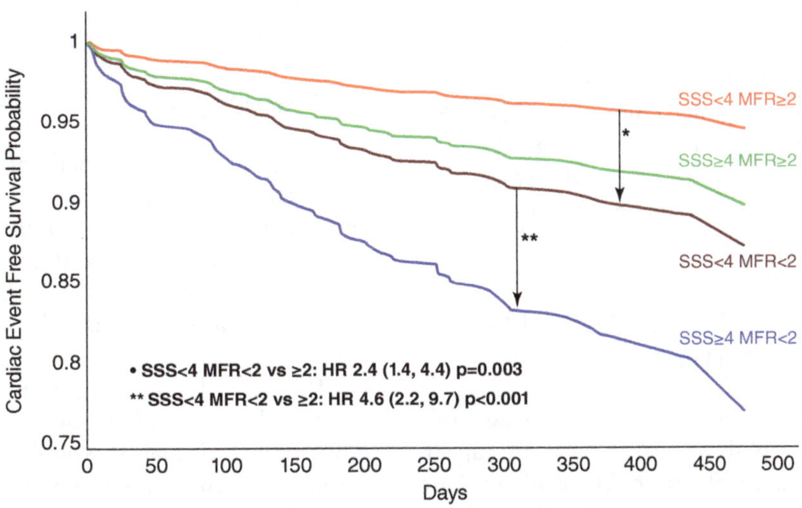

FIGURE 5-13 Adjusted Cardiac Event-Free Survival. This data shows how relatively short-term events track in relation to normal or abnormal spatially-relative perfusion scans. (Data from Ziadi MC, Williams K, Guo A, et al: Does quantification of myocardial flow reserve using rubidium-82 positron emission tomography facilitate detection of multivessel coronary artery disease? J Nucl Cardiol. 2012 Aug;19(4):670-680).

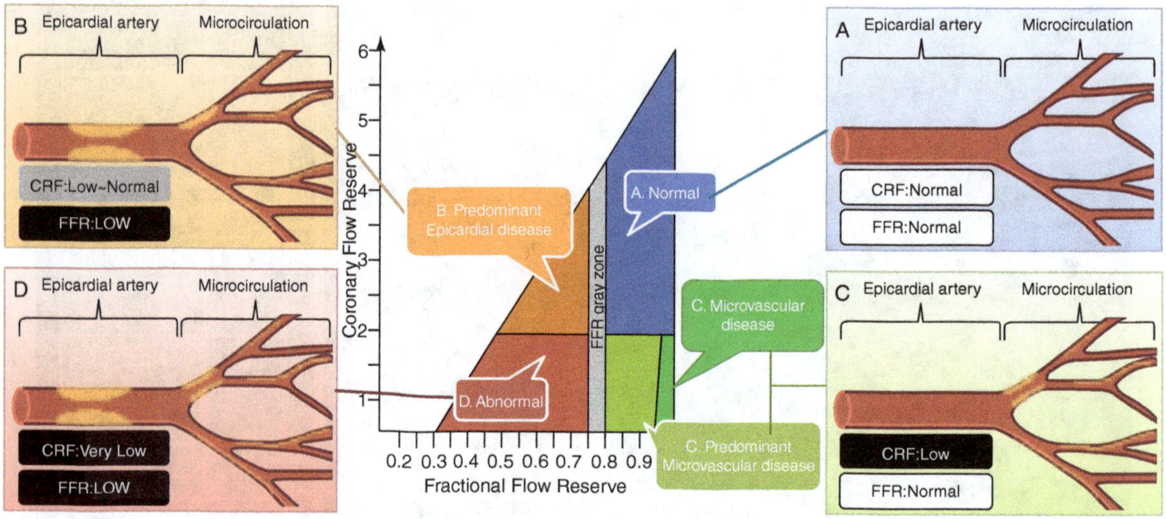

FIGURE 5-14 Interplay Between FFR and CFR (MBFR). (Derived from several articles primarily from Gould and DiCarli)

On the other hand, it is important to be forceful about the role of MBFR in appropriate situations. Consider, for example, a report based on a study with a mild apical reversible perfusion defect.

1. There is a small and mild reversible perfusion defect at the apex
2. Normal ventricular function segmentally and globally with LVEF (sic) 60%
3. LVEF 59% at peak hyperemia
4. Myocardial blood flow reserve is globally abnormal, averaging (sic) 1.5 baseline flows
5. The abnormally low global flow reserve places this study into a high-risk category despite the mild perfusion abnormality. Recommend further studies to determine whether patient has multivessel CAD.

CHALLENGES FOR MYOCARDIAL BLOOD FLOW QUANTIFICATION

The evidence-base for the value of PET flow quantification is growing rapidly. However, there are gaps in knowledge that require attention. The evidence base so far is entirely observational and based mostly on single-center retrospective analyses. As of yet, there are no prospective studies to address whether patient management in relation to MBFR confers better outcomes, reduced costs, or improved health status.

There exists a complex interplay of protocols, tracers, stressors, and equipment in the clinical and scientific community. In some sense, it is remarkable that the various centers using different techniques are finding commonalities in terms of cut-off ranges for flow measurements. For the field to move forward, there needs to be a deeper understanding of the factors that are important to acquiring robust data.

Even within single centers using the same equipment and protocols, there is relatively high test-retest variability in both rest and hyperemic flow measurements.[39, 40] This is likely partly reflective of the complexity of the underlying physiology that is being probed. However, poorly understood technical matters are likely also to influence measurement variability. Some of these include imperfect tracer delivery systems in relation to flow quantification, timing variances after vasodilator injection, dosing, and even the choice of tracer.

The field also needs greater convergence as to the models employed for measuring flow and to the development of quality assurance tools. There are a variety of software programs that claim superiority for different tracers and equipment; published data suggests that they mostly provide similar values,[36–38] but the differences are sufficient that multicenter trials based on flow measurements will be challenging. Currently, providers need to know the details of their specific software and equipment and optimize their own parameters and protocols.

CONCLUSIONS: CLINICAL MYOCARDIAL BLOOD FLOW

This chapter has reviewed many aspects of clinical myocardial blood flow with cardiac PET. This is a rapidly developing field. In the next few years, it is likely that there will be convergence on methodology, including acquisition differences according to tracers, equipment, and stressors; compartment modeling; quality assurance tools; and reporting guidelines. Currently, the evidence base is impressive that quantification of myocardial blood flow and the comparison between rest and stress has value, and will ultimately evolve to be a standard of practice for PET cardiac myocardial perfusion imaging.

REFERENCES

1. Murthy VL, Bateman TM, Beanlands RS, et al. Clinical quantification of myocardial blood flow using positron emission tomography: a joint position paper of the Cardiovascular Council (CVC) of the Society of Nuclear Medicine and Molecular Imaging (SNMMI) and the American Society of Nuclear Cardiology (ASNC). *J Nucl Cardiol.* 2018;25:269–297.
2. Hajjiri MM, Leavitt MB, Zheng H, Spooner AE, Fischman AJ, Gewirtz H. Comparison of positron emission tomography measurement of adenosine-stimulated absolute myocardial blood flow versus relative myocardial tracer content for physiological assessment of coronary artery stenosis severity and location. *J Am Coll Cardiol Imaging.* 2009;2:751–758.
3. Klocke FJ, Lee DC. Absolute myocardial blood flow. *J Am Coll Cardiol Imaging.* 2011;4:413–414.
4. Gupta A, Taqueti VR, van de Hoef T, et al. Integrated noninvasive physiologic assessment of coronary circulatory function and impact on cardiovascular mortality in patients with stable coronary artery disease. *Circulation.* 2017;136:2325–2336.
5. Hachamovitch R, Hayes SW, Friedman JD, Cohen I, Berman DS. Comparison of the short-term survival benefit associated with revascularization compared with medical therapy in patients with no prior coronary artery disease undergoing stress myocardial perfusion single photon emission computed tomography. *Circulation.* 2003;107:2900–2907.
6. Hachamovitch R, Rozanski A, Shaw LJ, et al. Impact of ischaemia and scar on the therapeutic benefit derived from myocardial revascularization vs medical therapy among patients undergoing stress-rest myocardial perfusion scintigraphy. *Eur Heart J.* 2011;32:1012–1024.
7. Bateman TM, O'Keefe JH Jr, Dong VM, Barnhart C, Ligon RW. Coronary angiography rates following stress SPECT scintigraphy. *J Nucl Cardiol.* 1995;2:217–223.
8. Lima RSL, Watson DD, Goode AR, et al. Incremental value of combined perfusion and function over perfusion alone by gated SPECT myocardial perfusion imaging for detection of severe three-vessel coronary artery disease. *J Am Coll Cardiol.* 2003;42:64–70.
9. Berman DS, Kang X, Slomka PJ, Gerlach J, de Yang L, Hayes SW. Underestimation of extent of ischemia by gated SPECT myocardial perfusion imaging in patients with left main coronary artery disease. *J Nucl Cardiol.* 2007;14:52–528.
10. Hendel RC, Corbett JA, Cullom SJ, DePuey EG, Garcia EV, Bateman TM. The value and practice of attenuation correction for myocardial perfusion SPECT imaging: a joint position paper from the American Society of Nuclear Cardiology and the Society of Nuclear Medicine. *J Nucl Cardiol.* 2002;9:135–143.
11. Heller GV, Links J, Bateman TM, et al. American Society of Nuclear Cardiology and Society of Nuclear Medicine Joint Position Statement: Attenuation correction of myocardial perfusion SPECT scintigraphy. *J Nucl Cardiol.* 2004;11:229–230.
12. Lertsburapa K, Ahlberg AW, Bateman TM, et al. Independent and incremental prognostic value of left ventricular ejection fraction determined by stress gated rubidium 82 PET imaging in patients with known or suspected coronary artery disease. *J Nucl Cardiol.* 2008;15:745–753.
13. Dorbala S, Hachamovitch R, Curillova Z, et al. Incremental prognostic value of gated Rb-82

positron emission tomography myocardial perfusion imaging over clinical variables and rest LVEF. *J Am Coll Cardiol Imaging*. 2009;2: 846–854.

14. Uren NG, Melin JA, De Bruyne B, Wijns W, Baudhuin T, Camici PG. Relation between myocardial blood flow and the severity of coronary-artery stenosis. *N Engl J Med*. 1994;330:1782–1788.
15. Di Carli M, Czernin J, Hoh CK, et al. Relation among stenosis severity, myocardial blood flow, and flow reserve in patients with coronary artery disease. *Circulation*. 1995;91:1944–1951.
16. Muzik O, Duvernoy C, Beanlands RS, et al. Assessment of diagnostic performance of quantitative flow measurements in normal subjects and patients with angiographically documented coronary artery disease by means of nitrogen-13 ammonia and positron emission tomography. *J Am Coll Cardiol*. 1998;31:534–540.
17. Anagnostopoulos C, Almonacid A, Fakhri G, et al. Quantitative relationship between coronary vasodilator reserve assessed by 82Rb PET imaging and coronary artery stenosis severity. *Eur J Nucl Med Mol Imaging*. 2008;35:1593–1601.
18. Kajander S, Joutsiniemi E, Saraste M, et al. Cardiac positron emission tomography/computed tomography imaging accurately detects anatomically and functionally significant coronary artery disease. *Circulation*. 2010;122:603–613.
19. Gould KL, Johnson NP, Bateman TM, et al. Anatomic versus physiologic assessment of coronary artery disease: role of coronary flow reserve, fractional flow reserve, and positron emission tomography imaging in revascularization decision-making. *J Am Coll Cardiol*. 2013;62:1639–1653.
20. Herzog BA, Husmann L, Valenta I, et al. Long-term prognostic value of 13N-ammonia myocardial perfusion positron emission tomography added value of coronary flow reserve. *J Am Coll Cardiol*. 2009;54(2):150–156.
21. Murthy VL, Naya M, Foster CR, et al. Improved cardiac risk assessment with noninvasive measures of coronary flow reserve. *Circulation*. 2011;124:2215–2224.
22. Ziadi MC, Williams KA, Guo A, et al. Impaired myocardial flow reserve on rubidium-82 positron emission tomography imaging predicts adverse outcomes in patients assessed for myocardial ischemia. *J Am Coll Cardiol*. 2011;58:740–748.
23. Naya M, Murthy VL, Taqueti VR, et al. Preserved coronary flow reserve effectively excludes high-risk coronary artery disease on angiography. *J Nucl Med*. 2014;55:248–255.
24. Ziadi MC, Williams K, Guo A, et al. Does quantification of myocardial flow reserve using rubidium-82 positron emission tomography facilitate detection of multivessel coronary artery disease? *J Nucl Cardiol*. 2012;19:670–680.
25. Dilsizian V, Bacharach SL, Beanlands RS, et al. ASNC imaging guidelines/SNMMI procedural standard for positron emission tomography nuclear cardiology procedures. *J Nucl Cardiol*. 2016;23:1187–1226.
26. Mishra RK, Dorbala S, Logsetty G, et al. Quantitative relation between hemodynamic changes during intravenous adenosine infusion and the magnitude of coronary hyperemia: implications for myocardial perfusion imaging. *J Am Coll Cardiol*. 2005;45:553–558.
27. Klein R, Ocneanu A, Renaud JM, Ziadi MC, Beanlands RS. Consistent tracer administration profile improves test-retest repeatability of myocardial blood flow quantification with 82Rb. *J Nucl Cardiol*. 2018;25:929–941.
28. Cremer PC, DiFilippo FP, Jamber WA . Moving towards a better understanding of potential pitfalls dynamic PET imaging. *J Nucl Cardiol*. 2017 Feb 22. doi:10.1007/s12350-017-0828-9.
29. Hunter CRRN, Klein R, Beanlands RS, deKemp RA. Patient motion effects on the quantification of regional myocardial blood flow with dynamic PET imaging. *Med Phys*. 2016;43:1829.
30. Rajaram M, Tahari AK, Lee AH, et al. Cardiac PET/CT Misregistration causes significant changes in estimated myocardial blood flow. *J Nucl Med*. 2013;54:50–54.
31. Votaw JR, Packard RRS. Technical aspects of acquiring and measuring myocardial blood flow: Method, technique, and QA. *J Nucl Cardiol*. 2017. Online first.
32. Moody JB, Lee BC. Precision and accuracy of clinical quantification of myocardial blood flow by dynamic PET: a technical perspective. *J Nucl Cardiol*. 2015;22:935–951.

33. Czernin J, Müller P, Chan S, et al. Influence of age and hemodynamics on myocardial blood flow and flow reserve. *Circulation*. 1993;88:62–69.
34. Chareonthaitawee P, Kaufmann PA, Rimoldi O, Camici PG. Heterogeneity of resting and hyperemic myocardial blood flow in healthy humans. *Cardiovasc Res*. 2001;50:151–161.
35. Omer M, Kureshi F, Muskula P, Patel KK, Kennedy K, Saeed I, et al. Development of a simple screening measure to approximate resting myocardial blood flow in Rb-82 PET: value of the rate-pressure product. *J Nucl Cardiol*. 2017;24:1890.
36. Murthy VL, Lee BC, Sitek A, et al. Comparison of prognostic validation of multiple methods of quantification of myocardial blood flow with 82Rb PET. *J Nucl Med*. 2014;55:1952–1958.
37. deKemp RA, Declerk J, Klein R, et al. Multi-software reproducibility study of stress and rest myocardial blood flow assessed with 3D dynamic PET/CT and a 1-tissue-compartment model of 82Rb kinetics. *J Nucl Med*. 2013;54:571–577.
38. Johnson NP, Gould KL. Regadenoson versus dipyridamole hyperemia for cardiac PET imaging. *J Am Coll Cardiol Imaging*. 2015;8:438–447.
39. Efseaff M, Klein R, Ziadi MC, Beanlands RS, deKemp RA. Short-term repeatability of resting myocardial blood flow measurements using rubidium-82 PET imaging. *J Nucl Cardiol*. 2012;19:997–1006.
40. Kitkugvan D, Johnson NP, Roby AE, Patel MB, Kirkeeide R, Gould KL. Routine clinical quantitative rest stress myocardial perfusion for managing coronary artery disease clinical relevance of test-retest variability. *J Am Coll Cardiol Imaging*. 2017;10:565–577.

EDITOR'S PERSPECTIVE

Gary V. Heller

The clinical use of cardiovascular PET imaging has been on the rise for several years with new applications and demonstrated value. Many clinical nuclear cardiology laboratories have begun cardiac PET myocardial imaging programs, successfully adopting this exciting technology for their patients. In contrast, few beyond academic centers have incorporated myocardial blood flow (MBF) into their procedures. However, with the recent joint SNMMI/ASNC position paper, the understanding of blood flow is at the point of clinical implementation.[1]

While the data supporting myocardial blood flow with cardiac PET are extensive,[1] the clinical application and interpretation are challenging, requiring a different mind-set than with myocardial perfusion imaging. Very few documents are available for guidance in the interpretation of MBF in a clinical setting as well as its relevance to clinical decisions.[2] This chapter as well as Chapter 4 contain the first detailed descriptions of MBF for clinicians, providing not only guidance to the validity of the collected data, but also what to do with the information and how it applies to clinical decisions. As such, the authors are to be congratulated on providing tools to help understand the value of myocardial blood flow and provide proper interpretation.

This clinical blood flow chapter carefully delineates the patient value and the circumstances in which MBF assessment can be of considerable assistance. Somewhat analogous to calcium scoring (discussed in Chapter 2), the value of MBF in making a diagnostic and prognostic decision for patients with suspected CAD is very high, and differs in those patients with known CAD and cardiomyopathies. The negative predictive value of normal perfusion/normal MBF is very high and should result in fewer unnecessary cardiac catheterizations. This is fundamentally important in an era in which there are consequences for catherization of patients with no disease, especially from the perspective of the referring healthcare provider. It also provides an opportunity to regain lost confidence for referring healthcare providers who become frustrated when a patient with a normal nuclear study is subsequently found to have disease or worse, suffers a coronary event. With advances in technologies in other imaging fields such as MR and CT, the value of MBF for PET is very important in keeping nuclear cardiac imaging in the forefront of noninvasive procedures.

There are other circumstances in which MBF is very helpful. Previously, a conundrum of pharmacologic stress has been the inability to assess the adequacy of the injected agent, unlike exercise and the use of a predictive heart rate. Now, with MBF, if a patient does not demonstrate a change in global blood flow between rest and stress, this indicates a lack of physiologic response to the administered stress agent such as adenosine, dipyridamole, or regadenoson. This is generally due to something that interferes with the drug such as caffeine ingestion, or similar, and is reported as a nonresponder in the presence of normal PET perfusion. This indicates to the referring healthcare provider that the normal study does not exclude CAD and the study should be repeated after appropriate measures aretaken.

The positive test showing moderate to severe reduction in blood flow is confirmatory of CAD and perhaps severity of stenosis. These data are very complementary to the PET MPI data. In addition, global reduction of MBF reserve is an indication of small vessel disease, which carries a risk of cardiac events independent of epicardial CAD.

The experience in clinical laboratories with PET MBF is growing as is the confidence by interpreting physicians and referring health care providers that these data are very helpful in clinical decisions, and should be a routine part of the cardiac PET study. It is no wonder that the recent ASNC/SNMMI Position Statement specificied a cardiac PET study as the provision of myocardial blood flow data.[3]

As this chapter also points out, quality control evaluation is very important for the interpreting physician to ensure that the numbers presented are valid. In contrast to imaging data in which the reader sees the data and can confirm it, the MBF data are only as good as the quality of the data acquired. Thus, there can be discrepancies between imaging data and myocardial blood flow. In such cases, which are rare, the interpreter should rely upon what he or she knows best, namely the perfusion and function data. As the eminent philosopher Kenny Rogers once said: "You've got to know when to hold 'em, know when to fold 'em."[4]

References for Editor's Perspective

1. Murthy VL, Bateman TM, Beanlands RS, et al. Clinical quantification of myocardial blood flow using positron emission tomography: a joint Position paper of the Cardiovascular Council (CVC) of the Society of Nuclear Medicine and Molecular Imaging (SNMMI) & the American Society of Nuclear Cardiology (ASNC). *J Nucl Cardiol.* 2018;25:269-297.
2. Bateman MB, Gould KL, Di Carli MF. Proceedings of the Cardiac PET Summit, May 12, 2014, Baltimore, MD; 2015.
3. Bateman TM, Dilsizian V, Beanlands RS, DePuey EG, Heller GV, Wolinsky DA American Society of Nuclear Cardiology and Society of Nuclear Medicine and Molecular Imaging Joint Position Statement on the Clinical Indications for Myocardial Perfusion PET. *J Nucl Cardiol.* 2016; 23(5):1227-31.
4. Kenny Rodgers, "The Gambler," 1979.

SECTION

4

TECHNICAL DEVELOPMENTS IN CARDIOVASCULAR PET

Latest Innovations in Cardiovascular PET Instrumentation

CHAPTER 6

Piotr J. Slomka

INTRODUCTION

PET instrumentation has undergone several incremental improvements in recent years. This chapter will discuss recent technology advances for PET/CT and PET/MR, which include improved sensitivity, new detectors, digital PET, improved electronics advanced reconstructions, implementation of time-of-flight (TOF), and motion compensation methods. We also review how these high-quality CT component and hybrid PET/MR systems enable some additional potential applications for advanced hybrid cardiac imaging.

3D PET

Historically, PET scanners operated in 2D mode, with interplane septa between slices and with each slice reconstructed independently. This technique had the advantage of reducing the scatter, randoms, and singles rate of the PET scanner. This improvement in image quality came at the expense of system sensitivity. In 3D PET, there are no interplane septa that physically separate detector rings along the axial dimension, which improves count sensitivity by a factor of 4–6, as compared to traditional 2D PET scanners with interplane septa. However, the disadvantage of 3D acquisitions is an increased scatter fraction, with the number of scattered events detected as a percentage of all coincidence events in the 30%-40% range.[1] As the technology for reducing system dead time and scatter correction improved, most instrumentation providers embraced the 3D imaging mode, with many modern PET/CT systems being built without a 2D option.

Importantly for first-pass cardiac imaging, with short-lived tracers such as ^{82}Rb or ^{15}O water, the number of single events is very high, and consequently so is the number of multiple random coincidence events (random events), which are primarily produced by the simultaneous occurrence of a true coincidence event and a single event or two single events in the detectors. This may lead to event pileups and saturation during initial phases of the first-pass cardiac imaging with PET. Clinical PET studies optimize the injected doses of ^{82}Rb for the new 3D PET scanners, thereby avoiding the saturation issues.[2] Manufacturers also introduced specially designed high-count rate detectors to withstand the high-count rates during initial phases of dynamic ^{82}Rb imaging. However, challenges still remain with analog PET systems for the high-count rate with ^{82}Rb.[3] Despite these potential technical difficulties with 3D PET kinetic imaging, the advantages of lower injected doses and a lower overall radiation burden for the patient make 3D PET protocols preferred.

When performing 3D PET imaging with short-lived tracers such as ^{82}Rb, attention must be paid to the approximately 13% of nuclear decays associated with a 776 keV prompt-gamma emission. These prompt gammas occur when the ^{82}Rb nucleus decays into an unstable final state, which then decays to its ground state releasing the 776 keV photon. These prompt-gamma photons can downscatter into the

511 keV PET energy window. Prompt-gamma corrections have been now incorporated in the 3D reconstruction process together with corrections for standard scattered events. This was not necessary for 2D PET imaging, but is very important for cardiac 3D PET ^{82}Rb imaging with the new generation of scanners.[4]

PET DETECTOR CRYSTALS

An important aspect of the PET system is the choice of the scintillation crystal used for annihilation photon detection. The density of the detector crystal will affect its ability to stop incoming 511 keV radiation completely on the first interaction. The high light yield (expressed as the number of light photons emitted for each MeV of energy absorbed) is desirable to improve signal-to-noise and scatter photon discrimination characteristics. Finally, the speed of the scintillation and the decay of the light impulse after absorbing the annihilation photon will affect PET system count-rate capability, which will be important in first-pass dynamic acquisitions with short-lived tracers and time of flight (TOF) capabilities. A summary of common PET scintillators is given in Table 6-1. Active research is currently underway with the goal to develop superior PET scintillation crystals, which feature high-density and high-atomic numbers, necessary for an efficient photoelectric conversion of the annihilation photons, and short decay time of the scintillation light.[5,6]

The size of the individual scintillation crystals in a block of the detector ranges typically from $4 \times 4 \times 20$ mm^3 to $6.3 \times 6.3 \times 30$ mm^3 for the PET/CT scanners listed in Table 6-2. Most traditional PET scanners use analog photomultiplier tubes (PMT), which are much larger than the individual detectors in the detector block to which the tubes are coupled; therefore the interpolation of the signals between neighboring PMTs (Anger principle) is needed to determine the γ-ray's original impact. Because of this, the use of analog PMTs limits possible improvement of spatial resolution in PET imaging, by the use of smaller crystals.

DIGITAL PET

Digital imaging systems replace the analog photomultiplier tubes with silicon digital photomultipliers (SiPMs),[7]blocks of avalanche photodiodes (APCs),[8] or analog SiPMs.[9] More compact size of digital detectors allows to achieve one-to-one coupling of the between digital photomultipliers and scintillation crystal blocks (Table 6-2, Figure 6-1). In addition, these digital detectors are not affected by magnetic fields, making them particularly useful in PET/MR systems.

SiPMs are built from APCs and will detect light events in serially connected APCs. The total gain in the light signal in the SiPM is similar to that obtained in the analog PMT (approximately 10^6). One design used in digital PET connects multiple SiPM pixels together and adds the signals from each pixel for a summed output, which requires so-called application-specific integrated circuits (ASICs) to condition the signal and minimize the interference from the electronic noise or unstable baseline currents (present without any counts). This type of design is sometimes referred to as the analog SiPM. Analog SiPM tends to consume more power and generate more heat than digital SiPM.[10] True digital SiPM incorporates electronics to each photodiode

Table 6-1

Characteristics of Inorganic Scintillating Materials Used in PET

Material	Density [g/cm3]	Effective Atomic # (Z)	Light Yield [% NaI(Tl)]	Decay [ns]
BGO	7.1	74	8	300
GSO	6.7	59	16	60
LSO	7.4	66	75	40
LYSO	5.4	54	75	53

Table 6-2

Specifications and key parameters for modern, commercially available PET/CT and PET/MR systems by Philips (Ingenuity TF and Vereos), GE (Discovery and IQ, MI, Signa) and Siemens (Biograph mCT, and Vision 600). Biograph mMR specification from work by Delso et al. [93]. Biograph Vision 600 obtained from vendor specification sheet 06/2018

Model	Ingenuity TF	Vereos	Discovery IQ (5-ring)	Discovery MI (4-ring)	Biograph mCT	Biograph Vision 600	Signa PET/MR	Biograph mMR
Patient port [cm]	70	70	70	70	78	78	60	60
CT [slices]	64-128	64-128	16	32-128	20-128	64-128	N/A	N/A
Maximum patient weight [kg (lbs)]	195 (430)	195 (430)	226 (500)	226 (500)	226 (500)	226 (500)	226 (500)	200 (441)
Plane spacing [mm]	2 or 4	1, 2, or 4	3.3	2.8	2	1.6	2.8	2
Crystal size [mm^3]	4.0 x 4.0 x 22	4.0 x 4.0 x 22	6.3 x 6.3 x 30	3.95 x 5.3 x 25	4.0 x 4.0 x 20	3.2 x 3.2 x 20	4.0 x 5.3 x 25	4.0 x 4.0 x 20
Number of crystals	28,336	23,040	19,200	19,584	32,448	60,800	20,160	28,672
PMTs	Analog	Digital SiPM	Analog	SiPM	Analog	SiPM	SiPM	APD
Physical axial FOV [cm]	18	16.3	26	20	21.8	26	25	25.8
Detector material	LYSO	LYSO	BGO	LxSO**	LSO	LSO	LxSO**	LSO
System sensitivity %	0.74	0.57*	2.2	1.35	0.95	1.6	2.1	1.5
Transaxial resolution @ 1 cm [mm]	4.7	4.0	4.9	4.5	4.4	3.2	4.2	4.1
Transaxial resolution @ 10 cm [mm]	5.2	4.5	5.5	4.5	4.9	3.8	5.2	5.2
Axial resolution @ 1 cm, [mm]	4.7	4.0	5.1	4.8	4.5	3.4	5.8	4.3
Axial resolution @ 10 cm, [mm]	5.2	4.5	5.5	4.7	5.9	3.7	7.1	6.6
Peak NECR [kcps] kBq/@ ml*	120 @ 19	171@50***	120 @ 9	180 @ 20	175 @ 28	300@30	210 @ 17.5	175 @ 21.8
Time-of-Flight resolution [picosecs]	550	345	N/A	385	540	214	400	N/A
Time-of-Flight localization [cm]	8.9	5.2	N/A	5.8	8.1	3.2	6.0	N/A
Coincidence window [nanosecs]	4.5	1.5	9.5	4.9	4.1	4.7	4.6	5.9

*NEMA 2001

**LxSO -lutetium based scintillators meeting specifications (LYSO, LGSO, LSO or LGYSO)

***Obtained from[119] as vendor published only effective numbers including TOF gain

to achieve a single readout for each photodiode. The digital SiPM design has been used in the preclinical system designed as a PET insert for the standalone MRI scanner[11] and in the Philips Vereos system.[12]

Both digital and analog SiPMs have very good intrinsic timing resolution, and are therefore well suited for use in conjunction with TOF PET acquisition (described further in the chapter), potentially

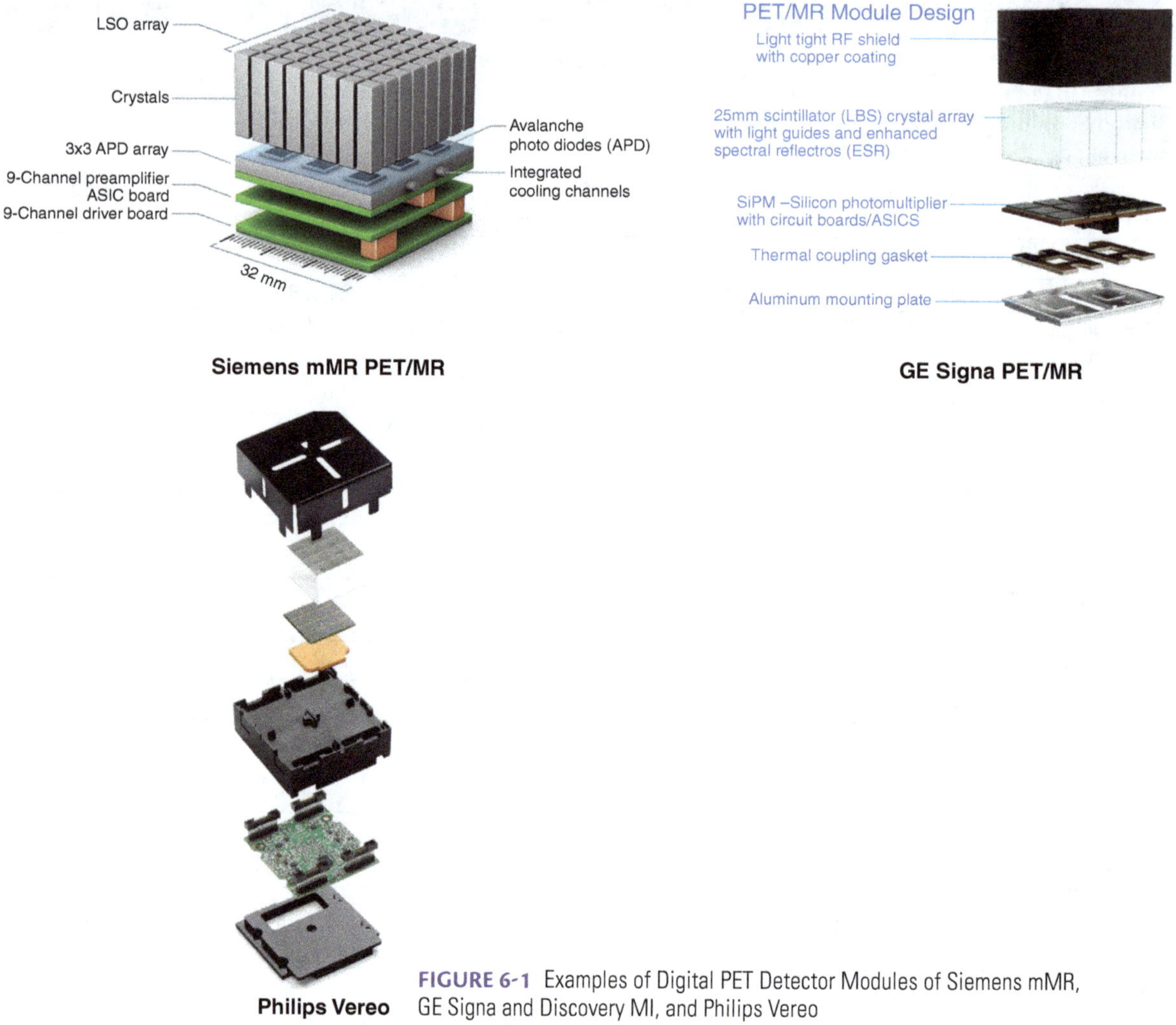

FIGURE 6-1 Examples of Digital PET Detector Modules of Siemens mMR, GE Signa and Discovery MI, and Philips Vereo

achieving simultaneous improvements in sensitivity, image resolution, and maximal count rate. Digital counting can potentially improve reading the digital signals from the detectors at the high-count rates. The maximal count rate is very important for the myocardial flow measurements with short-lived PET tracers, such as ^{82}Rb.[13] SiPMs in the clinical system can match crystal size, currently as low as 4 mm (Table 6-2). However, SiPM or avalanche photodiodes can be fabricated easily in even smaller sizes and could be matched in the future with much smaller size crystals, if required. In comparison, the size of conventional analog PMT will limit the accuracy of photon positioning detection for crystal element sizes of less than 4 × 4 mm. It is likely that the imaging resolution of digital PET is improved further with the use of smaller detector elements. In cardiovascular imaging, this is particularly important for vascular PET applications, device infection, and sarcoid imaging where high image resolution is of utmost importance. Examples of new digital PET detectors are shown in Figure 6-1.

All current digital PET designs still require scintillation crystals for the detection of the annihilation photons, because the digital detectors detect the scintillation photon rather than the annihilation photons directly. It is possible that in the future, fully digital PET detectors without photon conversion to visible light will provide even greater image quality benefits for PET.[14] However, such designs are currently hampered by the poor timing performance of CdTe and CZnTe solid state radiation detectors, which is currently about 10 ns (compared to the 0.3 ns of current state-of-the-art PET systems). Some novel solutions to this limitation for CdTe solid state detectors have been recently proposed.[15,16] However, none of the current clinical systems or clinical prototypes to date are using such direct radiation detection solid-state technology.

EXTENDED AXIAL COVERAGE

Typical axial coverage of PET in one bed position varies from 16 to 26 cm. The smallest 16 cm axial coverage is sufficient for the typical cardiac imaging protocols. Larger axial coverage may be sometimes required to include aorta in the field of view (FOV) for heart imaging, and for carotid imaging. The larger axial coverage is achieved in the hardware by extending more PET detector rings (so called 4-ring and 5-ring systems). These systems are primarily designed for oncology applications, since the extended axial coverage allows reduced number of bed positions for whole-body imaging and consequently faster overall imaging time. However, there is a trade-off: the longer axial FOV requires more detectors and more crystals, increasing the cost.

For cardiac applications, there are no obvious benefits of extended bore length since the standard coverage for the typical 3-ring system of about 16 cm in one bed position is typically sufficient to cover the heart region. In addition, there could be potentially negative consequences of longer bore in a PET scanner for cardiac imaging. Since the scatter fraction during PET imaging is typically increased with the longer bore, the effects such as gamma-prompt with ^{82}Rb imaging are dramatically increased. This limitation would not be present if an ^{18}F agent such as FDG or F-18-flurpiridaz were used. If not appropriately corrected, this may lead to significant artifacts, mimicking myocardial perfusion defects. In addition, extended coverage of the PET scanner may require acquisition of larger number of slices for the CT attenuation correction (AC) map, even if they do not cover the heart. This is because it is usually not possible to perform AC with a reduced FOV using the clinical software, since iterative 3D scatter correction algorithms require a match between the CT and PET axial coverage for accurate results. Thus, purely for cardiac applications, the shorter axial coverage of the PET scanner may be preferable.

NEW PET RECONSTRUCTION TECHNIQUES FOR CARDIOVASCULAR IMAGING

Iterative Reconstruction

All current PET/CT systems use iterative PET reconstruction. New reconstruction methods offer great potential for improved noise statistics[17] and improved image fidelity.[18] Ordered subset expectation maximization (3D-OSEM) has been implemented on all systems to reduce reconstruction time of iterative reconstruction algorithms.[19] Despite OSEM acceleration, computational time can still pose significant limitations, when using standard workstations, particularly for cardiac PET imaging utilizing dynamic and gated protocols. In a typical cardiac protocol, it is possible to have up to 20–30 dynamic and 8-bin gated stress/rest acquisitions in addition to the static stress/rest perfusion images. Thus, the reconstruction time for typical cardiac protocol can be in the order of two magnitudes longer than in standard static imaging. However, it has been shown that iterative techniques yield improved image accuracy and less noise, compared to filtered backprojection for kinetic myocardial flow imaging,[20] and, therefore, these techniques are recommended despite longer processing times, even for kinetic imaging with multiple dynamic frames.

Point Spread Function Modeling

During iterative reconstruction, various processes can be modeled, including photon attenuation, scatter, random events, and various resolution degrading defects. One of the most important corrections recently introduced by all vendors is point spread function (PSF) modeling, which corrects for various resolution-degrading effects in the PET system. The knowledge of the variation of the system PSF across the FOV is required for this correction. This could be obtained by recording a 3D map of measurements of moving point sources across the entire 3D FOV of the scanner.[21] The measured 3D maps of PSF responses can be stored for each specific PET scanner model. The PSF resolution in the PET scanner typically deteriorates towards the edge of the FOV. The PSF corrections can be built into the iterative reconstruction process. This method has been implemented on Siemens as the High-Definition option[22] and on GE as the SharpIR option[23] (Figure 6-2). On the Philips PET system, PSF modeling is implemented postreconstruction as a separate iterative computation using the Richardson-Lucy algorithm, designed previously for applications in astronomy.[24]

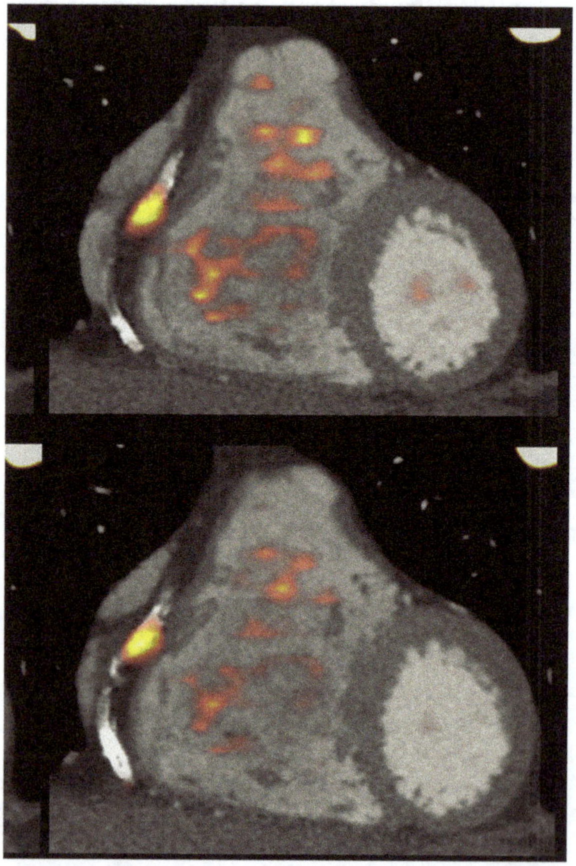

FIGURE 6-2 Cardiac Motion Corrected Coronary 18F-NaF PET Without (Top) and With SharpIR and Time-of-Flight Option on the GE 710 System

Similar to Siemens HD, the implementation of this technique also requires the estimation of the PSF 3D maps scanner in the FOV.

PSF correction or resolution recovery can dramatically increase the values of standardized uptake value (SUV) measurement of a lesion when the size of the lesion is smaller than the resolution of the imaging system. Effective tomographic image resolution as low as 2 mm (in the air) and significant improvements in image contrast have been achieved using resolution recovery,[25] and better definition of subtle myocardial perfusion defects have been reported in clinical settings with the use of this approach.[26]

In coronary PET studies with small lesions, the use of PSF correction is important to restore the signal and improve the signal-to-noise ratio (SNR) resulting in a signal increase of up to 4 times in small coronary lesions,[27] as seen in Figure 6-3. The use of PSF has also been studied for dynamic myocardial flow studies to reduce low-statistics bias in quantitative dynamic PET.[28] The effect of the new reconstruction techniques with PSF on dynamic PET imaging is discussed in detail in a comprehensive technical review.[29]

Typically, the use of iterative reconstruction requires postfiltering to reduce image noise. This is usually accomplished by 3D Gaussian smoothing with kernels, such as 4 or 5 mm, to match the desired imaging resolution. An advancement in the techniques for noise suppression recently implemented by some (but not all) vendors is noise regularization

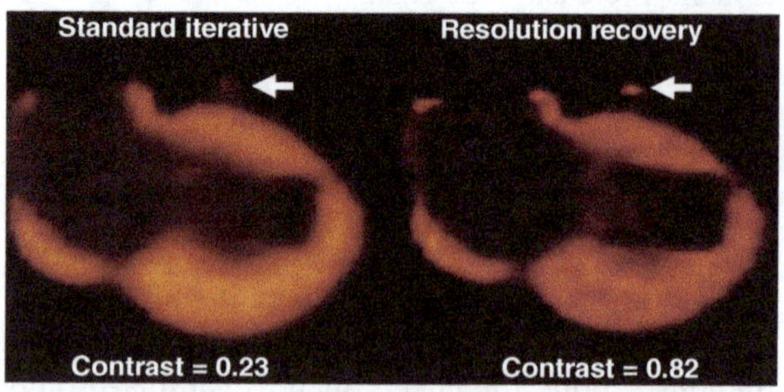

FIGURE 6-3 Coronary Phantom Study of Resolution Resolution Recovery With Point Spread Function (PSF). Static phantom acquisition of simulated cylindrical coronary lesion (arrows): 2 mm diameter, volume 44 mm^3, 6 mm from myocardium on a Siemens scanner with HD reconstruction (resolution recovery). The lesion/myocardium 18F concentration was 4:1. In this example, contrast improved 4 times with HD resolution recovery reconstruction.

during iterative reconstruction by statistical modeling. One example is Bayesian penalized likelihood, which utilizes additional constraints and knowledge about the image data to suppress noise while preserving details. Bayesian penalized likelihood regularization is implemented in the Q.Clear reconstruction method from GE.[30] This relatively new approach has not yet been used widely in cardiovascular imaging and is not available for all scanners. In preliminary studies, it has been reported that Bayesian penalized likelihood techniques result in less noise than comparable reconstructions obtained with filtered back projection (FBP) and OSEM, and do not cause bias in the estimation of the input function, during cardiac dynamic imaging.[31] Further work is required to validate these advanced techniques for various cardiovascular PET protocols.

TIME-OF-FLIGHT IMAGING

One of the notable improvements in the next-generation PET scanners is the use of TOF information, achieved by the fast decay time of the new crystals (LSO and LYSO) combined with fast coincidence electronics. The principle of TOF PET was investigated and proposed early in PET development,[32] but until recently has not been implemented in clinical PET scanners.

The TOF principle is based on estimating the time difference between two events of annihilation photons hitting the crystal at opposite sides of the detector ring (Figure 6-4). If Δt is the difference in the detection times of two photons originating from the same positron annihilation and c is the velocity of light (3×10^8 m/sec), the positron annihilation location along the path (called line of response) of two photons with the reference to the center of the detector can be estimated as $P = \Delta t \times c/2$.

The accuracy of the estimation of the positron annihilation position is related to the timing resolution of the detector and front-end electronics. The TOF localization accuracy of current TOF clinical PET system ranges from 5.2 to 8.2 cm corresponding to the TOF timing resolution of 345–544 picoseconds (Table 6-2). This estimation of the location of the event along the line of response can be then used in the reconstruction algorithm to reduce noise and scatter, resulting in higher SNR in the TOF-reconstructed images. It has been demonstrated that for large objects, the gain of the SNR with TOF, as compared to images reconstructed without TOF information, can be approximated by the $g = \sqrt{(D/a)}$ where D is the detector field of view (usually 60 to 80 cm) and a is TOF positioning accuracy.[33] From Table 6-2, we can see that typical TOF SNR gains could be approximately in the 3-4 range.

Vendors have used this estimated SNR gain attributed to TOF to provide an *effective* net equivalent count rate (NECR) and *effective* system sensitivity, by simply multiplying the non-TOF baseline NECR or sensitivity by the TOF gain. This can lead to confusion when comparing the characteristics of TOF and non-TOF PET scanners. Because of vendor differences in measuring TOF NECR numbers, direct comparison of these values is not possible (Table 6-2). Furthermore,

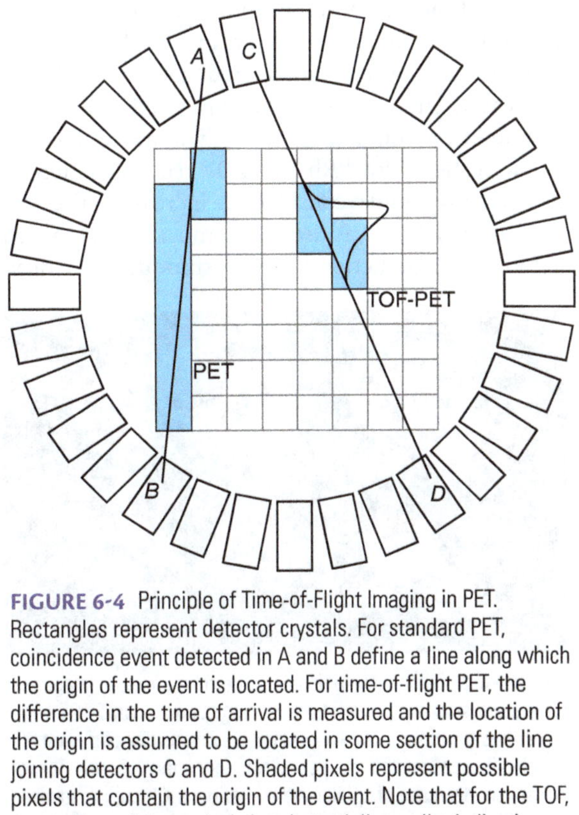

FIGURE 6-4 Principle of Time-of-Flight Imaging in PET. Rectangles represent detector crystals. For standard PET, coincidence event detected in A and B define a line along which the origin of the event is located. For time-of-flight PET, the difference in the time of arrival is measured and the location of the origin is assumed to be located in some section of the line joining detectors C and D. Shaded pixels represent possible pixels that contain the origin of the event. Note that for the TOF, the number of these pixels is substantially smaller indicating more precise localization. (Reproduced with permission from Sitek A: Data analysis in emission tomography using emission-count posteriors, Phys Med Biol. 2012 Nov 7;57(21):6779-6795)

the absolute sensitivity of the TOF scanner (percent of detected events) is not changed as compared to the non-TOF scanner. Similarly, TOF gain will not guard against potential system saturation with ^{82}Rb scanner, and therefore raw NECR number should be considered for these applications.

The strongest clinical advantage of TOF seen when it is used in combination with PSF correction.[34,35] However, the effects TOF and PSF in cardiac imaging differ significantly between vendors[36] because their implementations of these corrections are unique and proprietary. It has been recently shown that TOF imaging results in contrast improvement and increased uptake in the lateral wall for N-13 ammonia myocardial perfusion PET imaging[37](Figure 6-5). Estimation of TOF SNR gains for 18-FDG cardiac viability patients has been reported recently.[38] The average overall clinical SNR increases were in the order of 21% when TOF was used. Clinically, these gains may be of most importance in obese patients, where SNR is low.[39] For cardiac ^{82}Rb myocardial blood flow imaging, it has been demonstrated that the use of TOF can lead to more consistent reconstruction results.[40] A note of caution is needed for dynamic blood flow quantification with ^{82}Rb and TOF reconstruction. A recent study found a considerable increase in the flow values when TOF was used, as compared to standard iterative reconstruction.[41] TOF techniques have been

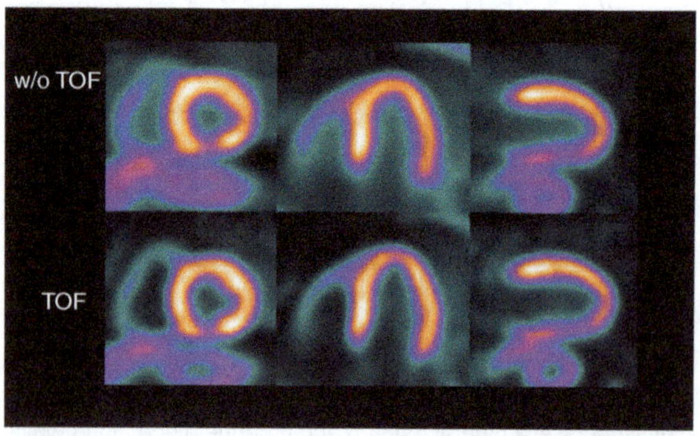

FIGURE 6-5 Comparison of Images. The comparison of images is between standard 3D iterative reconstruction (top) and TOF reconstruction (bottom) for N-13 ammonia myocardial perfusion PET imaging in a case with three-vessel coronary artery disease. There is a severe decrease of uptake in the inferior wall more pronounced with TOF. (Reproduced with permissions from Tomiyama T, Ishihara K, Suda M, et al: Impact of time-of-flight on qualitative and quantitative analyses of myocardial perfusion PET studies using (13) N-ammonia, J Nucl Cardiol. 2015 Oct;22(5):998-1007)

primarily developed for different tracers and ^{82}Rb could require special considerations because of longer positron range and prompt-gamma corrections.[4] TOF imaging may be of particular importance for the high-resolution PET imaging vascular imaging or imaging with high-resolution myocardial perfusion tracers, such as 18F-flurpiridaz. Advanced coronary PET imaging with 18NaF has been reported with TOF system[42–45]; however, to date it has not yet been compared to non-TOF imaging.

ATTENUATION CORRECTION ON 3D PET/CT SYSTEMS

AC for PET is mandatory owing to the need to record both the forward traveling and backward traveling photons to record a true coincidence event. The result is that the total attenuation of a true event is the total attenuation along the line of site (as opposed to SPECT where the attenuation begins where the nucleus decay, inside the patient and continues to the detector face). AC for PET was originally implemented with radionuclide transmission rod-sources, which were used to create patient photon attenuation maps. However, all modern commercial systems now use CT-based AC or MR-based -AC. High-quality CT-based attenuation maps can be obtained within few seconds on current PET/CT scanners.[46] There are significant quantitative PET differences between traditional AC by transmission sources with ^{68}Ge or ^{137}Cs sources and CT-based AC. These differences may remain even after alignment of the CT maps to the emission data, particularly when there are metal-induced artifacts caused by, for example, pacemakers or implantable cardioverter defibrillators in the CT images.[47,48] Vendors employ various software algorithms for the correction of metal artifacts in the CT scans.[49] When these methods are applied to the CT attenuation maps, they result in increased quantitative accuracy of PET.

When CT maps are used for the AC, one issue is the potential misalignment between CT and PET images caused by respiratory or patient motion,[50] a particularly important factor in imaging of the heart.[47,51] It has been demonstrated that PET/CT AC map misalignment can affect the results in about 40 to 60% of myocardial perfusion imaging.[47,52,53] Careful visual verification of the alignment is needed to minimize misregistration artifacts. Automatic correction of the misalignment registration of CT and PET maps to reduce these artifacts have been developed by vendors.[54] In a recent study, it has been demonstrated that the automatic alignment of the CT-based AC maps is superior to the clinically performed manual quality control (QC) and alignment by the PET technologists.[53] Figure 6-6 shows an example of potential misdiagnosis caused by misregistration in the cardiac ^{82}Rb study.

Another possibility to reduce the misalignment artifacts caused by respiration for cardiovascular PET is averaging the cine CT data acquisition over one breath cycle (about 4 to 5 seconds) to match the respiratory blurring during CT and PET acquisition. This technique has been implemented on some commercial PET scanners. The attenuation maps obtained by the cine CT acquisition could significantly reduce the frequency and magnitude of the spatial misregistration between CT and PET.[47] The dose of cine CT is higher than the CT acquisition obtained without respiratory gating. Nevertheless, low-dose cine CT with a 0.8 mSv effective radiation dose is possible.[55]

CT IN PET/CT FOR CALCIUM SCORING AND CT ANGIOGRAPHY

The current maximum number of detector rows for the CT scanner component of a PET/CT is 128. Typically, the lowest number of slices offered is 16, which is sufficient for standard CT calcium scoring imaging.[56] Calcium scoring plays an important role in cardiovascular risk assessment. It has been demonstrated that the calcium scan information can be integrated with the cardiac PET perfusion information, increasing overall accuracy of hybrid PET/CT for the obstructive stenosis.[57] In clinical cardiac PET/CT protocols the PET/CT are routinely used to obtain s CT calcium scan during the time the patient undergoes a PET scan.

One concern is that the additional noncontrast CT calcium scan adds to the overall radiation burden. Therefore, for cardiac PET, researchers have evaluated repurposing separately obtained CT calcium scans for AC[58] after manual or automatic alignment. This approach would allow the overall dose reduction for the cardiac PET/CT exam, which includes

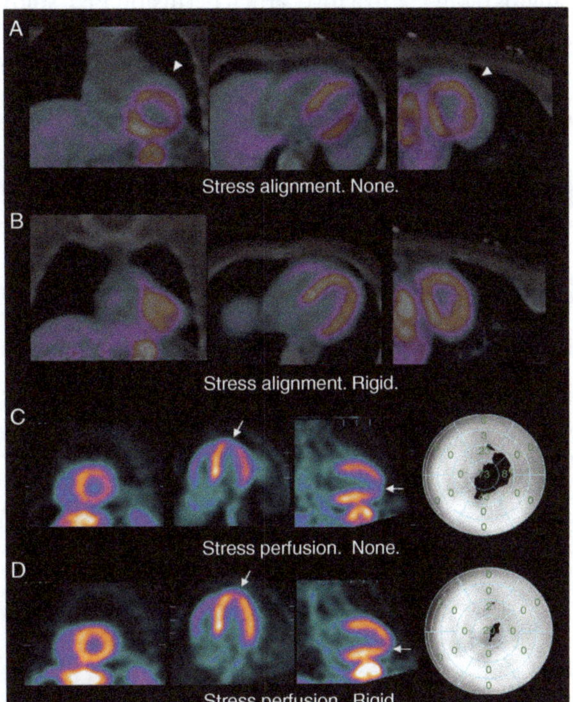

FIGURE 6-6 False-Positive Nuclear Scan. The false-positive result is caused by the CT attenuation correction (CTAC) scan registration error resolved by the automatic correction in a 44-year-old male presenting with shortness of breath. PET and CTAC images fused before alignment (A) and after rigid alignment (B). Misalignment is indicated by the white arrow head (A). Stress perfusion PET images before alignment (C) and after alignment (D) and polar maps are shown with the white arrow indicating the perfusion artifact caused by misalignment. Quantitative plese delete mask green text on figure was 11% (C right), when no correction for alignment was performed (ITPD after manual verification was also 11%) compared to a normal scan (ITPD 1.8%) after automatic registration (D right). Invasive coronary angiography did not show significant coronary artery disease. (Reproduced with permission from Slomka PJ, Diaz-Zamudio M, Dey D, et al: Automatic registration of misaligned CT attenuation correction maps in Rb-82 PET/CT improves detection of angiographically significant coronary artery disease, J Nucl Cardiol. 2015 Dec;22(6):1285-1295)

the calcium scan. However, unlike the ungated CT scan obtained for the AC, the calcium scan is cardiac gated, so care must be taken with regard to the possible misregistration of the data. It has been demonstrated that the automated software utilized for the correction of misregistration of CT attenuation maps could be also used for the purposes of alignment of the CT calcium scans with PET.[59] It has been demonstrated that deformable registration of CT calcium scans can be used to adjust for differences in respiratory patterns, yielding excellent correlations of myocardial perfusion flow values as compared to PET corrected with standard attenuation maps.[59] Conversely, it may also be possible to estimate coronary calcium from nongated low-dose CT attenuation maps[60–62]; however, noise and lack of cardiac gating may present challenges.

CT component of PET/CT scanner can be also used for CT-angiography imaging. High-end PET/CT scanners from most vendors are equipped with 64- or 128-slice CT with gantry rotation of 0.33 to 0.35 second. High-quality coronary angiography will require 64 slices or higher to minimize breath-hold or scan time with less iodinated contrast injection. Such systems permit adding a high-quality coronary CT angiography[63,64] to a myocardial perfusion PET study without moving the patient from the bed. PET/CT scanners with high-end 64-slice or higher CT also allow the localization of small coronary plaque lesions using accurate superposition with high-resolution CT angiography.[65–68] However, cardiac or coronary PET and coronary CT angiography images obtained on a hybrid PET/CT scanner are still obtained at different times and in different breathing patterns: free-breathing in PET and typically breath-hold in coronary CT angiography. This results in significant misregistration between PET and CT angiography scans even if the patient remains in the same position on the scanner bed. This misregistration can be corrected with software registration.[53]

CARDIORESPIRATORY MOTION TRACKING AND CORRECTION WITH PET

One of the major challenges in cardiovascular imaging with PET is loss of resolution caused by cardiorespiratory and patient motion during the PET scan, during scan time of at least several minutes. This becomes more important with the latest-generation scanners with PSF correction and small detector elements. With high resolution of the static images possible with the new PET scanners, motion becomes a dominant effect, degrading quality during imaging of the heart.

Cardiac and respiratory motion can be mitigated with PET gating, dividing the raw PET signal in subsets or bins. Such gating is typically performed as either phase gating (binning signal into same time bins within a cycle) or as amplitude gating (binning signal into identical displacement locations). Cardiac gating is typically performed as phase gating (dividing average cardiac cycle into equal timings with the use of ECG signal) because heart wall displacements are fairly consistent from beat to beat. However, for respiratory gating, amplitude gating has been found to be more robust, especially in patients with variable respiration.[69,70]

The concept of amplitude gating has been used by Siemens to form respiratory gated images designed to keep the 35% of the PET counts in one optimal respiratory gate (ORG), in which the breathing motion was minimal[71] (Figure 6-7). Respiratory gating can be performed in an inductive respiration monitor with an elastic bellows/pressure sensor[72] or by an infrared camera, which is tracking the reflective marker on the chest of the patient.[73] These systems send trigger signals at the beginning of a respiratory phase and/or displacement level in order to organize data into specific bins. Vendors provide tools on the PET/CT scanners to perform either phase-based gating and motion correction (Philips, GE -Q.Static/Q.Freeze) or amplitude based gating (Siemens HD. Chest).

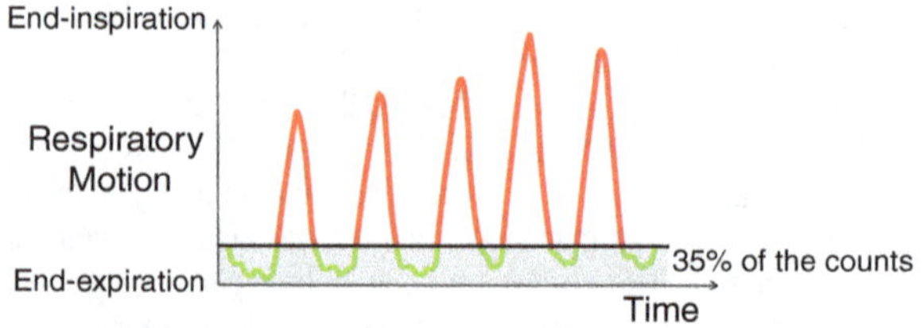

FIGURE 6-7 Optimal Respiratory Gating. An example of a breathing pattern showing the optimal gating window. The optimal respiratory gate method selects the narrowest bandwidth (green curve, shaded area) containing 35% of the total counts.

Cardiac gating is routine in cardiovascular PET/CT protocols, but respiratory gating is uncommon in cardiovascular PET. In cardiac PET imaging, the simultaneous cardiac and respiratory gating (so called dual-gating) is technically challenging. The need for additional respiratory gating devices adds to the complexity of the already demanding cardiac imaging protocols. Some solutions have been proposed for simultaneous acquisition of both respiratory and cardiac gating signals by signals obtained from standard ECG electrodes during cardiac PET[74] and techniques based on accelerometers.[75] These techniques have the potential to simplify the challenging logistics of dual-gating for cardiac imaging.

Several self-gated, data-driven respiratory gating techniques have also been proposed, which estimate the respiratory motion directly from the raw PET acquisition data.[76–78] The advantages of self-gated data are that there is no need for additional devices and there is the possibility of retrospective application of the existing data, which may make them more suitable for cardiovascular applications. Derivation of the respiratory motion of the myocardium directly from the PET is usually accomplished by tracking the centroid of the myocardial activity. This method has shown to be comparable to techniques based on monitoring with external devices, and has been applied to cardiac imaging.[76] The limitation of data-driven techniques is that they depend on the tracer uptake in the organs of interest. Data-driven techniques are not yet commercially offered by vendors.

Dual cardiorespiratory gating has been shown to improve the spatial resolution and discrimination of the myocardial walls when compared to an ungated cardiac acquisition.[74] Data-driven respiratory motion correction of cardiac gated studies has been shown to improve the accuracy of ejection fraction measurement in clinical cardiac PET imaging.[79] Dual cardiorespiratory gating presents greater challenges because count statistics in individual bins are much lower. For example, if eight cardiac bins and four respiratory bins are used, each dual-gated bin will have less than 3% of the counts. Therefore, the compromise between the amount of motion in the images and the image noise must be carefully considered.[80] Dual cardiorespiratory gating from image data alone has been proposed as a solution.[81]

Although motion-tracking techniques allow improvement of the effective image resolution, the individual gates usually have poor count statistics. One solution is to detect spatial displacements between each bin and subsequently correct for motion between the individual bins, without rejecting any counts. If the myocardium is relatively well defined, the heart motion could be computed directly by tracking myocardial contours. Techniques based on the application of nonlinear warping algorithms for "motion-frozen" correction of cardiac motion have been proposed.[82,83] This motion correction method showed improvements compared to classical reconstruction techniques regarding apparent static myocardial wall thickness and contrast-to-noise ratio.[83] In coronary PET imaging, where image resolution is of key importance, there may be no uptake in the myocardium, presenting challenges for motion tracking. In a ^{18}F-NaF coronary PET study,[84] a motion-correction method was employed to enhance image quality and improve uptake estimates guided by the coronary arteries extracted from the CT angiography. The motion-corrected data resulted in a significantly higher target to background ratio and greatly reduced noise (-50%) caused by the use of counts from all the cardiac gates, as seen in Figure 6-8. Cardiac motion correction was also applied to PET/MR ^{18}F-NaF PET imaging of aortic stenosis.[45]

Vendors are developing advanced schemes where motion correction is built into the reconstruction of PET. Potentially, a reconstruction method utilizing the motion information directly during the iterative image formation[85]should result in less noise and image bias, compared to the motion correction performed as a postreconstruction step.[86,87] Additionally, when motion correction is incorporated in the reconstruction, the potential misregistration of CT attenuation maps with PET emission data caused by cardiorespiratory motion can be simultaneously handled during the reconstruction and, in general, other imaging effects can be more optimally accounted for. Preliminary studies of motion correction built into reconstruction have been reported. Hong et al.[88,89] used a mass preservation optical flow method[90] initially to reconstructed PET cardiac gated images determining the motion vectors. These motion vectors were then fed into the repeated reconstruction process. They demonstrated superior signal-to-noise

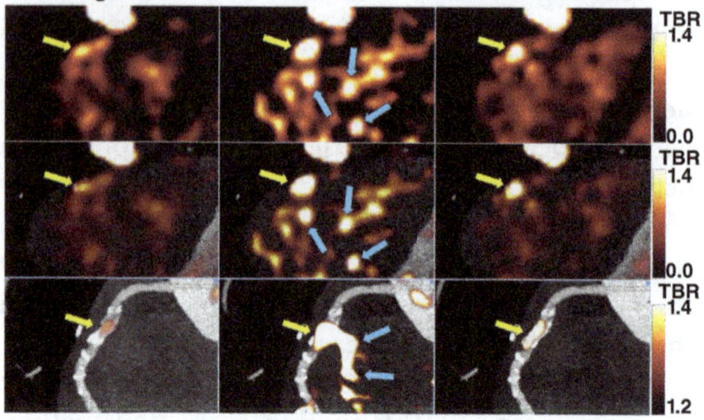

FIGURE 6-8. High-Resolution Coronary PET Imaging. The imaging is reconstructed with TOF and PSF without motion correction, in one cardiac gate and with cardiac motion correction. Superimposed on CT coronary angiography. Cardiac motion correction with TOF and PSF. Right coronary artery (RCA) vulnerable plaque, PET images (top row), fused PET and coronary CTA (middle row) and multiplanar-reformatted views PET/coronary CTA (bottom row) of the RCA lesion (red arrows) with exponential color table. The images show the low lesion signal in ungated image (first column), significant noise in one-bin images (blue arrows, second column) and high lesion signal with reduced noise in motion corrected image (third column). (Reproduced with permission from Rubeaux M, Joshi NV, Dweck MR, et al: Motion Correction of 18F-NaF PET for Imaging Coronary Atherosclerotic Plaques, J Nucl Med. 2016 Jan;57(1):54-59)

ratio, without deterioration of spatial resolution by this approach. The potential superiority of motion correction performed during PET reconstruction, as compared to the postprocessing approach need to be further evaluated.

Dual cardiorespiratory motion-correction techniques have been investigated on phantom[91] and patient data.[92] In a recent study, cardiorespiratory motion correction was applied to dual-gated 18F-flurpiridaz cardiac PET data. The dual-gated PET consisted of eight cardiac and four respiratory bins. The cardiorespiratory motion-correction algorithm was then applied in 2 consecutive steps. Initially, the cardiac gated images (but not respiratory gated) were warped to the end-diastolic gate by tracking of the detected left ventricle endocardial and epicardial borders.[83] Then, to compensate for respiratory motion, the four respiratory gates, already corrected for cardiac motion, were registered to the end-inspiration bin using a rigid transform. A final motion-free end-diastole/end-inspiration static images of the myocardium demonstrated better contrast-to-noise ratio and decreased wall thickness as compared to ungated data (Figure 6-9). This final motion-corrected myocardial PET includes all counts from the full cardiac and respiratory cycles. The data in this study was obtained with the PSF reconstruction, which allows high-resolution static images. These results demonstrate that motion in cardiac imaging remains the dominating effect when the static resolution of new scanners surpasses is significantly below extent of the motion of the heart.

HYBRID PET/MR SYSTEMS

Recently, several clinical hybrid PET/MR systems have entered clinical use. One vendor, Philips, offers sequential scanning of the patient in two modalities (Philips Ingenuity TF PET/MR). Two vendors offer PET/MR systems, which acquire PET and MR image data simultaneously.[93] Some engineering challenges exist in the scanner design performing simultaneous acquisition, owing to potential cross-interference of PET and MR systems. The digital PMT designs

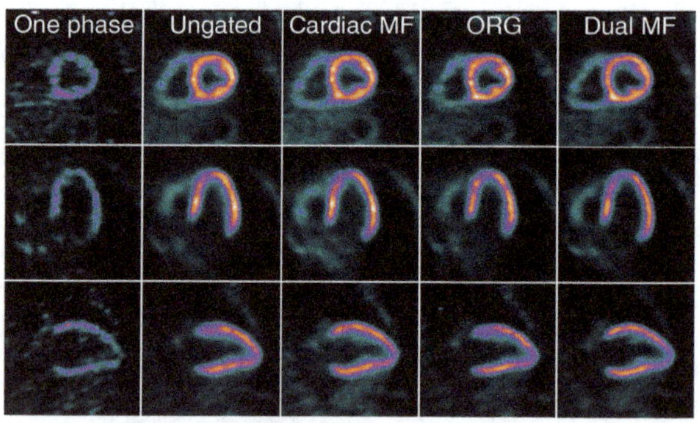

FIGURE 6-9 Dual-Gated 18F-Flurpiridaz PET. A 42-year-old female patient with a low likelihood of coronary disease (weight: 190 lbs, BMI: 34.7) is injected with 7.7 mCi of 18F-flurpiridaz during exercise stress and acquired in dual-cardiac and respiratory mode. Short axis, vertical and horizontal axis views of adenosine stress images. One phase-one cardiac gate in end-inspiration. MF—cardiac motion frozen no respiratory gating, ORG—optimal respiratory gating. Dual MF—dual (cardiac/respiratory) motion frozen. (Reproduced with permission from Slomka PJ, Rubeaux M, Le Meunier L, et al: Dual-Gated Motion-Frozen Cardiac PET with Flurpiridaz F 18, J Nucl Med. 2015 Dec;56(12):1876-1881)

described in this chapter allow this cross-modality interference to be minimized, because they are insensitive to magnetic fields unlike analog PMTs. The high-speed solid-state avalanche photodiode detectors (APDs) in mMR (Siemens) or SiPMs (GE Signa)[94] use such digital detection of scintillation light. The static magnetic field generated by the MR system can reduce the effective positron range and potentially improve the PET image resolution for these systems. However, this effect will not help when imaging with ^{18}F-based tracers because the effective path of this tracer is already very short. This could potentially be helpful with other tracers with longer positron range, for example, such as ^{82}Rb used in cardiac imaging, because this tracer has positrons with much higher average kinetic energy.

Siemens introduced the clinical (FDA-approved) Biograph mMR simultaneous PET/MR system in 2011. It uses Verio 3T MR scanner as an MR component with a modified body radiofrequency coil, a gradient coil, and a patient-handling system. The PET detector system fits into the MR gantry reducing the effective diameter of the bore from 70 to 60 cm[95] (Figure 6-10). Technical details of this system are given in Table 6-2. LSO scintillator crystals are arranged in blocks (8 × 8 crystals), are combined into a cylinder of detector blocks with 8 axial x 56 circumferential blocks. Therefore, the PET component has 25.8 cm axial field of view. Each of the 446 PET detector blocks consists of 64 crystals and a 3 × 3 array of silicon APDs, and electronics for amplification and pulse shaping. The MR gradient component is cooled and the PET detectors are shielded with copper to reduce electromagnetic interference. The APDs do not distort the main magnetic field of the MR, and the acquisitions of the MR and PET systems are synchronized to reduce any possible distortion of the detected PET signals by the MR radiofrequency and gradient pulses. Although the PET system has the improved sensitivity compared to their PET/CT systems, the mMR system does not offer the TOF capability because of the relatively low timing resolution of APDs. Note that the Siemens mMR system was introduced more than 6 years ago and an update to PET technology is likely.[96]

In 2016, GE introduced the Signa PET/MR hybrid scanner, which utilizes digital SiPM for their PET/MR system. This allows TOF implementation with a coincidence timing resolution of 390–400 picoseconds. The GE scanner has a PET axial field of 25 cm and a photon sensitivity of 2.1%. The PET detector is fitted into the MR gradient set based on the GE MR750w 3 Tesla (3T) scanner on the outer diameter of the RF body coil[97] (Figure 6-10). It has

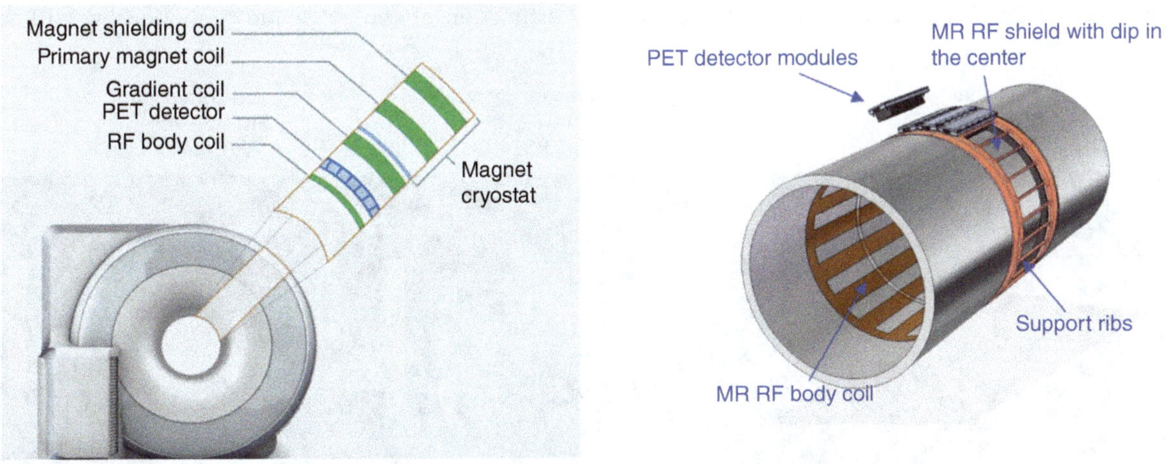

FIGURE 6-10 Integration of the PET Detectors in the MR Hardware Structure of the Biograph mMR (Left) and GE Signa (Right). The inner most element is MR radiofrequency body coil and then PET detector. The MR/PET integration as shown requires that the PET detector works within strong static and dynamic magnetic fields, and does not disturb any of the associated electromagnetic MR fields. The PET detector must not disturb the static magnetic field, the gradient fields, nor the RF transmission and reception. Additionally, in this configuration the RF body coil needs to be "PET transparent" with little photon attenuation.[100] (©Siemens Healthlineers 2018, with permission and courtesy GE Healthcare.)

5 rings of 112 detector blocks (each a 4 × 9 array of LYSO crystals, 3.95 × 5.3 × 25 mm^3) coupled to 1 × 3 arrays of SiPM devices. Thus, each SiPM obtains signals from four crystal elements (Figure 6-1).

Potential clinical cardiovascular applications for PET/MR have been discussed in reviews.[98–101] The MR is able to provide much better soft tissue contrast compared to CT, which makes PET/MR potentially preferable to PET/CT for some cardiovascular applications, such as imaging of myocardium and intravascular plaque. One promising application of PET/MR in the cardiovascular field is with cardiac sarcoidosis. Initial reports were performed on separate PET and MR scanners,[102,103] but recent studies have utilized PET/MR for this application. The advantage of the PET/MR over PET/CT is a better ability to outline the myocardial scar with the late gadolinium enhancement (LGE) imaging. PET/MR can also play an important role in the imaging of myocarditis, where 18F-FDG-PET can be performed together with MR to provide complementary information about disease activity.[106] Another example of recent a cardiovascular application of PET/MR is imaging of aortic valve disease[45] (Figure 6-11). Here, the advantage of MR is a better ability to depict the anatomy and motion of the aortic valves, which can be used for the correction of the PET images. PET/MR can be also exploited as a powerful research tool for direct cross-validation of advanced PET and MR cardiovascular techniques.[107]

In comparison to PET/CT, PET/MR can reduce the overall patient's radiation dose significantly, depending on the protocol, because it does not require CT acquisition. For cardiac imaging, especially with low-dose 3D cardiac protocols,[108] the radiation from the CT component can represent a significant portion of the overall radiation dose. However, there are significant challenges for cardiac PET/MR imaging with short-lived tracers such as ^{82}Rb, owing to the need of the generator and/or the tracer delivery systems; for example, it is not possible to use the ^{82}Rb generator in the 3T magnetic field. These difficulties will need to be resolved before clinical utilization of PET/MR for these applications is possible. Additionally, the main PET/MR disadvantage as compared to PET/CT is its significantly higher cost, typically more than 5 million US dollars for the hybrid PT/MR system. Furthermore, the MR electromagnetic field may prevent imaging of patients with pacemakers, implantable cardioverter defibrillators, or other implanted devices susceptible to electromagnetic interference.

CARDIAC MOTION CORRECTION WITH PET/MR AND PET/CTA

New PET/MR scanners offer a unique possibility of simultaneous acquisition of PET and exact estimation of cardiorespiratory motion by MRI to

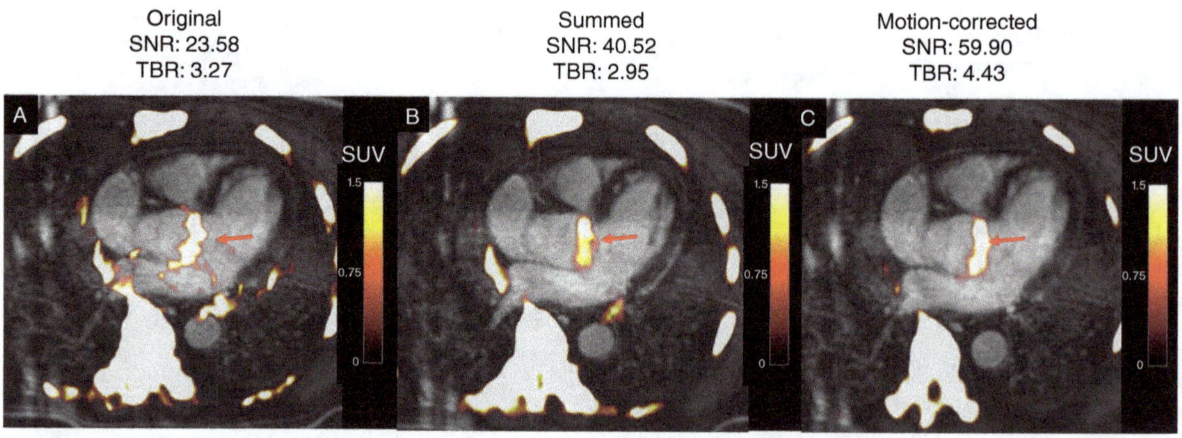

FIGURE 6-11 Fused ^{18}F-Fluoride PET and Contrast-Enhanced Magnetic Resonance Angiography of the Aortic Valve in 60-Year-Old Male With Aortic Stenosis Images display the original diastolic gate (A), summed image (B) and motion-corrected image (C) with focal ^{18}F-fluoride uptake (red arrows). (Reproduced with permission from Doris MK, Rubeaux M, Pawade T, et al: Motion-Corrected Imaging of the Aortic Valve with 18F-NaF PET/CT and PET/MRI: A Feasibility Study, J Nucl Med. 2017 Nov;58(11):1811-1814)

compensate for motion-induced quantitation inaccuracies. This is currently not possible with sequential imaging with CT and PET on a PET/CT scanner. The respiratory signal (similar to that obtained from an external sensor) can be acquired by MRI by setting a virtual marker in the scanning field of view, such as a 1D navigator to acquire a vertical data slab in the superior-inferior direction through the diaphragm. The excitation, 1-dimensional MR readout and reconstruction can be obtained in a very short time (<20 milliseconds).[109] These simple sequences can be combined easily with other types of MR imaging.[110]

Potentially, the 3D motion of the heart could be directly measured by the MR system during a simultaneous PET/MR session; however, such sequences would require continuous MR scanning during the whole PET acquisition. Patient motion (respiratory, cardiac, or gross) can be measured by MR in real time, for example, by tagging. In MR tagging, a sequence of radiofrequency pulses is applied, marking a series of parallel strips (tags), in a 3D field of view. The 3D deformation fields of the tags can be then measured and directly used to estimate motion of the tissue at an arbitrary 3D point. The real-time 3D motion field derived from tagged acquisition can be synchronized with PET data and the position of PET events can be shifted during the iterative reconstruction according to the motion field.[111] This approach has been demonstrated for cardiac imaging.[112] Motion correction based on MR tagging has been shown to improve the image quality of high-resolution F18-flurpiridaz studies obtained on hybrid PET/MR systems in animal studies.[113] This issue is currently the focus of intense research of vendors and research PET/MR sites.

PET-only self-gated methods for motion correction have been compared with MR-based methods.[110] In general, MR-based methods are more robust than self-gated PET approaches; however, PET data-driven techniques are more universal and potentially much simpler in clinical application. The same data-driven methods also can be utilized for PET/CT and PET/MR. The advantage of using PET data alone for patient motion correction on the PET/MR would also free the MR scanning time for some relevant and clinically important imaging sequences during PET acquisition. PET data-driven methods can be comprehensively validated with MR-derived motion data on the PET/MR scanners. The PET-only approach, however, will be likely compromised for low-dose (high-noise) scans, where the MR signal could be utilized to correct for patient motion.

ATTENUATION CORRECTION FOR PET/MR

The PET/MR system may offer advantages in AC because potentially the attenuation maps can be obtained at the same time and with the same respiratory pattern as PET acquisition, minimizing the misalignment often seen in sequential PET/CT scanning; however, unlike CT, MR cannot measure photon attenuation directly. Therefore, in PET/MR systems, the PET photon attenuation maps must be estimated indirectly from the MR data. Various software approaches have been proposed for MR-based AC. These methods are based on image segmentation or co-registration to templates with assumed attenuation coefficients for different tissue classes. An exact AC is particularly crucial for cardiac PET applications.

A method proposed by Martinez-Moeller et al.[114] has been utilized by vendors, with a two-point Dixon VIBE MR sequence to obtain fat and water compartments for calculating attenuation. Lung tissue in the MR images is identified by computational segmentation algorithms. Typically, only a few tissue classes can be defined by such approaches. The true photon attenuation coefficients may be different than the assumed values, especially in the lungs.[98] MR-based AC for cardiac imaging has been now reported in several studies.[115–117] Although CT and MR-based AC uses different information, the initial clinical studies of myocardial blood flow show a high correlation between PET/CT and PT/MR obtained flow values.[118]

SUMMARY

PET is an important cardiovascular imaging modality. New PET scanner hardware and reconstruction software have allowed significant improvement of image quality in cardiovascular applications. The most significant hardware improvements include the use of digital photomultipliers of avalanche photodiodes for the detection of scintillation events, smaller crystal size, and fast electronics enabling TOF imaging. New digital PET detector modules with SiPM enable higher sensitivity and accurate positioning accuracy for coincidence photon detection, and allow for the improvement of spatial resolution without loss of sensitivity. Advanced reconstruction algorithms for PET allows point spread function correction and optimal regularization techniques to reduce image noise. Cardiac motion remains one of the biggest challenges for high-resolution cardiovascular PET imaging. New reconstruction techniques are being proposed for PET to correct for respiratory and cardiac patient motion during PET imaging. These techniques have been shown to increase image quality in cardiac and coronary PET imaging. Software corrections have been developed by vendors to improve the co-registration of PET and CT for AC. New PET/MR allow new cardiovascular with potential advantages over PET/CT such as accurately aligned attenuation maps, MR-based motion correction and better soft-tissue contrast than CT for anatomical imaging.

REFERENCES

1. Fahey FH. Data acquisition in PET imaging. *J Nucl Med Technol.* 2002;30(2):39–49. PubMed PMID: MEDLINE:12055275.
2. Tout D, Tonge C, Muthu S, Arumugam P. Assessment of a protocol for routine simultaneous myocardial blood flow measurement and standard myocardial perfusion imaging with rubidium-82 on a high count rate positron emission tomography system. *Nucl Med Comm.* 2012;33:1202–1211.
3. Renaud JM, Yip K, Guimond J, et al. Characterization of 3-dimensional PET systems for accurate quantification of myocardial blood flow. *J Nucl Med.* 2017;58(1):103–109. Epub 2016 Aug 20. doi:10.2967/jnumed.116.174565. PubMed PMID: 27539843.
4. Esteves FP, Nye JA, Khan A, et al. Prompt-gamma compensation in Rb-82 myocardial perfusion 3D PET/CT. *J Nucl Cardiol.* 2010;17(2):247–253. doi:10.1007/s12350-009-9170-1. PubMed PMID: 19937169.
5. Lecomte R. Novel detector technology for clinical PET. *Eur J Nucl Med Mol Imaging.* 2009;36 Suppl1:S69–85.doi:10.1007/s00259-008-1054-0. PubMed PMID: 19107476.
6. Miyaoka RS, Li X, Lockhart C, Lewellen TK. Design of a high resolution, monolithic crystal, PET/MRI detector with DOI positioning capability. *IEEE Nucl Sci Symp Conf Rec* (1997). 2008;4688–4692. doi:10.1109/NSSMIC.2008.4774469. PubMed PMID: 20607144; PubMed Central PMCID: PMCPMC2895620.
7. van Dam HT, Seifert S, Schaart DR. The statistical distribution of the number of counted scintillation photons in digital silicon photomultipliers: model and validation. *Phys Med Biol.* 2012;57(15):4885–4903. doi:10.1088/0031-9155/57/15/4885. PubMed PMID: 22796633.
8. Pichler B, Boning C, Lorenz E, et al. Studies with a prototype high resolution PET scanner based on LSO-APD modules. *IEEE Trans Nucl Sci.* 1998;45(3):1298–1302.
9. Hsu DFC, Ilan E, Peterson WT, Uribe J, Lubberink M, Levin CS. Studies of a next-generation silicon-photomultiplier-based time-of-flight PET/CT system. *J Nucl Med.* 2017;58(9):1511–1518. Epub 2017 Apr 30. doi:10.2967/jnumed.117.189514. PubMed PMID: 28450566.
10. Frach T, Prescher G, Degenhardt C, de Gruyter R, Schmitz A, Ballizany R. The digital silicon photomultiplier–principle of operation and intrinsic detector performance. IEEE Nuclear Science Symposium conference record. 2009;1961–1965.
11. Schug D, Lerche C, Weissler B, et al. Initial PET performance evaluation of a preclinical insert for PET/MRI with digital SiPM technology. *Phys Med Biol.* 2016;61(7):2851–2878. Epub Mar 19, 2016. doi:10.1088/0031-9155/61/7/2851. PubMed PMID: 26987774; PubMed Central PMCID: PMCPMC5362057.
12. Brunner S, Gruber L, Hirtl A, Suzuki K, Marton J, Schaart D. A comprehensive characterization of the time resolution of the Philips Digital Photon Counter. *J Instrum.* 2016;11(11):P11004.
13. Klein R, Beanlands RS, deKemp RA. Quantification of myocardial blood flow and flow reserve: technical aspects. *J Nucl Cardiol.* 2010;17(4):555–570.

14. Gu Y, Matteson JL, Skelton RT, et al. Study of a high-resolution, 3D positioning cadmium zinc telluride detector for PET. *Phys Med Biol.* 2011;56(6):1563–1584. Epub Feb 22, 2011. doi:10.1088/0031-9155/56/6/004. PubMed PMID: 21335649; PubMed Central PMCID: PMCPMC3274175.
15. Nakhostin M. Optimizing timing performance of CdTe detectors for PET. *Phys Med Biol.* 2017. Epub Aug 16, 2017. doi:10.1088/1361-6560/aa8664. PubMed PMID: 28809758.
16. Macias-Montero JG, Sarraj M, Chmeissani M, Puigdengoles C, Lorenzo GD, Martinez R. Toward VIP-PIX: a low noise readout ASIC for pixelated CdTe gamma-ray detectors for use in the next generation of PET scanners. *IEEE Trans Nucl Sci.* 2013;60(4). Epub Nov 5, 2013. doi:10.1109/tns.2013.2270115. PubMed PMID: 24187382; PubMed Central PMCID: PMCPMC3814062.
17. Chen GP, Branch KR, Alessio AM, et al. Effect of reconstruction algorithms on myocardial blood flow measurement with 13N-ammonia PET. *J Nucl Med.* 2007;48(8):1259–1265. doi:10.2967/jnumed.106.038232
18. Di Carli MF, Dorbala S, Meserve J, El Fakhri G, Sitek A, Moore SC. Clinical myocardial perfusion PET/CT. *J Nucl Med.* 2007;48(5):783–793. PubMed PMID: 17475968.
19. Hudson HM, Larkin RS. Accelerated image reconstruction using ordered subsets of projection data. *IEEE Trans Med Imaging.* 1994;13(4):601–609. Epub Jan 1, 1994. doi:10.1109/42.363108. PubMed PMID: 18218538.
20. Søndergaard HM, Madsen MM, Boisen K, et al. Evaluation of iterative reconstruction (OSEM) versus filtered back-projection for the assessment of myocardial glucose uptake and myocardial perfusion using dynamic PET. *Eur J Nucl Med Molecul Imaging.* 2007;34(3):320–329. doi:10.1007/s00259-006-0198-z.
21. Jakoby BW, Bercier Y, Conti M, Casey ME, Bendriem B, Townsend DW. Physical and clinical performance of the mCT time-of-flight PET/CT scanner. *Phys Med Biol.* 2011;56(8):2375–2389. doi:10.1088/0031-9155/56/8/004. PubMed PMID: 21427485.
22. Jakoby BW, Bercier Y, Watson CC, Bendriem B, Townsend DW. Performance characteristics of a new LSO PET/CT scanner with extended axial field-of-view and PSF reconstruction. *IEEE Trans Nucl Sci.* 2009;56(3):633–639.
23. Yoon HJ, Jeong YJ, Son HJ, Kang D-Y, Hyun K-Y, Lee M-K. Optimization of the spatial resolution for the GE discovery PET/CT 710 by using NEMA NU 2-2007 standards. *J Korean Phys Soc.* 2015;66(2):287-294. doi:10.3938/jkps.66.287
24. Lucy LB. An iterative technique for the rectification of observed distributions. *Astron J.* 1974;79:745.
25. Panin VY, Kehren F, Michel C, Casey M. Fully 3-D PET reconstruction with system matrix derived from point source measurements. *IEEE Trans Med Imaging.* 2006;25(7):907–921. Epub Jul 11, 2006. PubMed PMID: 16827491.
26. L. Le Meunier SP, Germano G, Dey D, Berman DS. Motion frozen of dual gated (cardiac and respiratory) PET image. *J Nucl Med.* 2010;50:294P (abstract).
27. Le Meunier L, Slomka P, Dey D, et al., eds. Feasibility of coronary plaque imaging with FDG high-definition PET: phantom study. *Soc Nucl Med Ann Meet Abs.* 2008: Society of Nuclear Medicine.
28. Walker MD, Asselin MC, Julyan PJ, et al. Bias in iterative reconstruction of low-statistics PET data: benefits of a resolution model. *Phys Med Biol.* 2011;56(4):931–949. Epub Jan 21, 2011. doi:10.1088/0031-9155/56/4/004. PubMed PMID: 21248391.
29. Moody JB, Lee BC, Corbett JR, Ficaro EP, Murthy VL. Precision and accuracy of clinical quantification of myocardial blood flow by dynamic PET: a technical perspective. *J Nucl Cardiol.* 2015;22(5):935–951. Epub Apr 15, 2015. doi:10.1007/s12350-015-0100-0. PubMed PMID: 25868451.
30. Teoh EJ, McGowan DR, Macpherson RE, Bradley KM, Gleeson FV. Phantom and clinical evaluation of the Bayesian penalized likelihood reconstruction algorithm Q.Clear on an LYSO PET/CT system. *J Nucl Med.* 2015;56(9):1447–1452. Epub Jul 15, 2015. doi:10.2967/

jnumed.115.159301. PubMed PMID: 26159585; PubMed Central PMCID: PMCPMC4558942.

31. J OD, McGowan DR, Abreu C, Barrington S. Effect of Bayesian-penalized likelihood reconstruction on [13N]-NH3 rest perfusion quantification. *J Nucl Cardiol.* 2017;24(1):282–290. Epub Jul 21, 2016. doi:10.1007/s12350-016-0554-8. PubMed PMID: 27435278; PubMed Central PMCID: PMCPMC5084874.
32. Mullani N, Markham J, Ter-Pogossian M. Feasibility of time-of-flight reconstruction in positron emission tomography. *J Nucl Med.* 1980;21(11):1095–1097.
33. Conti M. Focus on time-of-flight PET: the benefits of improved time resolution. *Eur J Nucl Med Mol Imaging.* 2011;38(6):1147–1157. Epub Jan 14, 2011. doi:10.1007/s00259-010-1711-y. PubMed PMID: 21229244.
34. Schaefferkoetter J, Ouyang J, Rakvongthai Y, Nappi C, El Fakhri G. Effect of time-of-flight and point spread function modeling on detectability of myocardial defects in PET. *Med Phys.* 2014;41(6):062502. Epub Jun 1, 2014. doi:10.1118/1.4875725. PubMed PMID: 24877836; PubMed Central PMCID: PMCPMC4032408.
35. Presotto L, Gianolli L, Gilardi MC, Bettinardi V. Evaluation of image reconstruction algorithms encompassing time-of-flight and point spread function modelling for quantitative cardiac PET: phantom studies. *J Nucl Cardiol.* 2015;22(2):351–363. Epub Nov 5, 2014. doi:10.1007/s12350-014-0023-1. PubMed PMID: 25367452.
36. Matheoud R, Lecchi M, Lizio D, et al. Comparative analysis of iterative reconstruction algorithms with resolution recovery and time of flight modeling for 18F-FDG cardiac PET: a multi-center phantom study. *J Nucl Cardiol.* 2017;24(3):1036–1045. Epub Jan 14, 2016. doi:10.1007/s12350-015-0385-z. PubMed PMID: 26758376.
37. Tomiyama T, Ishihara K, Suda M, Kanaya K, et al. Impact of time-of-flight on qualitative and quantitative analyses of myocardial perfusion PET studies using 13N-ammonia. *J Nucl Cardiol.* 2014. Epub ahead of print Dec 3.
38. Armstrong IS, Tonge CM, Arumugam P. Assessing time-of-flight signal-to-noise ratio gains within the myocardium and subsequent reductions in administered activity in cardiac PET studies. *J Nucl Cardiol.* 2017. Epub May 13, 2017. doi:10.1007/s12350-017-0916-x. PubMed PMID: 28497418.
39. DiFilippo FP, Brunken RC. Impact of time-of-flight reconstruction on cardiac PET images of obese patients. *Clin Nucl Med.* 2017;42(2):e103-e108. Epub Nov 2, 2016. doi:10.1097/rlu.0000000000001441. PubMed PMID: 27801740.
40. Chilra P, Gnesin S, Allenbach G, et al. Cardiac PET/CT with Rb-82: optimization of image acquisition and reconstruction parameters. *EJNMMI Phys.* 2017;4. doi:10.1186/s40658-017-0178-3. PubMed PMID: 28205113; PubMed Central PMCID: PMCPMC5311016.
41. Armstrong IS, Tonge CM, Arumugam P. Impact of point spread function modeling and time-of-flight on myocardial blood flow and myocardial flow reserve measurements for rubidium-82 cardiac PET. *J Nucl Cardiol.* 2014;21(3):467–474. doi:10.1007/s12350-014-9858-8.
42. Dweck MR, Doris MK, Motwani M, et al. Imaging of coronary atherosclerosis—evolution towards new treatment strategies. *Nature Rev Cardiol.* 2016;13(9):533–548. Epub May 27, 2016. doi:10.1038/nrcardio.2016.79. PubMed PMID: 27226154.
43. Krishnan S, Otaki Y, Doris M, et al. Molecular imaging of vulnerable coronary plaque: a pathophysiologic perspective. *J Nucl Med.* 2017;58(3):359–364. Epub Feb 12, 2017. doi:10.2967/jnumed.116.187906. PubMed PMID: 28183988.
44. Rubeaux M, Doris MK, Alessio A, Slomka PJ. Enhancing cardiac PET by motion correction techniques. *Curr Cardiol Rep.* 2017;19(2):14. Epub 2017 Feb 12, 2017. doi:10.1007/s11886-017-0825-2. PubMed PMID: 28185169.
45. Doris MK, Rubeaux M, Pawade T, et al. Motion-corrected imaging of the aortic valve with 18F-NaF PET/CT and PET/MR: a feasibility study. *J Nucl Med.* 2017. Epub May 27, 2017. doi:10.2967/jnumed.117.194597. PubMed PMID: 28546334.
46. Xia T, Alessio AM, De Man B, Manjeshwar R, Asma E, Kinahan PE. Ultra-low dose CT attenuation correction for PET/CT. *Phys Med Biol.* 2012;57(2):309–328. Epub Dec 14, 2011. doi:10.1088/0031-9155/57/2/309. PubMed

PMID: 22156174; PubMed Central PMCID: PMCPMC3353418.

47. Gould KL, Pan T, Loghin C, Johnson NP, Guha A, Sdringola S. Frequent diagnostic errors in cardiac PET/CT due to misregistration of CT attenuation and emission PET images: a definitive analysis of causes, consequences, and corrections. *J Nucl Med.* 2007;48(7):1112–1121. PubMed PMID: 17574974.
48. Slomka PJ, Le Meunier L, Hayes SW, et al. Comparison of myocardial perfusion 82Rb PET performed with CT- and transmission CT-based attenuation correction. *J Nucl Med.* 2008;49(12):1992–1998. Epub Nov 29, 2008. doi:10.2967/jnumed.108.056580. PubMed PMID: 19038996.
49. van der Vos CS, Arens AI, Hamill J, et al. Metal artifact reduction of CT scans to improve PET/CT. *J Nucl Med.* 2017:jnumed. 117.191171.
50. Pan T, Mawlawi O, Nehmeh SA, et al. Attenuation correction of PET images with respiration-averaged CT images in PET/CT. *J Nucl Med.* 2005;46(9):1481–1487.
51. Bacharach SL. PET/CT Attenuation correction: breathing lessons. *J Nucl Med.* 2007;48(5):677–679. PubMed PMID: 17475952.
52. Klingensmith WC, 3rd, Noonan C, Goldberg JH, Buchwald D, Kimball JT, Manson SM. Decreased perfusion in the lateral wall of the left ventricle in PET/CT studies with 13N-ammonia: evaluation in healthy adults. *J Nucl Med Technol.* 2009;37(4):215–219. Epub Nov 17, 2009. doi:10.2967/jnmt.109.062059. PubMed PMID: 19914976.
53. Slomka PJ, Diaz-Zamudio M, Dey D, et al. Automatic registration of misaligned CT attenuation correction maps in Rb-82 PET/CT improves detection of angiographically significant coronary artery disease. *J Nucl Cardiol.* 2015;22(6):1285–1295. doi:10.1007/s12350-014-0060-9. PubMed PMID: 25698471.
54. Bond S, Kadir T, Hamill J, et al., eds. Automatic registration of cardiac PET/CT for attenuation correction. Nuclear Science Symposium Conference Record, 2008 NSS'08 IEEE; 2008 19–25 October 2008; Dresden, Germany: IEEE.
55. Pan T, Mawlawi O, Luo D, et al. Attenuation correction of PET cardiac data with low-dose average CT in PET/CT. *Med Phys.* 2006;33(10):3931–3938. Epub Nov 9, 2006. PubMed PMID: 17089855.
56. Hong C, Becker CR, Schoepf UJ, Ohnesorge B, Bruening R, Reiser MF. Coronary artery calcium: absolute quantification in nonenhanced and contrast-enhanced multi-detector row CT studies. *Radiology.* 2002;223(2):474–480. PubMed PMID: 11997555.
57. Brodov Y, Gransar H, Dey D, et al. Combined quantitative assessment of myocardial perfusion and coronary artery calcium score by hybrid 82Rb PET/CT improves detection of coronary artery disease. *J Nucl Med.* 2015;56(9):1345–1350. Epub Jul 15, 2015. doi:10.2967/jnumed.114.153429. PubMed PMID: 26159582.
58. Burkhard N, Herzog BA, Husmann L, et al. Coronary calcium score scans for attenuation correction of quantitative PET/CT 13N-ammonia myocardial perfusion imaging. *Eur J Nucl Med Mol Imaging.* 2010;37(3):517–521. doi:10.1007/s00259-009-1271-1. PubMed PMID: 19774376.
59. Zaidi H, Nkoulou R, Bond S, et al. Computed tomography calcium score scan for attenuation correction of N-13 ammonia cardiac positron emission tomography: effect of respiratory phase and registration method. *Int J Cardiovasc Imaging.* 2013;29(6):1351–1360. Epub Mar 19, 2013. doi:10.1007/s10554-013-0207-9. PubMed PMID: 23504215.
60. Einstein AJ, Johnson LL, Bokhari S, et al. Agreement of visual estimation of coronary artery calcium from low-dose CT attenuation correction scans in hybrid PET/CT and SPECT/CT with standard Agatston score. *J Am Coll Cardiol.* 2010;56(23):1914–1921.
61. Mylonas I, Kazmi M, Fuller L, et al. Measuring coronary artery calcification using positron emission tomography-computed tomography attenuation correction images. *Eur Heart J Cardiovasc Imaging.* 2012;13(9):786–792.
62. Isgum I, de Vos BD, Wolterink JM, et al. Automatic determination of cardiovascular risk by CT attenuation correction maps in Rb-82 PET/CT. *J Nucl Cardiol.* 2017. Epub Apr 6, 2017. doi:10.1007/s12350-017-0866-3. PubMed PMID: 28378112.

63. Danad I, Raijmakers PG, Appelman YE, et al. Hybrid imaging using quantitative H215O PET and CT-based coronary angiography for the detection of coronary artery disease. *J Nucl Med.* 2013;54(1):55–63.
64. Di Carli MF, Dorbala S, Hachamovitch R. Integrated cardiac PET-CT for the diagnosis and management of CAD. *J Nucl Cardiol.* 2006;13(2):139–144.
65. Cheng VY, Slomka PJ, Le Meunier L, et al. Coronary arterial 18F-FDG uptake by fusion of PET and coronary CT angiography at sites of percutaneous stenting for acute myocardial infarction and stable coronary artery disease. *J Nucl Med.* 2012;53(4):575–583. Epub Mar 16, 2012. doi:10.2967/jnumed.111.097550. PubMed PMID: 22419753.
66. Joshi NV, Vesey AT, Williams MC, et al. 18F-fluoride positron emission tomography for identification of ruptured and high-risk coronary atherosclerotic plaques: a prospective clinical trial. *Lancet.* 2014;383(9918):705–713. doi:10.1016/S0140-6736(13)61754-7. PubMed PMID: 24224999.
67. Tawakol A, Migrino RQ, Bashian GG, et al. In vivo 18F-fluorodeoxyglucose positron emission tomography imaging provides a noninvasive measure of carotid plaque inflammation in patients. *J Am Coll Cardiol.* 2006;48(9):1818–1824. Epub Nov 7, 2006. doi:S0735-1097(06)01980-2 [pii]10.1016/j.jacc.2006.05.076. PubMed PMID: 17084256.
68. Tawakol A, Migrino RQ, Hoffmann U, et al. Noninvasive in vivo measurement of vascular inflammation with F-18 fluorodeoxyglucose positron emission tomography. *J Nucl Cardiol.* 2005;12(3):294–301. PubMed PMID: 15944534.
69. Dawood M BF, Lang N, Schober O, Schäfers KJMP. Respiratory gating in positron emission tomography: a quantitative comparison of different gating schemes. *Med Phys.* 2007;34(7):3067–3076.
70. Tsutsui Y, Kidera D, Taniguchi T, et al. Accuracy of amplitude-based respiratory gating for PET/CT in irregular respirations. *Ann Nucl Med.* 2014;28(8):770–779. Epub Jun 22, 2014. doi:10.1007/s12149-014-0870-5. PubMed PMID: 24950753.
71. van Elmpt W, Hamill J, Jones J, De Ruysscher D, Lambin P, Ollers M. Optimal gating compared to 3D and 4D PET reconstruction for characterization of lung tumours. *Eur J Nucl Med Mol Imaging.* 2011;38(5):843–855. Epub Jan 12, 2011. doi:10.1007/s00259-010-1716-6. PubMed PMID: 21222120; PubMed Central PMCID: PMCPMC3070073.
72. Li XA, Stepaniak C, Gore E. Technical and dosimetric aspects of respiratory gating using a pressure-sensor motion monitoring system. *Med Phys.* 2006;33(1):145–154.
73. Nehmeh SA, Erdi YE. Respiratory motion in positron emission tomography/computed tomography: a review. *Semin Nucl Med.* 2008;38(3):167–176. Epub Apr 9, 2008. doi:10.1053/j.semnuclmed.2008.01.002. PubMed PMID: 18396177.
74. Koivumaki T, Nekolla SG, Furst S, et al. An integrated bioimpedance - ECG gating technique for respiratory and cardiac motion compensation in cardiac PET. *Phys Med Biol.* 2014;59(21):6373–6385. Epub Oct 9, 2014. doi:10.1088/0031-9155/59/21/6373. PubMed PMID: 25295531.
75. Jafari Tadi M, Koivisto T, Pankaala M, Paasio A. Accelerometer-based method for extracting respiratory and cardiac gating information for dual gating during nuclear medicine imaging. *Int J Biomed Imaging.* 2014;2014:690124. Epub Aug 15, 2014. doi:10.1155/2014/690124. PubMed PMID: 25120563; PubMed Central PMCID: PMCPMC4120481.
76. Büther F, Dawood M, Stegger L, et al. List mode–driven cardiac and respiratory gating in PET. *J Nucl Med.* 2009;50(5):674–681.
77. Kesner AL, Chung JH, Lind KE, et al. Validation of software gating: a practical technology for respiratory motion correction in PET. *Radiology.* 2016;281(1):239–248. doi:10.1148/radiol.2016152105. PubMed PMID: 27027335.
78. Manber R, Thielemans K, Hutton BF, et al. Practical PET respiratory motion correction in clinical PET/MR. *J Nucl Med.* 2015;56(6):890–896. Epub May 9, 2015. doi:10.2967/jnumed.114.151779. PubMed PMID: 25952740.
79. Tang J, Wang X, Gao X, Paul Segars W, Lodge MA, Rahmim A. Enhancing ejection fraction

measurement through 4D respiratory motion compensation in cardiac PET imaging. *Phys Med Biol.* 2017;62(11):4496–4513. Epub Mar 3, 2017. doi:10.1088/1361-6560/aa6417. PubMed PMID: 28252451.

80. Teras M, Kokki T, Durand-Schaefer N, et al. Dual-gated cardiac PET-clinical feasibility study. *Eur J Nucl Med Mol Imaging.* 2010;37(3):505–516. Epub Oct 1, 2009. doi:10.1007/s00259-009-1252-4. PubMed PMID: 19789872.
81. Feng T, Wang J, Fung G, Tsui B. Non-rigid dual respiratory and cardiac motion correction methods after, during, and before image reconstruction for 4D cardiac PET. *Phys Med Biol.* 2016;61(1):151–168. Epub Dec 2, 2015. doi:10.1088/0031-9155/61/1/151. PubMed PMID: 26624887.
82. Slomka PJ, Nishina H, Berman DS, et al. "Motion-frozen" display and quantification of myocardial perfusion. *J Nucl Med.* 2004;45(7):1128–1134. PubMed PMID: 15235058.
83. Le Meunier L, Slomka PJ, Dey D, et al. Motion frozen (18)F-FDG cardiac PET. *J Nucl Cardiol.* 2011;18(2):259–266. Epub Dec 17, 2010. doi:10.1007/s12350-010-9322-3. PubMed PMID: 21161704; PubMed Central PMCID: PMCPMC3069314.
84. Rubeaux M, Joshi NV, Dweck MR, et al. Motion correction of 18F-NaF PET for imaging coronary atherosclerotic plaques. *J Nucl Med.* 2016;57(1):54–59. Epub Oct 17, 2015. doi:10.2967/jnumed.115.162990. PubMed PMID: 26471691.
85. Qiao F, Pan T, Clark JW Jr., Mawlawi OR. A motion-incorporated reconstruction method for gated PET studies. *Phys Med Biol.* 2006;51(15):3769–3783. doi:10.1088/0031-9155/51/15/012. PubMed PMID: 16861780.
86. Livieratos L, Stegger L, Bloomfield PM, Schafers K, Bailey DL, Camici PG. Rigid-body transformation of list-mode projection data for respiratory motion correction in cardiac PET. *Phys Med Biol.* 2005;50(14):3313–3322. Epub Sep 24, 2005. doi:10.1088/0031-9155/50/14/008. PubMed PMID: 16177511.
87. Chun SY, Fessler JA. Noise properties of motion-compensated tomographic image reconstruction methods. *IEEE Trans Med Imaging.* 2013;32(2):141–152. Epub Jul 5, 2012. doi:10.1109/TMI.2012.2206604. PubMed PMID: 22759442; PubMed Central PMCID: PMCPMC3821946.
88. Hong I, Furst S, Jones J, Casey M, editors. The strategy of elastic motion corrections. Nuclear Science Symposium and Medical Imaging Conference (NSS/MIC); 2013: IEEE.
89. Hong I, Jones J, Casey M, eds. Elastic motion correction for cardiac PET studies. Nuclear Science Symposium and Medical Imaging Conference (NSS/MIC); 2013: IEEE.
90. Dawood M, Gigengack F, Jiang X, Schafers KP. A mass conservation-based optical flow method for cardiac motion correction in 3D-PET. *Med Phys.* 2013;40(1):012505. Epub Jan 10, 2013. doi:10.1118/1.4770276. PubMed PMID: 23298116.
91. Lamare F, Le Maitre A, Dawood M, et al. Evaluation of respiratory and cardiac motion correction schemes in dual gated PET/CT cardiac imaging. *Med Phys.* 2014;41(7):072504. Epub Jul 6, 2014. doi:10.1118/1.4881099. PubMed PMID: 24989407.
92. Slomka PJ, Rubeaux M, Le Meunier L, et al. Dual-gated motion-frozen cardiac PET with flurpiridaz F 18. *J Nucl Med.* 2015;56(12):1876–1881. Epub Sep 26, 2015. doi:10.2967/jnumed.115.164285. PubMed PMID: 26405171.
93. Delso G, Fürst S, Jakoby B, et al. Performance measurements of the Siemens mMR integrated whole-body PET/MR scanner. *J Nucl Med.* 2011;52(12):1914–1922.
94. Judenhofer MS, Wehrl HF, Newport DF, et al. Simultaneous PET-MRI: a new approach for functional and morphological imaging. *Nature Med.* 2008;14(4):459–465.
95. Quick HH, Ladebeck R, Georgi J. Whole-body MR/PET hybrid imaging: technical considerations, clinical workflow, and initial results. MAGNETOM Flash 1/2011 · [Internet]. 2011; 1(1):88–100. Available from: www.siemens.com/magnetom-world.
96. Casey M, Burbar Z, Rothfuss H, Panin V, Bharkhada D. A next generation SiPM based PET/CT system with improved time and spatial resolution. *J Nucl Med.* 2017;58(suppl 1):1332.
97. Levin C, Glover G, Deller T, McDaniel D, Peterson W, Maramraju SH. Prototype time-of-flight

PET ring integrated with a 3T MRI system for simultaneous whole-body PET/MR imaging. *J Nucl Med Meet Abstr.* 2013;54(2_MeetingAbstracts):148.

98. Rischpler C, Nekolla SG, Dregely I, Schwaiger M. Hybrid PET/MR imaging of the heart: potential, initial experiences, and future prospects. *J Nucl Med.* 2013;54(3):402–415.
99. Ratib O, Nkoulou R, Schwaiger M. Cardiovascular clinical applications of PET/MRI. *Clin Transl Imaging.* 2013:1–7.
100. Quick HH. Integrated PET/MR. *J Magn Reson Imaging.* 2014;39(2):243–258. doi:10.1002/jmri.24523. PubMed PMID: 24338921.
101. Adenaw N, Salerno M. PET/MRI: current state of the art and future potential for cardiovascular applications. *J Nucl Cardiol.* 2013;20(6):976–989.
102. Schneider S, Batrice A, Rischpler C, Eiber M, Ibrahim T, Nekolla SG. Utility of multimodal cardiac imaging with PET/MRI in cardiac sarcoidosis: implications for diagnosis, monitoring and treatment. *Eur Heart J.* 2014;35(5):312. Epub Aug 27, 2013. doi:10.1093/eurheartj/eht335. PubMed PMID: 23975480.
103. Zandieh S, Bernt R, Mirzaei S, Haller J, Hergan K. Image fusion between 18F-FDG PET and MRI in cardiac sarcoidosis: a case series. *J Nucl Cardiol.* 2016. Epub Sep 9, 2016. doi:10.1007/s12350-016-0653-6. PubMed PMID: 27604109.
104. Wada K, Niitsuma T, Yamaki T, et al. Simultaneous cardiac imaging to detect inflammation and scar tissue with (18)F-fluorodeoxyglucose PET/MRI in cardiac sarcoidosis. *J Nucl Cardiol.* 2016;23(5):1180–1182. Epub Dec 3, 2015. doi:10.1007/s12350-015-0348-4. PubMed PMID: 26626783.
105. Dweck MR, Abgral R, Trivieri MG, et al. Hybrid magnetic resonance imaging and positron emission tomography with fluorodeoxyglucose to diagnose active cardiac sarcoidosis. *JACC Cardiovasc Imaging.* 2017. Epub Jun 19, 2017. doi:10.1016/j.jcmg.2017.02.021. PubMed PMID: 28624396.
106. Nensa F, Kloth J, Tezgah E, et al. Feasibility of FDG-PET in myocarditis: comparison to CMR using integrated PET/MRI. *J Nucl Cardiol.* 2016. Epub Sep 18, 2016. doi:10.1007/s12350-016-0616-y. PubMed PMID: 27638745.
107. Yang HJ, Dey D, Sykes J, et al. Arterial CO2 as a potent coronary vasodilator: a preclinical PET/MR validation study with implications for cardiac stress testing. *J Nucl Med.* 2017;58(6):953–960. Epub Mar 4, 2017. doi:10.2967/jnumed.116.185991. PubMed PMID: 28254864; PubMed Central PMCID: PMCPMC5450368.
108. Slomka PJ, Berman DS, Germano G. Low-dose 3D (82)Rb PET. *J Nucl Cardiol.* 2012;19(6):1110–1112. Epub Nov 7, 2012. doi:10.1007/s12350-012-9637-3. PubMed PMID: 23129187.
109. Ouyang J, Li Q, El Fakhri G, eds. Magnetic resonance-based motion correction for positron emission tomography imaging. *Semin Nucl Med.* 2013;43(1):60–67.
110. Furst S, Grimm R, Hong I, et al. Motion correction strategies for integrated PET/MR. *J Nucl Med.* 2015;56(2):261–269. Epub Jan 13, 2015. doi:10.2967/jnumed.114.146787. PubMed PMID: 25572092.
111. Ouyang J, Li Q, El Fakhri G. Magnetic resonance-based motion correction for positron emission tomography imaging. *Semin Nucl Med.* 2013;43(1):60–67. doi:10.1053/j.semnuclmed.2012.08.007. PubMed PMID: 23178089; PubMed Central PMCID: PMCPMC3508789.
112. Huang C, Petibon Y, Ouyang J, et al. Accelerated acquisition of tagged MRI for cardiac motion correction in simultaneous PET-MR: phantom and patient studies. *Med Phys.* 2015;42(2):1087–1097. Epub Feb 6, 2015. doi:10.1118/1.4906247. PubMed PMID: 25652521; PubMed Central PMCID: PMCPMC4312342.
113. Petibon Y, Guehl NJ, Reese TG, et al. Impact of motion and partial volume effects correction on PET myocardial perfusion imaging using simultaneous PET-MR. *Phys Med Biol.* 2017;62(2):326–343. Epub Dec 21, 2016. doi:10.1088/1361-6560/aa5087. PubMed PMID: 27997375; PubMed Central PMCID: PMCPMC5241952.
114. Martinez-Möller A, Souvatzoglou M, Delso G, et al. Tissue classification as a potential approach for attenuation correction in whole-body PET/MRI: evaluation with PET/CT data. *J Nucl Med.* 2009;50(4):520–526.

115. Kershah S, Partovi S, Traughber BJ, et al. Comparison of standardized uptake values in normal structures between PET/CT and PET/MRI in an oncology patient population. *Mol Imaging Biol.* 2013;15(6):776–785. doi:10.1007/s11307-013-0629-8. PubMed PMID: WOS:000327216300016.
116. Marshall HR, Patrick J, Laidley D, et al. Description and assessment of a registration-based approach to include bones for attenuation correction of whole-body PET/MRI. *Med Phys.* 2013;40(8):082509. doi:10.1118/1.4816301. PubMed PMID: 23927354.
117. Lau JM, Sharma S, Laforest R, et al. Feasibility of MRI attenuation correction in cardiac FDG-PET. *J Cardiovasc Mag Reson.* 2013;15(Suppl 1): O61.
118. Kero T, Nordstrom J, Harms HJ, Sorensen J, Ahlstrom H, Lubberink M. Quantitative myocardial blood flow imaging with integrated time-of-flight PET-MR. *EJNMMI Phys.* 2017;4(1):1. Epub Jan 7, 2017. doi:10.1186/s40658-016-0171-2. PubMed PMID: 28058674; PubMed Central PMCID: PMCPMC5216001.
119. Miller M, Zhang J, Binzel K, et al. Characterization of the vereos digital photon counting PET system. *J Nucl Med.* 2015;56(supplement 3):434.
120. Sitek A. Data analysis in emission tomography using emission-count posteriors. *Phys Med Biol.* 2012;57(21):6779–6795. doi:10.1088/0031-9155/57/21/6779. PubMed PMID: WOS:000310528700008.

EDITOR'S PERSPECTIVE

James A. Case

The rapid introduction of new technology in the cardiovascular PET arena has offered a wide variety of options for clinicians. In the past 20 years, image resolution has improved almost three-fold, from 15-20 mm to sub 5 mm, with time of flight and digital imaging systems. These improvements in resolution make the detection and localization of coronary artery disease easier and more precise and, when combined with new tracers, they have the potential for revolutionizing the care of heart disease.

As this chapter illustrates, there are several approaches to improving resolution with PET. The simplest approach is to use more sophisticated multidimensional reconstruction approaches: 3D and 4D iterative reconstruction. Hardware solutions also improve resolution further. Time of flight reconstruction creates better separation between the organs, creating a nonlinear improvement in image resolution, and digital imaging can improve resolution and system sensitivity. As the resolution improves, cardiac pathology is being visualized in ways never thought possible. In addition to improvements in image resolution, the combination of PET with CT or MR opens the door to new imaging procedures, such inflammation and sarcoidosis imaging.

In some ways, the new technology is extending image quality beyond what we can currently understand. Much like when the Hubble telescope first looked at the universe, we are initially presented with more questions than answers, but as we dive into those questions, we gain a much deeper understanding. Some of this new technology will be essential to day-in and day-out practice, while others will stimulate researchers to a better understanding of the processes of heart disease.

For the present, when considering all the technological advancements in cardiac PET instrumentation, it is often difficult to identify those innovations that can make the difference in day-in and day-out practice. Each nuclear laboratory has different needs, capabilities, and expectations. The cost of technology can oftentimes drive the decision-making process, however, it should not be the exclusive determinant.

Identification of the right instrumentation for an individual nuclear cardiology laboratory begins by defining the overall practice goal. At the beginning of this process, each practice should establish its guiding principle, for example: providing a robust cardiac PET program, providing an advanced imaging service, or providing state-of-the-art instrumentation for clinical practice and research. By defining the goal of the cardiac PET program, decisions about what type of instrumentation and options are needed become clearer. Clinical practices should not let the diversity of options available for cardiac PET instrumentation be an impediment to implementation of a cardiac PET program. Many features are not necessary to begin a cardiac PET program, but may become important as the program evolves. These options and upgrades should be considered advancements to the program as needs change.

When transitioning from cardiac SPECT to cardiac PET, robustness and versatility of the system is essential for beginning a cardiac PET program.[1] All cardiac PET systems should be capable of acquiring high quality perfusion, gated, and dynamic acquisitions. These systems should also be able to acquire a high-quality attenuation map either using radionuclide- or CT-based transmission imaging. Systems must also have the capability of processing the data, making corrections for misregistration, assessing the quality of the examination, and, finally, presenting that data in an environment for accurate image interpretation. Physicians should be able to easily assess the relative perfusion, wall motion thickening and ejection fraction, and absolute myocardial blood flow and blood flow reserve. These basic needs can be accomplished both with a refurbished dedicated system all the way to the latest digital PET/CT system (see Figure 1).

As the needs and technical abilities of a laboratory increase, hybrid PET/CT instrumentation should be considered as an upgrade path from radionuclide-based attenuation correction. Several publications have demonstrated the value of quantitatively and qualitatively assessing patient coronary calcium. In addition, hybrid instrumentation can be helpful for assessing sarcoidosis and inflammation.[4]

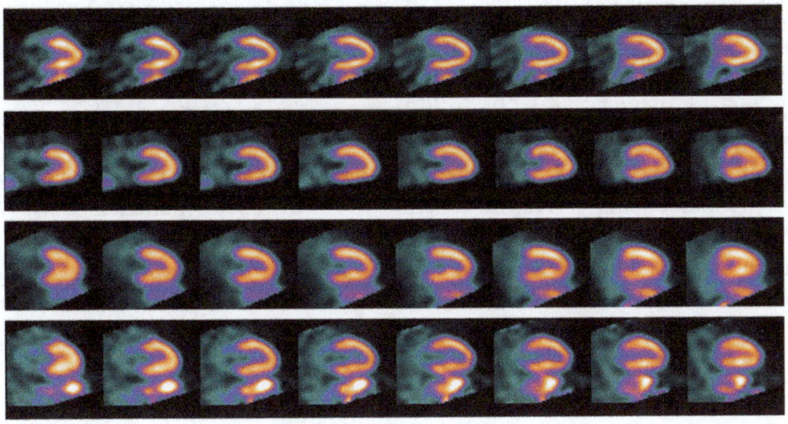

FIGURE 1: High Quality Cardiac PET Perfusion Studies Can Be Obtained Across a Wide Variety of Instrumentation. Images of normal stress Rb-82 PET studies from differing patients and instrumentation: (A) 2D Siemens ACCEL dedicated PET scanner, (B) 2D GE NXi dedicated PET scanner, (C) Siemens 64 slice Biograph PET/CT, and (D) Siemens 128 slice Time of Flight PET/CT.

State-of-the-art cardiac PET imaging has seen considerable effort in improving resolution and reducing patient-specific artifacts. Time-of-flight PET instrumentation has proven to be very useful in oncologic studies—however, data demonstrating value in cardiac studies has been slow to accumulate. The latest time-of-flight PET scanners can achieve sufficient temporal resolution to realize the potential of scanners in the cardiac arena. These scanners have the potential to improve separation of noncardiac activity in the lungs or bowel from cardiac uptake, as well as improving images in obese patients.[5] For laboratories interested in distinguishing themselves, these state-of-the-art PET scanners can offer significant advantages in terms of image quality and usability across a wide range of body habitus.

The next generation of cardiac PET scanners will be defined by digital PET. These scanners offer consistent resolution of less than 5 mm. With these scanners, it will be possible to detect ischemia beyond the great vessels, into the distal and smaller vessels, and perhaps even into the myocardium itself. This has the potential for visualizing the entire blood supply mechanism from the myocardium down to the capillary bed.

Cardiac PET instrumentation covers a wide range of technologies ranging from dedicated, 2-D PET scanners through the latest digital PET/CT scanners. Clinical laboratories should not let this diversity in instrumentation be an impediment to beginning a cardiac PET program. High-tracer extraction fraction, attenuation and scatter correction, perfusion gating and absolute flow, laboratory efficiency, and reduced patient radiation exposure can be achieved with almost all PET scanners. Each laboratory should assess their own individual goals for their cardiac PET program and then choose the instrumentation that best achieves those goals. As their program grows, these goals should be periodically reevaluated to assess if the next generation of technology better meets their new goals.

References for Editor's Perspective

1. Dilsizian V, Bacharach SL, Beanlands SR, et al. Imaging guidelines/SNMMI procedure standard for positron emission tomography (PET) nuclear cardiology procedures. *J Nucl Cardiol.* 2016;23(5):1187- 1226.
2. Chang S, Nabi F, Xu J, et al. The coronary artery calcium score and stress myocardial perfusion imaging provide independent and complementary prediction of cardiac risk. *J Am Coll Cardiol.* 2009;54(20):1872-1882.

3. Einstein AJ, Johnson LL, Bokhari S, et al. Agreement of visual estimation of coronary artery calcium from low-dose CT attenuation correction scans in hybrid PET/CT and SPECT/CT with standard Agatston Score. *J Am Coll Cardiol. 2010;56(23)*:1914-1921.
4. Slart RHJA, Glaudemans AWJM, Lancellotti P, et.al. A joint procedural position statement on imaging in cardiac sarcoidosis: from the Cardiovascular and Inflammation & Infection Committees of the European Association of Nuclear Medicine, the European Association of Cardiovascular Imaging, and the American Society of Nuclear Cardiology. *J Nucl Cardiol. 2018*;25:298-319.
5. DiFilippo FP, Brunken RC. Impact of time-of-flight reconstruction on cardiac PET images of obese patients. *Clin Nucl Med.* February 2017;42(2):e103-e108.
6. Pan TS. Respiratory gating in PET/CT: a step in the right direction. *J Nucl Cardiol.* 2018;25: 416-418.

New Developments in Cardiac PET Radionuclide Production: Tracers, Cyclotrons, Generators, and Delivery Systems for Cardiac PET Imaging

CHAPTER 7

James A. Case

INTRODUCTION

The field of cardiovascular PET imaging is constantly evolving, and this includes all aspects of tracers, production of tracers, and delivery to the patient. This chapter discusses the new developments in cardiac PET tracers, cyclotrons, and delivery systems.

PHYSICS OF TRACERS

Positrons are the stable antiparticle of the electrons. Despite being stable, they are extremely rare in nature. When positrons combine with electrons, they quickly annihilate, leaving behind nothing but photon energy. The positrons that are used in nuclear cardiology originate from the decay of radionuclides, the most common of these being fluorine-18 (^{18}F), carbon-11 (^{11}C), oxygen-15 (^{15}O), nitrogen-13 (^{13}N), and rubidium-82 (^{82}Rb). These radionuclides an excess number of protons; when the proton is converted to a neutron, an energetic positron is ejected from the nucleus of the atom.

PHYSICS OF POSITRONS

Positron emission tomography (PET) relies on the annihilation of a positively charged particle (an anti-electron or positron) with a conventional electron to produce two high-energy gamma rays traveling 180 degrees from each other. The existence of positrons was first proposed by Paul Dirac in 1928,[1] and ultimately discovered in 1932 by Carl D. Anderson.[2] Positrons, though stable in vacuum, annihilate almost immediately when they come in contact with electrons, producing a complete conversion of the mass of the two particles (511 keV/c^2) into energy. This unique property of positrons, the complete conversion of the positron-electron pair into two photons of identical energies (511 keV), was recognized as potentially revolutionary for medical imaging. The first application of positron annihilation medical imaging was first explored by Brownell et al in 1953 for imaging brain tumors.[3] This technique was later expanded to tomographic imaging in 1971.[4]

Before a positron can annihilate, it needs to come to rest in the medium (thermalization). This thermalization drift from the parent atom reduces the overall resolution of the image. For ^{18}F, the maximum energy of the emerging positron is 633 keV, leading to a thermalization length of 0.239 cm.[5] However for ^{82}Rb, the maximum energy of the positron is 3.148 MeV, leading to a maximum thermalization length of 1.561 cm (Table 7-1).

Though many atoms, such as ^{18}F and ^{13}N, decay to a stable nuclear state, some atoms, such as ^{82}Rb, can decay to an unstable nuclear state. For these atoms, the decay to an unstable state results in the emission

Table 7-1

PET Radionuclide Properties: F-18, N-13, Rb-82, O-15, C-11

	Half-Life	Beta Energy (max, mean) in MeV	Max Range (mm)	Mean Range (mm)
^{11}C	20.4 min	0.96, 0.386	4.2	1.2
^{13}N	9.93 min	1.199, 0.492	5.5	1.8
^{15}O	2.0 min	1.732, 0.735	8.4	3.0
^{18}F	110 min	0.634, 0.25	2.4	0.6
^{82}Rb (no prompt, 81%)	75 sec	3.38, 1.535	17.0	7.1
^{82}Rb (0.777 MeV prompt, 13%)	75 sec	2.601, 1.168	13.0	5.0

Half-life, max and mean beta particle energies, mean thermalization length

of a nuclear gamma ray (a "prompt gamma") in addition to the two photons produced by the positron annihilation. In the case of ^{82}Rb, 13% of all decays result in a prompt gamma ray (776 keV).[5] These gamma rays can influence the scatter correction algorithms of the imaging system, producing significant artifacts.[6,7]

PET TRACERS

Several tracers are currently in use for measuring myocardial perfusion and blood flow, myocardial viability infection and inflammation including sarcoidosis. Unlike SPECT tracers, the radionuclides used have a relatively short half-life, ranging from ^{82}Rb (75 seconds) to ^{18}F (110 minutes). Because of these short half-lives, isotope production often must be produced on-site or at a nearby radio pharmacy.

^{82}Rb

The most common tracer used in cardiac PET nuclear cardiology is ^{82}Rb. This agent has a 75-second half-life and is a potassium analog. As a potassium analog, ^{82}Rb is used as a myocardial blood flow agent with similar biokinetics as thallium-201.[8] Because of the short half-life of ^{82}Rb, the agent must be produced using a generator encased in an infusion system. These generator infusion systems are capable of eluting the generator, performing the radioassay of the product and infusing the ^{82}Rb directly into the patient with a single-button process (Figure 7-1).

^{82}Rb is produced as a by-product of the decay of strontium-82 (^{82}Sr). Because the atom itself is a blood flow tracer, no further radiochemistry is required before is it ready to use. ^{82}Sr has a long half-life of 28 days, allowing clinical nuclear laboratories to use the generator for 4–6 weeks before needing to replace the expired generators.

The production of the ^{82}Sr source requires a larger cyclotron capable of accelerating protons to more than 63 MeV. The process creates ^{82}Sr, and two contaminants: ^{85}Sr and ^{89}Sr.[9] These contaminants have a shorter half-life than ^{82}Sr and must be allowed to decay before the ^{82}Sr can be shipped.

^{13}N-Ammonia Production and Delivery

^{13}N-ammonia is a myocardial blood flow tracer that has been extensively studied for use in myocardial perfusion testing.[10] With a 9.93-minute half-life, it either has to be produced on-site or within a short delivery distance from a radiopharmacy. For these reasons, it is a reasonable alternative to ^{82}Rb only for those centers with a nearby cyclotron (Figure 7-2).

The most common method for producing ^{13}N-ammonia is a process known as internal chemistry. In this process, a solution of water and ethanol are placed directly in the beam line of a cyclotron. ^{13}N-ammonia is produced as a by-product of the reaction[11]:

$$^{16}O + p \rightarrow {}^{13}N + \alpha$$

Because this process is very simple, the high doses (>250 mCi) ^{13}N-ammonia can be quickly extracted

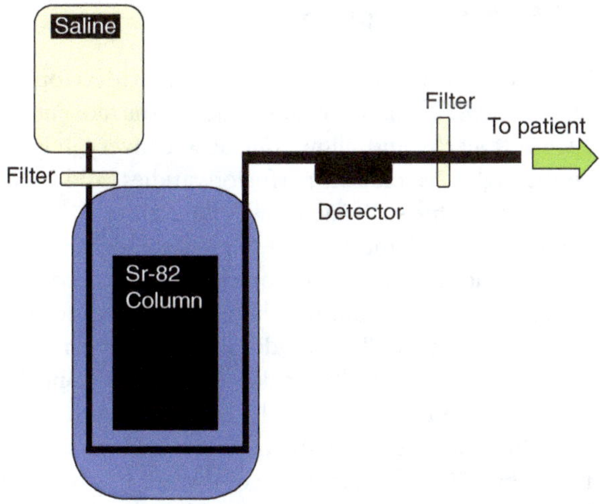

FIGURE 7-1 Rb-82 Generator Provides a One-Button Process for Delivering a Radionuclide Dose to Patient. The system draws saline over the ^{82}Sr coumn, collecting the free ^{82}Rb ions. This solution is passed over a detector that assays the solution and the is transferred direction into the patient's IV line.

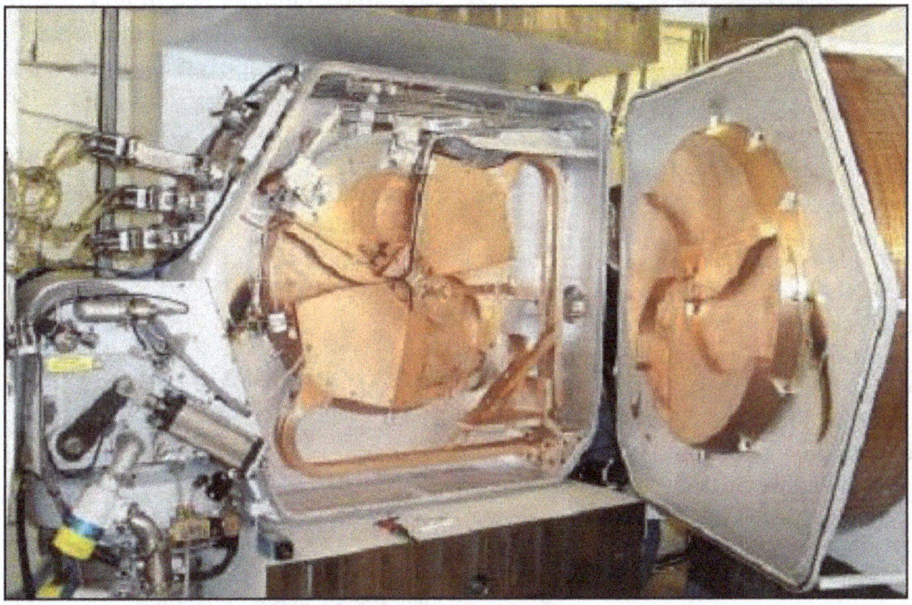

FIGURE 7-2 Inside of a GE PETtrace Cyclotron System (18MeV)

from the cyclotron, quality inspected, and packaged for delivery in minutes. This high dose at the time of packaging gives radiopharmacies up to 20 minutes to transport the product to a nuclear laboratory.

A process has also been introduced that uses a carbon target for producing the ^{13}N. Though the process involves a more complicated chemistry, it has the advantage of requiring a lower energy cyclotron.[11] Recent introduction of low energy, minicyclotrons using automated radiochemistry packages have opened the possibility of on-site production of ^{13}N-ammonia without a full radiopharmacy (Figure 7-3). This option is discussed later.

^{18}F-FDG

^{18}F-labeled compounds have the advantage of a relatively long nuclear half-life (110 minutes), allowing for longer distance delivery from the nuclear pharmacy. ^{18}F-FDG synthesis begins with

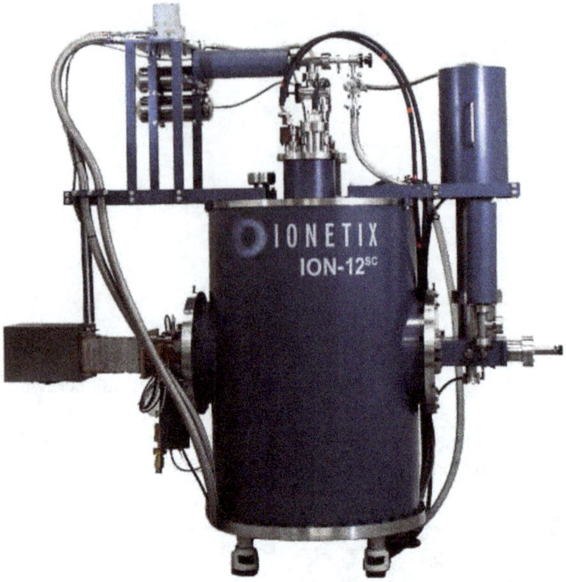

FIGURE 7-3 Ionetix Cyclotron. This system is a single isotope system that stands only 196 cm high with a diameter of 108 cm.

a cyclotron capable of producing protons with an energy >2 MeV. The high-energy protons produce ^{18}F by bombardment of an ^{18}O target. The ^{18}F is then extracted from the ^{18}O target using an anion separation process.[11,12]

The chemistry for FDG involves nucleophilic substitution using potassium carbonate. Finally, the FDG extract is purified to remove chelating agents and unreacted ^{18}F. This entire process is performed in a chemistry synthesis box that automates the production. Given the long half-life of ^{18}F, it can be shipped longer distances either by ground or air transportation.

^{18}F-FDG (fluorodeoxyglucose) is a glucose analog capable of tracking glucose metabolism.[13,14] Its most common application is in detection of cancer and following therapies. In nuclear cardiology, it can be used for the detection of myocardial viability, sarcoidosis, and infections, including devices or surrounding pockets.[14–17]

To use FDG for the detection of myocardial viability, glucose pathways often require activation via a process known as glucose loading. The methodology of clinical use of FDG for this purpose is discussed in Chapters 9, 10, and 11.

^{18}F-labeled Flurpiridaz

There has been considerable interest in developing an ^{18}F myocardial perfusion tracer. The advent of such a tracer would allow unit dose delivery, higher count-higher resolution perfusion studies, and exercise testing. One such agent is ^{18}F-flurpiridaz.[18–21] This agent has been demonstrated to produce high-quality studies and that are well correlated with coronary anatomy.[18] In addition, it is highly extracted at high flow rates, potentially exceeding the performance of ^{13}N-ammonia.[19] ^{18}F-flurpiridaz is a mitochondrial Complex 1 inhibitor that freely diffuses from the capillary bed into the cell with and extraction fraction of more than 90%.[19] Once inside of the cell it is trapped in mitochondrial Complex 1. In addition to its favorable uptake in the myocardium, it also has favorable noncardiac uptake with moyocardial uptake exceeding liver uptake for rest, exercise, and pharmacological stress studies.[20,21] The combination of favorable uptake characteristics, imaging properties, and convenience for ^{18}F-flurpiridaz has the potential for revolutionizing cardiac PET. The greatest challenge for this agent will be expanding the network of radiopharmacies capable of production. The clinical data are discussed in Chapter 1.

AMYLOID IMAGING WITH PET

There also has been considerable interest in the imaging of beta amyloid plaques. In particular florbetapir, visamyl and pyramil all have been FDA-approved for the imaging of beta amyloid plaques in the brain.[22,23] Though these agents are currently not approved for use for cardiac applications, they do hold considerable promise in the management of heart failure patients.

GENERATOR DELIVERY FOR RUBIDIUM

The majority of cardiac PET centers around the world utilize a generator to produce the positron emitting nuclei that are used for cardiac PET imaging. The most common generator uses a column of radioactive ^{82}Sr to produce a constant flux of ^{82}Rb atoms that are trapped in a saline bath[24,25] (Figure 7-6). The rubidium is then extracted from the generator, assayed for radioactive strength and quality controlled. The product is transferred to the patient using a continuous infusion system.

The first generator was introduced to the US market in 1989 by Bracco Diagnostic.[24] This system achieved widespread acceptance in 2000 with the introduction of high-sensitivity PET scanners. These newer systems allowed for high-quality perfusion and gated imaging exceeding the image quality and diagnostic accuracy of SPECT cardiac perfusion.[26–28]

Basic Generator Design

In the absence of an on-site cyclotron, many laboratories have utilized a generator to produce the short half-life PET tracers. Radionuclide generators use a column of a longer-lived radionuclide to produce the shorter half-life daughter radionuclide that is used for clinical imaging. The most common generator used in cardiac PET is the ^{82}Rb generator. These generators use a column of ^{82}Sr to produce the short half-life ^{82}Rb atoms that are used for imaging. The 28-day half-life of ^{82}Sr is ideal for many laboratories, providing an easily dispensed blood flow tracer over its 4–6 week generator in front of life cycle. ^{82}Sr decays via beta emission. The conversion of a neutron to a proton results in the unstable ^{82}Rb atom that is collected in the column. ^{82}Rb is maintained as an ion in the saline bath. As a potassium analog, no further chemistry is required to use it as a blood flow agent with similar chemical properties as thallium.

The ^{82}Rb infusion system consists of three major components: the ^{82}Sr generator, the infusion pump system, and the quality control systems. At the heart of the ^{82}Rb system is a column of ^{82}Sr. This column consists of a tin-oxide column that binds the ^{82}Sr. The tin column has low affinity for the ^{82}Rb and allows the ^{82}Rb to be dissolved in a NaCl bath. By eluting the system, the ^{82}Rb can be carried with the saline into the patient.

The assay of the patient dose must be done quickly because of the short half-life of the tracers. This is typically performed by allowing the tracer to pass over a photodiode and measure the counts in the diode. These counts are a function of time times the flow rate and are proportional to the activity delivered to the patient. By determining the proportionality constant, an accurate measurement of the dose delivered to the patient can be measured. More sophisticated systems have been created that are accurate over a wider range of count rate and for variable flow rates.[28,29]

Quality control steps must also be performed regularly to ensure the safety of the system. The most important of these quality tests is the measurement of ^{82}Sr breakthrough. As a generator is used, the filtration system containing the ^{82}Sr column can degrade, allowing ^{82}Sr to be included in the elute. This contaminant is of concern because strontium is an iron analog and is retained in the bone marrow.[24,25] For all generator systems, daily monitoring for ^{82}Sr breakthrough is required. In addition, the US FDA has placed limits on the total volume that can be passed over the ^{82}Sr, specifically requiring additional monitoring after 14 liters of use and complete expiration of the generator after 17 liters.[24]

The detection of ^{82}Sr breakthrough is performed by first eluting a volume of ^{82}Rb from the delivery system into a test vial then monitoring it as it decays. Because of the short half-life of ^{82}Rb, negligible amounts should remain in the vial after a long decay if strontium is present. In contrast, the concentration of ^{82}Sr will remain constant in the vial (28-day half-life). In the event that ^{82}Sr has broken through the column, a residual background of 511 keV emission should be detectable after a certain period of time. ^{82}Sr breakthrough represents a significant patient risk and nuclear cardiology laboratories must follow manufacturer recommendations for use of the ^{82}Rb systems and safety monitoring.

Currently, there are two commercially available rubidium generator systems: the CardioGen system from Bracco Diagnostics, and the RubyFill system from Drax Image. Both the CardioGen and RubyFill systems have at their core a ^{82}Sr generator. The differences between these two delivery systems are in the rate at which they deliver the rubidium to the patient, and their quality control procedures.

The CardioGen system uses a constant flow rate delivery system, meaning that it delivers the rubidium at a constant mL/sec delivery rate.[24] The system also uses a printout of the delivery of the activity to the patient as measured by a built-in activity meter. Users are then required to record the activity delivered to the patient as well as the milliliters of saline used by hand into a log sheet. These log sheets are then used to determine if and when alert thresholds for saline usage have been reached. In addition, strontium breakthrough must be measured using a separate dose calibrator and by performing a decay test.

The RubyFill system can deliver the rubidium in either a constant flow rate or constant activity rate mode.[25] The constant activity rate mode for delivery maintains a constant delivery of activity per second by varying the flow rate of the system. For most imaging protocols, a constant flow rate or constant activity rate delivery of the activity will make little difference in the final perfusion images. However, recent studies have indicated that there may be improved accuracy in myocardial blood flow estimates when using a constant activity rate delivery system.[30] The QC protocols for the RubyFill system are largely automated. Because of this, QC logs are maintained digitally by the generator system. In addition, the RubyFill system can be rapidly recalibrated for different activity dosages. This allows for weight-based patient dosing and potentially reducing patient radiation exposure.

The rapid growth in rubidium usage for myocardial perfusion imaging has placed strains on the worldwide network of high-energy cyclotrons that produce the strontium for rubidium generators, leading to the difficulty of getting strontium. Because most of the production centers in the world are government run, scientific enterprises, these government facilities had to share cyclotron use with other scientific and commercial needs. More recently, Zevacor began production of commercial strontium at its facility in Indiana. This facility was commissioned in 2017 and began producing strontium for distribution. This facility has greatly increased the amount of available strontium for use in cardiac PET and will allow for more predictable growth in cardiac PET. Additional improvements in process efficiency will continue to improve the availability of strontium and the shortages that have been occurred in the past should be considerably less frequent.

CYCLOTRON SYSTEMS

Positron-emitting isotopes typically have a very short half-life and must be produced in the laboratory. The most common approach is to use a particle accelerator to force additional protons into the nucleus of parent atoms to create an unstable, positron-emitting product. Cyclotron systems are a type of particle accelerator that accelerates particles using a system of static and oscillating electromagnetic fields to successively bump the charged particles to higher and higher energy.[31] Originally developed in the 1930s to study the subatomic properties of atoms, cyclotron systems have become an indispensable tool for producing medical isotopes.

Cyclotrons function by using a system of magnets to increase the velocity of protons in the system (Figure 7-4). At first, protons are injected into the center of the cyclotron and then, by oscillating the electromagnetic field, the electrons move in a

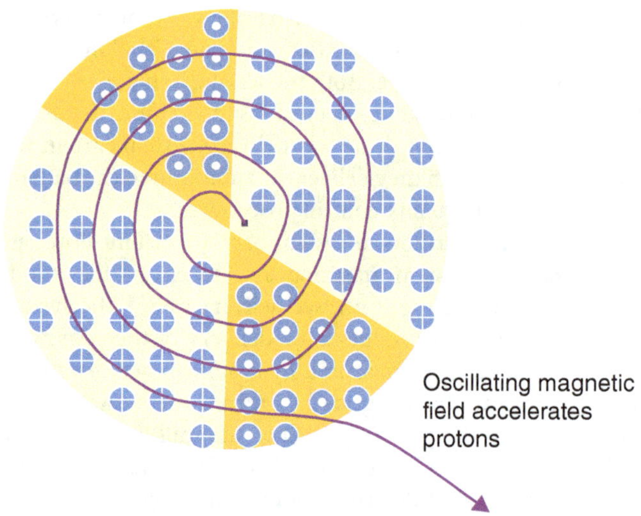

FIGURE 7-4 Cyclotrons Produce High-Energy Protons by Using a System of Oscillating Magnetic Fields. As the protons gain energy, their radius increases until the reach the edge of the system and can be extracted.

circle around the magnetic field. The field is then oscillated to force the protons to move from one side of the magnet to the other. As the protons move back and forth their energy increases, and thereby the radius from the center increases. This process is repeated over and over until the protons reach the edge of the cyclotron and they can be extracted into a high-energy beam. Finally, the beam of high-energy protons is directed onto a target with a system of magnets to produce the new radiative nuclei.

The energy of the extracted protons from a cyclotron is related to the strength of the magnetic field and the size of the cyclotron. Specifically, the maximum energy of the extracted protons is given by:

$$K = \frac{(er_L B)^2}{2m_p}$$

where K is the kinetic energy of the proton, e is the charge of the proton, m_p is the mass of the proton, r_L is the radius of the cyclotron, and B is the strength of the magnetic field.

In order to produce positron-emitting isotopes, energetic protons must be forced into the nucleus of atoms. In order to accomplish this, protons must have sufficient energy to overcome the Coulomb repulsion of the protons inside the nucleus. This minimum energy is referred to as the activation energy of the desired nuclear reaction (Figure 7-5). Specific activation energies are given in Table 7-2.[5]

Early cyclotrons were massive machines, filling entire buildings. Over time these systems have become smaller and more user-friendly. Current cyclotron systems used at PET radiopharmacies can be sited in a single room and support multiple extraction ports.[32] More recently, specialized cyclotron systems have been developed for producing PET tracers, such as ^{13}N ammonia and ^{15}O water in office based settings.[33,34] The miniaturization of cyclotrons has reduced the cost of PET tracers and expanded availability.

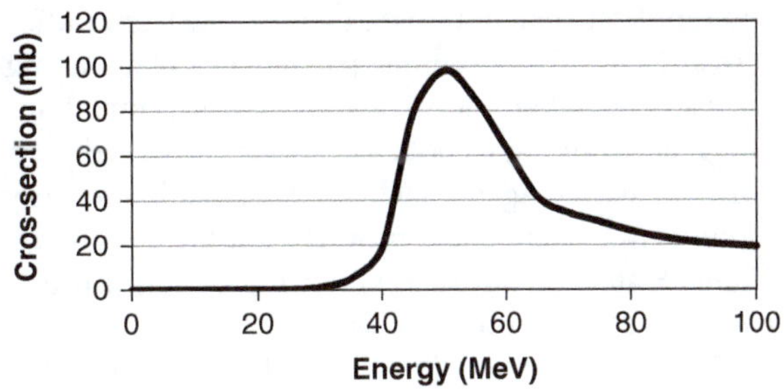

FIGURE 7-5 The Activation Energy of ^{82}Sr Is Well Above the Capabilities of Most Medical Cyclotrons. However, recent installation of a commercial, dedicate ^{82}Sr cyclotron could greatly improve the availability of ^{82}Sr in North America (Zevacor Inc. www.zevacor.com).

Table 7-2

Cyclotron Energies and Peak Cross-Section of ^{18}F, ^{13}N, ^{82}Rb, ^{15}O, ^{11}C

	Target	Proton Energy
^{82}Sr	RbCl or Rb metal	40-90 MeV
^{18}F	^{18}O	11-17 MeV
^{18}F	^{nat}Ne	8-14 MeV
^{13}N	^{16}O	19 MeV
^{13}N	^{13}C	11 MeV
^{15}O	^{15}N	11 MeV
^{11}C	^{14}N	11-17 MeV

Conventional Large Cyclotron

Most of the medical cyclotron systems in use today have a maximum beam energy of 12 to 20 MeV. At this energy, cross-sections for ^{18}F and ^{13}N are large and the production of these radionuclides is highly efficient. The challenge of these systems is the technical know-how and expense of setting up a cyclotron for producing PET tracers exceeds the capabilities of most clinical facilities. These conventional production type cyclotrons are typically based in commercial radio pharmacies or large academic/research institutions.

Another challenge in setting up a cyclotron for producing ^{18}F and ^{13}N for in-house use is regulatory compliance. The production of radionuclides for use in patients is managed by the current good manufacturing practice (cGMP) regulations of the US FDA. Compliance with these regulations is necessary even if the agents being produced are to be used in-house. For all of these reasons, there is little prospect for these large conventional cyclotrons to be used in most clinical settings.

To produce these agents and deliver them to clinical practices, radio pharmacies must have responsive and rapid delivery systems to avoid waste from radioactive decay. This becomes particularly challenging for users of ^{13}N ammonia, with its 9.93-minute half-life greatly limiting its potential for unit dose delivery. For longer-lived agents such as ^{18}F FDG, the delivery radius is much larger and most clinical facilities in the United States can have access to ^{18}F products through networks of radio pharmacies.

The introduction of ^{18}F-labeled perfusion agents will greatly increase pressure on existing cyclotron networks. Most radiopharmacies that are equipped with PET-producing cyclotrons, are currently working at near capacity to produce FDG for oncologic studies. Adding potentially tens of thousands of new orders of ^{18}F-labeled perfusion agents will not be possible without significant investment in the cyclotron infrastructure. It is likely that ^{18}F-labeled radiotracers may have limited availability until cyclotron capacity is increased.

Mini Cyclotrons

Highly specialized cyclotrons have recently been introduced to provide hospitals and smaller radiopharmacies the capability to create single radionuclide/single-dose radionuclides. Specifically, PET tracers ^{15}O-water or ^{13}N-ammonia and 18F-18-FDG could be produced on an as-needed basis. One such system that has become available is a dedicated ^{13}N-ammonia production.[34] This cyclotron uses a H^- (negative-ion) 14 MeV beam, and a superconducting magnet. Another system has been proposed for producing ^{15}O-water only. Though this system could only be used for the measurement of myocardial or cerebral blood flow, this minicyclotron uses a ^{2}H (deuteron) 3 MeV beam (35) to produce ^{15}O-gas, making it ideal for smaller settings. ^{18}F, with its more complicated chemistry, is more challenging. Despite this, investigators have tested a "generator system" using a 7.5 MeV proton beam,[35] capable of producing 1 mCi/min of ^{18}F. This could be revolutionary in filling the isotope needs if an ^{18}F PET perfusion agent is approved for use.

CONCLUSIONS

As the demand for cardiac PET tracers increases, so has innovation in their production. In the past 10 years, there has been a revolution in new cyclotron designs, novel isotope chemistry, and delivery. In addition, new tracers will challenge radiopharmacies to meet the demands of more disease specific tracers; however, with a wide spectrum of cyclotron energies and delivery models, clinicians should be able to have reliable access to a wide variety of tracers for varying indications. The greatest challenge for radiopharmaceuticals for cardiac PET is expanding the network of production facilities for ^{82}Sr and ^{18}F to meet the demands of the practicing cardiac PET community.

REFERENCES

1. Dirac PAM. The quantum theory of the electron. *Proc R Soc. Lond A*, 1928; Feb1:610–624.
2. Anderson CD. The positive electron. *Phys Rev.* 1933;43(6):491–494.
3. Brownell GL, Sweet, WH. Localization of brain tumors with positron emitters. *Nucleonics.* 1953;11:40–45.
4. Brownell GL, Burnham CA, Hoop B, Bohning DE. Quantitative dynamic studies using short-lived radioisotopes and positron detection. In: Proceedings of the Symposium on Dynamic Studies with Radioisotopes in Medicine, Rotterdam. August 31-September 4, 1970. *IAEA.* 1971:161–172.
5. Conti M, Eriksson L. Physics of pure and non-pure positron emitters for PET: a review and a discussion. *EJNMMI Phy.* 2016;3:8.
6. Esteves FP, Nye JA, Khan A, et al. Prompt-gamma compensation in Rb-82 myocardial perfusion 3D PET/CT. *J Nucl Cario.* 2010;17(2):247–253.
7. Armstrong IS, Memmott MJ, Tonge CM, Arumugam P. The impact of prompt gamma compensation on myocardial blood flow measurements with rubidium-82 dynamic PET. *J Nucl Cardiol.* Sep 13, 2016.
8. Hunter CR, Hill J, Ziadi MC, Beanlands RS, deKemp RA. Biodistribution and radiation dosimetry of (82)Rb at rest and during peak pharmacological stress in patients referred for myocardial perfusion imaging. *Eur J Nucl Med Mol Imaging.* 2015;42:1032–1042.
9. International Atomic Energy Agency. *Production of long lived parent radionuclides for generators:*

^{68}*Ge*, ^{82}*Sr*, ^{90}*Sr and* ^{188}*W*. IAEA Radioisotopes and Radiopharmaceuticals Series no. 2. Vienna, Austria: IAEA; 2010.
10. Schelbert HR, Phelps ME, Hoffman EJ, Huang SC, Selin CE, Kuhl DE. Regional myocardial perfusion assessed with N-13 labeled ammonia and positron emission computerized axial tomography. *Am J Cardiol.*1979;43:209–218.
11. International Atomic Energy Agency. *Cyclotron produced radionuclides: principles and practice.* Technical Reports Seriesno. 465. Vienna, Austria; 2008.
12. Saha GB. *Fundamentals of Nuclear Pharmacy.* 5th ed. New York, NY: Springer; 2004.
13. Som P, Atkins HL, Bandoypadhyay D, et al. A fluorinated glucose analog, 2-fluoro-2-deoxy-D-glucose (F-18): nontoxic tracer for rapid tumor detection. *J Nucl Med.* 1980;21(7):670–675.
14. Bonow RO, Maurer G, Lee KL, et al. Myocardial viability and survival in ischemic left ventricular dysfunction. *N Engl J Med.* 2011;364:1617–1625.
15. Ishmaru S, Tsujino I, Takei T, et al. Focal uptake on 18F-fluoro-2 deoxyglucose positron emission tomography images indicates cardiac involvement of sarcoidosis. *Eur Heart J.* 2005;26:1538–1543.
16. Sarrazin JF, Philippon F, Tessier M, et al. Usefulness of fluorine-18 positron emission tomography/computed tomography for identification of cardiovascular implantable electronic device infections. *J Am Coll Cardiol.* 2012;59:1616–1625.
17. Slart RHJA, et al. A joint procedural position statement on imaging in cardiac sarcoidosis: from the Cardiovascular and Inflammation & Infection Committees of the European Association of Nuclear Medicine, the European Association of Cardiovascular Imaging, and the American Society of Nuclear Cardiology. *Eur Heart J Cardiovasc Imaging.* Oct 1, 2017;18(10):1073–1089.
18. Berman DS, Maddahi J, Tamarappoo BK, et al. Phase II safety and clinical comparison with single-photon emission computed tomography myocardial perfusion imaging for detection of coronary artery disease: flurpiridaz F 18 positron emission tomography. *J Am Coll Cardiol.* Jan 29, 2013;61(4):469–477.
19. Nekolla SG, RederS, Saraste A, et al. Evaluation of the novel myocardial perfusion positron-emission tomography tracer 18F-BMS-747158-02: comparison to 13N-ammonia and validation with microspheres in a pig model. *Circulation.* 2009;119:2333–2342.
20. Maddahi J, Czernin J, Lazewatsky J, et al. Phase I, first-in-human study of BMS747158, a novel 18F-labeled tracer for myocardial perfusion PET: dosimetry, biodistribution, safety, and imaging characteristics after a single injection at rest. *J Nucl Med.* 2011;52:1490–1498.
21. Maddahi J, Packard SSR, Schiepers C, et al. Myocardial and background kinetics of flurpiridaz F 18 after injection at rest and during exercise or pharmacological stress test in normal subjects. In press.
22. Dorbala S, Vangala D, Semer J, et al. Beta, imaging cardiac amyloidosis: a pilot study using ^{18}F-florbetapir positron emission tomography. *Eur J Nucl Med Mol Imaging.* Sep 2014;41(9):1652–1662.
23. Law WP, Wang WY, Moore PT, Mollee PN, Ng AC. Cardiac amyloid imaging with 18F-florbetaben PET: a pilot study. *J Nucl Med.* Nov 2016;57(11):1733–1739.
24. Bracco Diagnostics. [Prescribing Information] CardioGen-82 (Rubidium Rb 82 Generator), Bracco Diagnostics (NJ, USA) revised April 2013. Available at: http://imaging.bracco.com/sites/braccoimaging.com/files/technica_sheet_pdf/Cardiogen%20Full%20Prescribing%20Information.pdf. Accessed June 30, 2016.
25. Jubilant DRAXIMAGE. [Prescribing Information] Ruby-Fill® (rubidium Rb 82 generator), Jubilant DRAXIMAGE (Kirkland Quebec). Available at: http://www.draximage.com/DATA/TEXTEDOC/Approval-202153-Ruby-Fill-Labeling-30Sept-2016.pdf. Accessed October 1, 2016.
26. McArdle, BA, Dowsley TF, deKemp RA, et al. Does rubidium-82 have superior accuracy to SPECT perfusion imaging for the diagnosis of obstructive coronary disease? A systematic review and meta-analysis. *J Am Coll Cardiol.* 2012;60:1828–1837.
27. Bateman T, Heller GV, McGhie I, et al. Diagnostic accuracy of rest/stress ECG-gated rubidium-82 myocardial perfusion PET: comparison with ECG-gated Tc-99m-sestamibi SPECT. *J Nucl Cardiol.* 2006;12:24–33.

28. Dorbala S, Di Carli MF, Beanlands RS, et al. Prognostic value of stress myocardial perfusion positron emission tomography: results from a multicenter observational registry. *J Am Coll Cardiol.* 2013;15;61:176–184.
29. Klein R, Adler A, Beanlands RS, de Kemp RA. Precision-controlled elution of a 82Sr/82Rb generator for cardiac perfusion imaging with positron emission tomography. *Phys Med Biol* 2007;52:659–673.
30. Klein R, Ocneanu A, Renaud JM, Ziadi MC, Beanlands RS, deKemp RA. Consistent tracer administration profile improves test-retest repeatability of myocardial blood flow quantification with 82Rb dynamic PET imaging. *J Nucl Cardiol.* Nov 1, 2016. Epub ahead of print.
31. Lawrence, EO, Livingston, MS. The production of high speed light ions without the use of high voltages. *Phys Rev.* American Physical Society. April 1, 1932:40(1):19–35.
32. http://www3.gehealthcare.in/en/products/categories/pet-radiopharmacy/tracer-center-equipment/pettrace-800-series-cyclotron. Product brochure.
33. Smirnov VL, Vorozhtsov SB, Vincent J. H–superconducting cyclotron for PET isotope production. *Phys Part Nuclei Lett.* 2014:11(6):774–787.
34. Mckay DB, et al. Quality assurance for PET gas production using the Cyclone 3D oxygen-15 generator. Applied Radiation and Isotopes, October 1999.
35. Nutt R. Low-volume biomarker generator. US patent 7,884,340 B2. February 8, 2011.

EDITOR'S PERSPECTIVE

Gary V. Heller

For those laboratories beginning a cardiac PET program, an early decision needed is about which PET tracer or tracers are going to be used clinically now and in the future. This decision has ramifications for the instrumentation to be purchased as well as design of the PET room(s) and lead shielding. This excellent chapter gives a contemporary assessment of the technical choices needing to be made in establishing a cardiovascular PET laboratory, and gives vital information on tracers, cyclotrons, and the evolving picture of generator delivery systems. These choices made by the PET laboratory developers will fundamentally affect what imaging procedures can be utilized later on.

To this editor, this most important decision depends, ironically, on F-18 imaging tracers and what value the laboratory developers see in these agents. This book elucidates the many aspects of FDG that have clinical applications and could be part of a new PET laboratory. In addition, the future of an F-18 myocardial perfusion agent becoming clinically available is now closer to reality. Despite this, the driving engine of a current cardiac PET laboratory in development is with the myocardial perfusion imaging (MPI) tracer, either rubidium or ammonia. If the lab chooses to use either tracer (rubidium or ammonia) without F-18 imaging, lead shielding is minimal and less expensive, as are space considerations, primarily due to the very short half-lives. The choice between rubidium and ammonia is elucidated in this chapter and assists those beginning the process. To a large extent, close availability of a cyclotron is an important aspect of ammonia use and currently limits its use.

Currently, F-18 tracers, namely FDG, are used for ancillary (non-MPI) imaging. The addition of F-18 in a given laboratory immediately expands the use of the PET camera to viability, infection, and inflammation imaging. These uses are covered extensively in other chapters of this book, and those establishing a cardiac PET program will need to give consideration as to whether these procedures will be beneficial in their practice. The decision is important, as the lead shielding of PET rooms will need to factor in a longer half-life tracer (2 hours vs minutes). Consideration of a patient holding space once the tracer is injected is also necessary as it requires 45 minutes between injection of FDG and imaging.

An important thought process for the configuration of the PET laboratory is the potential for use of an F-18 myocardial perfusion agent, namely Flurpiridaz. While this agent is not currently FDA approved, it is in the second Phase 3 Trial and could be approved within 2 to 4 years. As with other F-18 agents, the half-life is two hours which provides the opportunity to perform not only pharmacologic stress testing, but also, easily, exercise stress testing as well. This could potentially facilitate an even greater shift from SPECT to PET, including laboratories that exclusively utilize PET for their perfusion testing. Thus, consideration should be given to the future use of this agent within the intermediate term with regard to space, shielding design, and even camera selection.

The last section in this chapter describes advancements made in the instrumentation of delivery systems for PET tracers. This primarily affects decisions with regard to rubidium use, although data also support value in ammonia delivery and potentially F-18 myocardial blood flow tracers. The author of this section discusses the advantages/disadvantages and these new advancements should be considered.

In summary, tracer choices, cyclotron availability, and delivery systems are important considerations for the establishment of a successful cardiac PET laboratory. These decisions need to be made early for proper design of the facility.

Radiation Exposure with Cardiovascular PET: New Data

CHAPTER

8

James A. Case

INTRODUCTION

The use of radionuclides for the assessment of cardiovascular disease is well-established as a very low-risk, high-sensitivity, and specificity technology for establishing the presence of coronary disease, hibernating myocardium, and other cardiac and cardiovascular syndromes.[1,2] Recently societies and professional medical organizations have expressed concern for radiation exposure to patients undergoing nuclear cardiology procedures.[3] It is important in addressing concerns of radiation exposure that the quality of nuclear cardiology procedures not be sacrificed for the purposes of reducing the patient's radiation dose alone. Nuclear cardiology procedures can confer life-saving benefits; however, the application of sensible radiation reduction techniques can maintain and even improve the diagnostic quality of nuclear cardiology images while reducing the patient dose.[3–6]

Current understanding of the influence of radiation on the patient's long-term risk assumes the effect of ionizing radiation is cumulative over a patient's lifetime. More recent genomic studies of double strand breakage and repair mechanisms may indicate a simple linear; no threshold model for the influence of radiation may overestimate the risk of carcinogenesis from diagnostic radiation.[7] Despite this, each procedure must take into account radiation-reducing steps to have an impact on the overall patient dose. However, radiation-reduction strategies should not come at the expense of diagnostic quality.

Imaging societies encourage nuclear laboratories and health-care providers to consider patient needs when prescribing imaging tests.[8] For example, elderly patients with known coronary disease have a different risk-to-benefit relationship than younger patients at a lower likelihood for coronary disease. Customizations of imaging protocols should take into account patients' needs for an accurate assessment of cardiovascular disease in addition to their own sensitivity to ionizing radiation, as well as the frequency of testing procedures being ordered.

Cardiac PET offers some unique advantages over SPECT by simultaneously providing improved image quality, diagnostic accuracy, and reducing patient dosage.[9] This chapter investigates the trade-offs of reducing patient dose, specific advantages of cardiac PET, and recommends strategies for optimizing patient dose and image quality with a cardiac PET procedure.

RADIATION EFFECTS

Photon ionizing radiation interacts with cells by depositing energy in a focal region, disrupting the cell's machinery. Of greatest concern is changes in the cell's DNA that could lead to carcinogenesis. At lower photon energies (ultraviolet radiation), radiation can cause focal breakages of DNA base pairs, resulting in pyrimidine dimers that then can be sites of incorrect or incomplete DNA repair.[10] These incomplete repairs have the potential for producing viable cancerous cells as is the case of melanoma.

At higher photon energies, the mechanism for carcinogenesis is the production of hydroxyl radicals.[11] When gamma radiation interacts with molecules inside of a cell, the result is a Compton scattered electron that thermalizes in the medium. This thermalization process produces free electrons that break the hydrogen-hydroxide bond leading to free hydroxyl radicals inside of the cell. These hydroxyl radicals interact with the DNA, typically by breaking either a single or double strand of the DNA. In most cases single or double strand breakages of the DNA do not result in a viable cell, or the DNA strand is repaired.

The most common model for estimating radiations role in carcinogenesis is the "linear no threshold model."[12,13] This model assumes that radiation risk and the potential for carcinogenesis can be linearly extrapolated from high-dose examples of carcinogenesis. These high-dose examples, such as the atomic bomb blast victims in Hiroshima and Nagasaki, the Chernobyl nuclear accident, Fukushima nuclear accident, and so on, represent the limited experience of direct causal relationship between ionizing radiation and carcinogenesis. The linear no threshold model assumes that the incidence of radiation-induced cancer at these high-dose exposures can be extrapolated to the very low doses observed in diagnostic radiological exams. This is generally accepted as an upper bound of the risks of radiation exposure. These high-dose models differ significantly from diagnostic radiological exams in a number of ways. First, the source of radiation in most of these models is neutron radiation not photon radiation. Neutron radiation has been shown to have significantly higher capacity for cellular damage because of the intense deposition of ionization in a very small region (high-linear energy transfer, LET). In addition, the high-dose radiation overwhelms the cells natural systems for repairing damaged DNA.

Recent investigation of carcinogenesis as a result CT radiation showed DNA damage at varying levels of CT exposure.[14] This study investigated particular biomarkers for DNA damage: phosphorylated H2AX, ataxia telangiectasia mutated (ATM), and tumor protein p53. The study also investigated markers of apoptosis and BCL2 associated X protein (BAX). This study concluded that radiation exposure typically results in cell death and activation of DNA repair processes. Although it did not evaluate carcinogenesis specifically, the authors were able to conclude that higher energy ionizing radiation most commonly results in noncancerous by-products. In addition to limited evidence of double strand breaks in Nguyen 2015, mutational signatures for both leukemia and lymphoma do not exhibit the broad mutational spectrum associated with double strand breakage (Figure 8-1). Additional whole genome data is needed to establish an upper bound on the prevalence of double strand breakage and repair in patients with leukemia and lymphoma.

These and other data suggest that nuclear laboratories should continue to strive to make reductions in patient radiation exposure whenever possible. However, because of uncertainty in the relationship between radiation, carcinogenesis and optimal patient care, efforts to reduce patient radiation exposure should not come at the expense or sacrifice of the diagnostic utility of an imaging test.

CARDIAC PET RADIATION SOURCES

Radiation Measurements: Techniques and Units

In order to describe ionizing radiation, it is necessary to first establish the units of measurement. For radioactivity these measurements are usually made in terms of Curie or Becquerel. Both Curie and Becquerel are measurements of the number of disintegrations of radioactive atoms per second, or activity. One Becquerel of radioactive material is defined as one atomic disintegration per second. The Curie is also based on the number of disintegrations per second (3.7×10^{10} disintegrations/sec). In nuclear cardiology, measurements are typically made in terms of millicurie (mCi) or megabequerel (MBq). One mCi is equal to 37 MBq.

Radiation dose is described in one of two ways: amount of energy deposited per cubic centimeter of

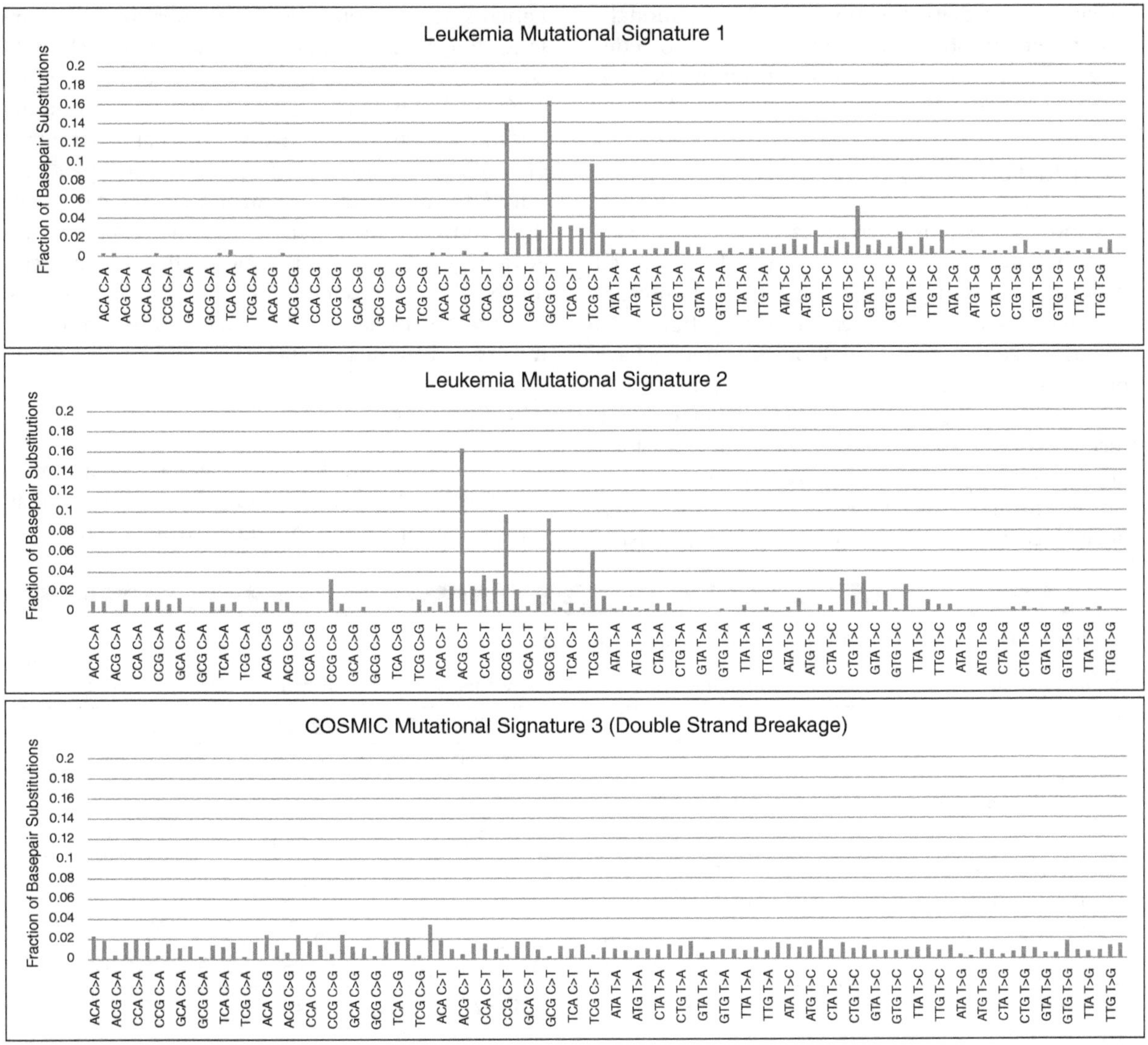

FIGURE 8-1 The Drivers Of Carcinogenesis Are Somatic Mutations To The DNA Of Patients Environmental Exposures leave specific signature on the characteristic mutations on DNA. For leukemia, there are only two particular mutations that are known to create these carcinomas and they do resemble the typical genetic markers associated with double strand breakage and repair.

tissue and amount of tissue damage per cubic centimeter of tissue. The measurement of the energy deposited per cubic centimeter is the Gy defined, which is 1 J per kilogram absorbed ionizing radiation. More common in diagnostic imaging is the rad, which is 1/100 of a Gy. Equivalent dose (H) takes into consideration the relative biological damage of ionizing radiation. It is the product of the absorbed dose (D), times a weighting factor for the source of radiation (1 for gamma rays), times a weighting factor for the sensitivity of the particular organ to ionizing radiation. The units of equivalent dose are Sieverts (Sv) or roentgen equivalent man (rem). For whole body, this can be summarized as the effective dose (E), which is a weighted sum of all of the individual dosages to the organs (ICRP). The adult organ and total body dosimetry values are usually based on an idealized 70 kg person.[15]

To compare radiation exposure between modalities or even radiotracers, most professional societies have adopted the mSv as a means of communication potential risk to patients.

PET Radiotracers

The most important current cardiac PET tracers are rubidium 82, ^{13}N-ammonia, and F-18 labeled FDG. In addition to these, several other important radionuclides are under research investigation: F-18 flurpiridaz and O-15 water. All of these tracers have the radiological advantage of a very short half-life. This short half-life is one of the key advantages PET tracers have over SPECT tracers in reducing patient radiation exposure. SPECT tracers, such as sestamibi and tetrofosmin, have biological half-lives (6 hours) much greater than the acquisition time, causing patients to continue receiving radiation exposure long after the conclusion of the diagnostic testing. In contrast, PET tracers typically decay to background soon after the conclusion of testing thus minimizing unused radioactive decays. A second advantage of cardiac PET tracers is 511 keV photon pair produced during positron annihilation travel in opposite directions, eliminating the need for collimation. This advantage provides much more efficient data collection thereby reducing the need for high injected activity. A summary of the radiation dose from PET tracers is given in Table 8-1.

^{82}Rb Rubidium

^{82}Rb is a 76-second half-life potassium that is produced by a ^{82}Sr-^{82}Rb generator that is eluted by an infusion pump system into the patient.[16,17] The eluate

Table 8-1

Radiation Dose from Common Nuclear Cardiology Procedures

Study Protocol	Isotope	Modality	Activity (mCi)†	E (mSv)††
Rest + Stress Perfusion	^{82}Rb-chloride	3D PET	25 + 25	2
		2D PET	50 + 50	4
Rest + Stress Perfusion	^{13}N-ammonia	3D PET	10 + 10	2
		2D PET	20 + 20	4
Rest Viability, Sarcoid or Inflammation (+ Perfusion)	^{18}F-FDG (+$^{13}NH_3$ or ^{82}Rb)	3D PET	5 (+10 or 25)	3.5 (+ 1)
		2D PET	10 (+20 or 50)	7 (+ 2)
Stress-only Perfusion (ultra-low-dose)	^{99m}Tc-sestamibi	CZT-SPECT	3.5	1
Stress-only Perfusion (full-dose)	^{99m}Tc-sestamibi	GC-SPECT	30	10
Rest + Stress Perfusion One-day (half-dose)	^{99m}Tc-sestamibi ^{99m}Tc-tetrofosmin	GC-SPECT	5 + 15	6.4 5.6
Rest + Stress Perfusion One-day (full-dose)	^{99m}Tc-sestamibi ^{99m}Tc-tetrofosmin	GC-SPECT	10 + 30	13 11

CZT = Cadmium Zinc Telluride, **GC** = Gamma Camera

Radiation effective dose (E): Activity (mCi) × 37 (MBq/mCi) × Effective Dose Constant (mSv/MBq) = Effective Dose (mSv).

Effective Dose Constants: ^{82}Rb-chloride = 1.1 × 10^{-3} mSv/MBq; ^{13}N-ammonia = 2.7 × 10^{-3} mSv/MBq; ^{18}F-FDG = 1.9 × 10^{-2} mSv/MBq; ^{99m}Tc-sestamibi = 8.0 × 10^{-3} mSv/MBq (stress), 7.9 × 10^{-3} mSv/MBq (rest) ; ^{99m}Tc-tetrofosmin = 8.0 × 10^{-3} mSv/MBq (stress), 6.3 x 10^{-3} mSv/MBq (rest).

†Doses listed are typical for cardiac PET and can vary for specific instrumentation and application. For specific dose recommendation, refer to the appropriate imaging guidelines[15] and manufacturer prescribing information.

††Effective doses listed are based on the ICRP Publication 128[10].

(Reproduced with permission from Case JA, deKemp RA, Slomka PJ, et al: Status of cardiovascular PET radiation exposure and strategies for reduction: An Information Statement from the Cardiovascular PET Task Force, J Nucl Cardiol. 2017 Aug;24(4):1427-1439)

from the ^{82}Sr-^{82}Rb generator must be checked daily to ensure that any contamination with long-lived ^{82}Sr and ^{85}Sr is below acceptable limits.

Radiation dosimetry measurements of ^{82}Rb have been difficult because of its very short half-life. Current estimates acquired on modern PET/CT imaging equipment and using improved kinetic modeling of ^{82}Rb now estimate the radiation dose from a typical rest stress perfusion ^{82}Rb study has been less than one-fourth the dose from Tc 99m myocardial perfusion SPECT studies (12–15 mSv for SPECT, 3–5 mSv for ^{82}RB PET[18–20]).

A significant contributor to the radiation dose from ^{82}Rb is the energetic positron that is emitted during decay (max energy 3.3 MeV). This positron's energy is deposited through thermalization in the tissue. This high-linear energy transfer of the positrons' kinetic energy increases the possibility of cellular damage. In addition to the high-kinetic energy of the admitted positron, 12% of ^{82}Rb decays also admit a secondary "prompt gamma" photon at 776 MeV. These additional contributors to ionizing radiation increase ^{82}Rb's potential for causing cellular damage.

^{13}N-Ammonia

^{13}N-ammonia is also commonly used for myocardial perfusion PET studies, and has several advantages of ^{82}Rb. ^{13}N-ammonia is a highly extracted tracer with a 9.93 minute half-life.[21] This longer half-life can enable both pharmacological and exercise testing, and can be delivered short distances as a unit dose.

The amount of ionizing radiation deposited in tissue per disintegration is less with ^{13}N-ammonia versus ^{82}Rb. The maximum kinetic energy of the emitted positron is 1.2 MeV with no prompt gamma. However, given the longer half-life of ^{133}ammonia the radiation dose from ^{13}N-ammonia is comparable to clinical doses of ^{82}Rb (Table 8-1).

^{18}F Fluorodeoxyglucose

^{18}F 2-fluorodeoxyglucose (^{18}F FDG) is also commonly used in cardiac PET procedures, but is not a blood flow tracer. Its most common application is for the detection of myocardial viability. In addition to viability studies, ^{18}F FDG is also used for the detection of sarcoidosis and inflammation. ^{18}F is usually produced in a cyclotron by proton irradiation of ^{18}O water and has a 109.8 minute half-life. The deoxyglucose is then labeled with ^{18}F to yield ^{18}F FDG, an analog of glucose.[22] Similar to ^{13}N-ammonia, FDG produces a low-energy positron (0.633 MeV), with no prompt gamma by-product.

New F-18 Labeled Perfusion Agents

Several PET perfusion tracers labeled with ^{18}F have been under active development for the past few years: a fluorinated perfusion agent, Flurpiridaz.[23,24]

The injected activity from ^{18}F-flurpiridaz tracer in phase II and phase III clinical trials has been approximately 1.9 mCi at rest and 6.5 mCi at stress for the exercise study and 2.9 mCi for rest and 6.8 mCi for the pharmacologic study (Figure 8-2). Phase 1 studies of Flurpiridaz[23] estimate the radiation dose as approximately 6.4 mSv and 4.8 mSv for

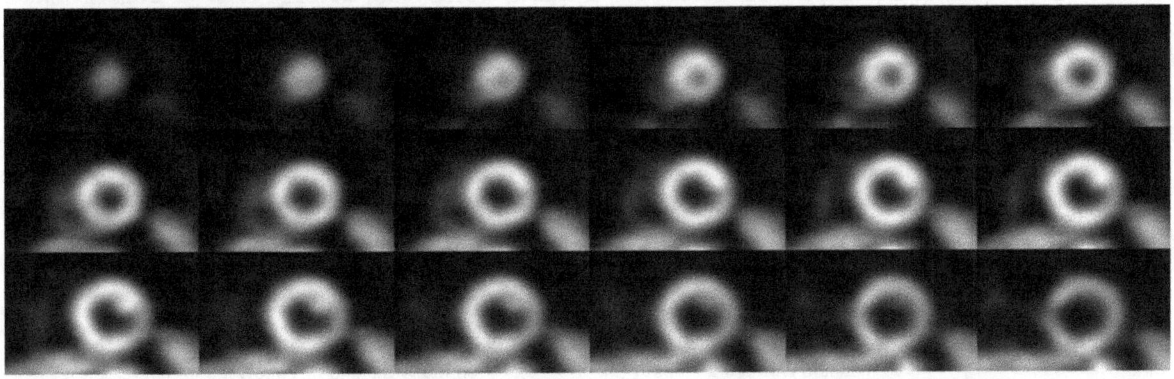

FIGURE 8-2 Flurpiridaz F-18 Has Substantially Improved Image Quality Characteristics When Compared With Other PET Agents. This comes at the expense of a modest increase in radiation dose. One approach would be to reduce injected dose to match the radiation dose of ^{82}Rb. However, if these improvements can yield better clinical outcomes, the modest increase in dose may be justified.

the pharmacologic and exercise rest/stress protocols, respectively. Because of the longer half-life of F-18, the radiation dose from flurpiridaz is higher than ^{82}Rb or ^{13}N-ammonia, although some studies have indicated that flurpiridaz could be effectively imaged using a lower injected dose. Even these levels of the radiation exposure is well below ASNC recommendations. In addition, exercise stress-only protocols will also be investigated to reduce dose. Either by using a low-dose stress high-dose rest study or by using a 2-day study, it may be possible to achieve a less than 2 mSv protocol in normal patients.

Radiation from Transmission Sources

In contrast to SPECT, myocardial perfusion PET studies are almost always corrected for nonuniform patient attenuation. Patient-specific attenuation maps can be acquired in two ways: using a low-resolution transmission computed tomogram of the patients or hybrid PET/CT systems of varying degrees of sophistication.[25–31] Depending on the protocol selected, radiation doses from these external sources can vary from a small fraction of the radiopharmaceutical dose to an amount exceeding the radiopharmaceutical dose.

Hybrid PET/CT systems are capable of acquiring diagnostic quality CT images; however, for many myocardial perfusion studies the acquisition of a diagnostic chest CT does not add meaningful clinical information to the study. For all patients who acquired only a PET/CT system, a full-field CT examination is required to perform the necessary attenuation correction. These studies are typically acquired in a low-resolution, low-dose configuration. Even when acquiring low-dose CT transmission data, these attenuation maps are often very high signal-to-noise. Despite the fact that CT studies have generally a better signal-to-noise than line source attenuation maps, CT specific artifacts, such as breathing artifacts and metal artifacts, can make PET/CT more challenging than line source attenuation correction.[28–33] Cine/CT has been demonstrated to be both robust and easy to implement and provides good compensation for respiratory motion, however, at the cost of increased radiation dose.[29] By using several passes over the diaphragm, the average position for the diaphragm can be obtained. Lowering the x-ray tube voltage (kVp) and tube current can help reduce the dose; however, these improvements still result in CTAC scans of over 2 mSv.[31] When using CT for attenuation correction, the radiation dose from the CT can be reduced by adjusting the acquisition parameters: kVp, mAs, scan length, FOV, and scan pitch (see Table 8-2).

Diagnostic quality CT scans in targeted populations can offer important additive information to the PET scan. In a study of 1126 asymptomatic patients with a quantitative coronary calcium score, the use of coronary calcium assessment in conjunction with myocardial perfusion assessment independently

Table 8-2

Recommended Strategies for Reducing the Radiation Dose from CT

CT Technique	Description	Techniques for Minimizing Dose
Shallow free breath	For scanners that require more than 10 secs to cover heart instruct the patient to breathe using small breaths though the study.	• Reduce current to <10 mAs • Reduce voltage to <100 kVp for lower BMI patients • Use dose modulation • Use high pitch acquisition (minimal slice overlap)
End expiration breath hold	For scanners that require less than 10 secs to cover heart instruct the patient to breathe out slightly then hold breath.	• Reduce current to <10 mAs • Reduce voltage to <100 kVp for lower BMI patients • Use dose modulation • Use high pitch acquisition (minimal slice overlap)
Cine-CT	For scanners with pre-installed cine-CT protocol.	• Proprietary technique. Follow manufacturers' recommendations.

(Reproduced with permission from Case JA, deKemp RA, Slomka PJ, et al: Status of cardiovascular PET radiation exposure and strategies for reduction: An Information Statement from the Cardiovascular PET Task Force, J Nucl Cardiol. 2017 Aug;24(4):1427-1439)

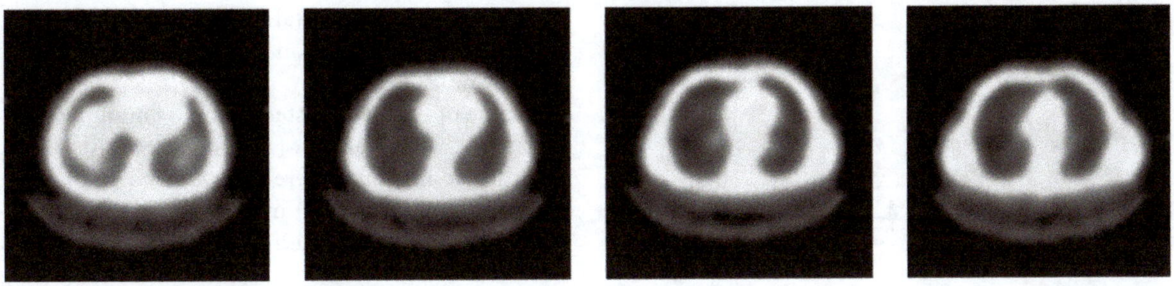

FIGURE 8-3 Iterative reconstruction of transmission studies can improve the image quality of attenuation maps and decrease the need for long acquisition times. The resulting images produce a very high quality transmission map with a very low radiation dose (0.01 mSv) and acquisition times can be as little as 60 seconds.

improved the prediction of future cardiac events.[34] In most cases, the added radiation exposure from a diagnostic CT (2.9 mSv for coronary calcium study on Siemens Biograph 64 PET/CT scanner,[35]) is not justified given its limited diagnostic value; however, in patients with no known coronary disease, low-dose, diagnostic CT image may add important clinical information.[35]

An external gamma line source can also be used for acquiring a patient-specific attenuation map.[24,25] When sufficient counts are present, this approach provides a very low-radiation dose, less than 0.01 mSv. Combining line source attenuation correction with iterative reconstruction methods can provide very high-quality attenuation maps using a relatively short transmission acquisition (Figure 8-3).

OPTIMIZING PET ACQUISITION PROTOCOLS

3D Imaging

The 511 keV photons used in PET are created when a positron annihilates with an electron creating two photons traveling in opposite directions. When these two photons are detected, a unique line of site can be determined. Unlike SPECT, this can be done without the use of collimation, thereby improving the overall system sensitivity by upward of 500%.[36] Despite the fact that PET imaging systems do not require collimation to determine the source of an annihilation event, many systems still use collimating septa (2D imaging) to reduce randoms, scatter, and singles events. The challenge in acquiring PET images with collimating septa (3D imaging) is the high singles count rate during the acquisition increases random coincidence events, losses owing to deadtime and increases scatter (Figure 8-4). In addition, the increased size of the dataset makes data processing more computationally intensive.

When 3D imaging is performed correctly, the increased system sensitivity can be used to enable lower dose imaging. ASNC recommends a 30 mCi dosage for rest and stress when 3D imaging is used and 50–60 mCi at rest and stress when 2D is used.[37] Comparisons of 2D and 3D protocols have demonstrated that equivalent accuracy can be obtained in 3D mode with a significantly lower radiation dosage.[38] In addition, absolute MBF measurements appear to be equivalent between 2D and 3D acquisitions. When 3D is available, clinicians should utilize imaging in 3D.

ADVANTAGES OF PET INSTRUMENTATION

PET scanners differ considerably from their SPECT counterparts in that collimation is not necessary to create an image. The main determinates of the maximum image quality that can be obtained from a PET scanner are: detector material, system dead-time, and field of view.

For the scintillator crystal, the denser the material, the higher is its photoelectric (PE) fraction, or its ability to stop the incoming 511 keV radiation completely on the first interaction. Also, high luminosity or light yield (expressed as the number of light

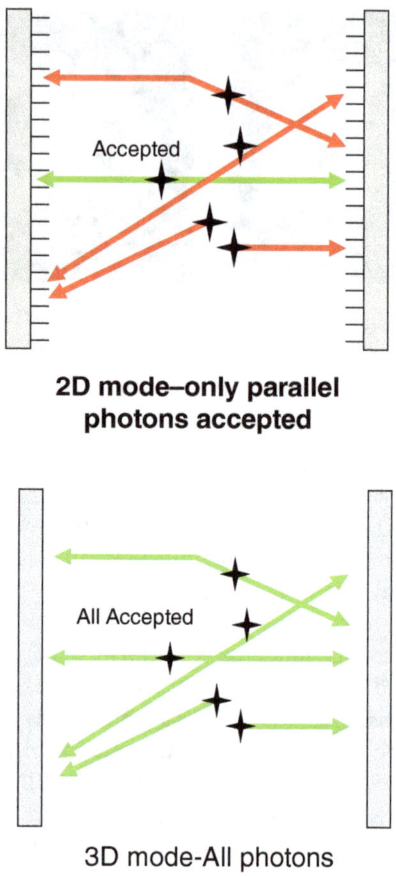

FIGURE 8-4 2D imaging use a system of septa to restrict the coincidence event to only those photons traveling perpendicular to the detector surface. By removing the septa, all true events are allowed to enter the system. In addition, the number of randoms, singles and scatter event are also increased, requiring additional processing steps to remove this additional signal.

photons emitted for each MeV of energy absorbed) is desirable for signal-to-noise and photon energy discrimination. Finally, the speed at which a detector emits visible light after absorbing a 511 keV γ-ray is directly proportional to its count-rate capability. This is essential when considering the very high count rates observed in 3D acquisitions.

The coincidence timing is also crucial in determining the system sensitivity and ultimate image quality. To enable 3D imaging, the system deadtime must be short enough that a single count can be fully recorded before the next photon arrives. This depends on the electronics of the system and the recovery time of the crystal to disperse all of the optical energy deposited by an interacting photon (light decay time).

Some of the latest systems employ multiple rings to extend the field of view (FOV) of the PET scanner. For cardiac imaging, there is little need to increase the FOV; however, in 3D mode, the increased number of rings increases the number of oblique planes that visualize the center of the FOV thus increasing sensitivity. See Table 8-3 for a summary of camera features and their effect on camera sensitivity.

Time of flight also has the potential for improving camera sensitivity. In phantom studies, this can assist in improving camera sensitivity. This improvement in sensitivity in patients translated in patient to an increase in sensitivity ranging from 15% in smaller patients to 40% in larger patients.[39]

Reconstruction algorithms. Current PET/CT systems employ an accelerated iterative reconstruction (OSEM) algorithm, incorporating CT attenuation maps, corrections for scatter, random events, spatial system response, and deadtime.[40, 41] Most PET/CT scanners offer isotropic spatial resolution only for the central FOV and resolution deteriorates in the transverse direction toward the edge of the FOV.

Using the point spread function (PSF) during image reconstruction can improve the uniformity of spatial resolution across the FOV. A penalized likelihood iterative reconstruction algorithm, incorporating PSF and suppression of large variations between the neighboring voxels in a large number of iterations, can be utilized to control noise.[40] PSF modeling has also been shown to provide better definition of subtle myocardial perfusion defects. The combination of TOF reconstruction and point-spread function correction has also been shown to improve image quality.[41,42]

All of these resolution enhancing techniques have the potential to reduce the need for high-dosage PET studies. Future studies are needed to determine whether using these advanced reconstruction techniques can enable clinics to use lower patient doses.

DOSE REDUCTION STRATEGIES

Cardiovascular PET myocardial perfusion imaging with ^{82}Rb, regardless of scanner type, is a low-radiation procedure, with total radiation doses of

Table 8-3

Effect of Instrumentation Choices on Radiation Dose

PET Scanner Feature	Description	Effect on Dose
3D (septa retracted)	The PET scanner retracts the septa allowing the system the record all 511 events. This allows more true events in, but increases scatter, randoms and singles events.	Can improve system sensitivity by up to 500%, reducing dose needed for study.
Newer scintillator crystal	Allows for better energy discrimination (reducing scatter) and shorter dead time.	Can improve SNR by reducing the contaminating signal.
Fast electronics	Reduces number of randoms and improves resolution. This improvement in resolution can improve SNR by reducing partial volume effect and random counts.	Can improve SNR by reducing the contaminating signal.
Time of Flight	Measures timing difference between coincidence events. This improve localization of the source of an annihilation event, thereby improving signal.	Improves SNR by improving resolution.

4 mSv for typical 2D protocols (50 mCi for each infusion) and 2 mSv for typical 3D protocols (25 mCi for each infusion). In addition, dose reductions can be achieved through: (1) the use of 3D imaging, (2) reducing the number of attenuation scans, and (3) the use of weight-adjusted radioactivity administration.

The most successful strategies for reducing patient dose are:

- **Use of 3D imaging when possible:** When well-validated 3D protocols are used, 3D imaging offers the greatest opportunity for reducing patient dose while maintaining or even improving image quality. Despite this, clinicians should carefully examine the quality of 3D images to ensure scatter correction, randoms correction, and 3D reconstruction algorithms that have been implemented corrected and do not introduce additional artifacts.
- **Optimize transmission scan settings:** Radiation dose from transmission scans can vary from 1/100 of the emission dose to nearly equivalent radiation dosages. For all transmission scanning approaches, single transmission scan approaches should be considered with optional repeat transmission scanning when patient motion is suspected. In addition, the laboratory should avoid high-dose diagnostic CT scanning on those patients where the addition of quantitative coronary calcium information would provide little value to the study.
- **Minimize FOV for CT studies:** Reducing the field of CT scout scans and the coverage of the CT study can also reduce the dose and should be considered when possible.
- **Avoid using ^{82}Rb positioning dosage:** In most cases, patients can be well positioned on dedicated and hybrid PET systems without using an emission scout scan. Because of the intrinsically lower radiation dose from the transmission scan, position should be verified using transmission scanning alone.
- **Use iterative reconstruction on all emission images:** Iterative reconstruction methods should be used in PET to improve the signal-to-noise in reconstructed images. Filtered backprojection techniques should be avoided.
- **Use weight-adjusted tracer doses:** Newer generator cart systems have been approved for use with a weight-adjusted dosing protocol. When possible, weight-adjusted patient doses should be used.

CONCLUSIONS

Radiation dose-reduction strategies should play a role in optimizing imaging protocols but should never reduce the diagnostic efficacy of an imaging test. Myocardial perfusion PET using ^{13}N-ammonia and ^{82}Rb offers a low radiation dose protocol for acquiring high-quality cardiac data. In addition, several new technologies have been introduced for reducing patient dose while maintaining and even improving overall image quality. These protocols can also be adapted to meet patient needs, including using the CT scanning to investigate coronary calcium in patients with no known coronary disease and weight-adjusted dosing protocols.

REFERENCES

1. Holly TA, Abbot BG, Mallah MA, et al. Single photon emission computed tomography. *J Nucl Card.* 2010;17(5): 941–973.
2. Dilsizian V, Bacharach SL, Beanlands RS, et.al. ASNC imaging guidelines for nuclear cardiology procedures: PET myocardial perfusion and metabolism clinical imaging. *J Nucl Cardiol.* 2009;16(4):651, http://www.asnc.org/imageuploads/ImagingGuidelinesPETJuly2009.pdf
3. Cerqueira MD, Allman KC, Ficaro EP, et al. American Society for Nuclear Cardiology Information Statement: recommendations for reducing radiation exposure in myocardial perfusion imaging. *J Nucl Cardiol.* 2010;17:709–718.
4. Piccinelli M, Garcia EV. Advances in software for faster procedure and lower radiotracer dose myocardial perfusion imaging. *Prog Cardiovasc Dis.* 2015;57:579–587.
5. Hill KD, Einstein AJ. New approaches to radiation exposure. *Trends Cardiovasc Med.* 2016;26: 55–65.
6. Einstein AJ, Blankstein R, Andrews H, et al. Comparison of image quality, myocardial perfusion, and left ventricular function between standard imaging and single-injection ultra-low-dose imaging using a high-efficiency SPECT camera: the MILLISIEVERT study. *J Nucl Med.* 2014;55:1430–1437.
7. Weber W, Zanzonico P. The controversial linear no-threshold model. *J Nucl Med.* Jan 1, 2017;58:1:7–8.
8. Image Wisely, Radiation Safety in Adult Medical Imaging, www.imagewisely.org, last 29 Apr, 2018.
9. Case JA, deKemp RA, Slomka PJ, Smith MF, Heller GV, Cerqueira MD. Status of cardiovascular PET radiation exposure and strategies for reduction: an information statement from the Cardiovascular PET Task Force. *JNucl Cardiol.,* 2017 Aug;24:4:1427–1439.
10. Alexandrov LB1, Nik-Zainal S, Wedge DC, Campbell PJ, Stratton MR. Deciphering signatures of mutational processes operative in human cancer. *Cell Rep.* 2013 Jan 31;3(1):246–259.
11. Reisz JA, Bansal N, Qian J, Zhao W, Furdui CM. Effects of ionizing radiation on biological molecules—mechanisms of damage and emerging methods of detection Antioxid Redox Signal. 2014 Jul 10;21(2):260-92.
12. Pierce DA, Preston DL. Radiation-related cancer risks at low doses among atomic bomb survivors. *Radiat Res.* 2000;154:178–186.
13. Brenner DJ, Doll R, Goodhead DT, et al. Cancer risks attributable to low doses of ionizing radiation: assessing what we really know. *Proc. National Aca. Sci.* 2003 Nov 25;100(24):13761–13766.
14. Nguyen PK , Lee WH, Li YF, et al. Assessment of the radiation effects of cardiac CT angiography using protein and genetic biomarkers. *JACC Cardiovasc Imaging.* 2015;8:873–884.
15. International Commission on Radiological Protection, 2015. Radiation dose to patients from radiopharmaceuticals: A compendium of current information related to frequently used substances. ICRP Publication 128. Ann. ICRP 44(2S).
16. Bracco Diagnostics. [Prescribing Information] CardioGen-82 (Rubidium Rb 82 Generator), Bracco Diagnostics (NJ, USA) revised April 2013. Available at: http://imaging.bracco.com/sites/braccoimaging.com/files/technica_sheet_pdf/Cardiogen%20Full%20Prescribing%20Information.pdf. Accessed June 30, 2016.
17. Jubilant DRAXIMAGE. [Prescribing Information] Ruby-Fill (rubidium Rb 82 generator), Jubilant DRAXIMAGE (Kirkland Quebec). Available at: http://www.draximage.com/DATA/TEXTEDOC/Approval-202153-Ruby-Fill-Labeling-30Sept-2016.pdf. Accessed October 1, 2016.
18. Senthamizhchelvan S, Bravo PE, Esaias C, et al. Human biodistribution and radiation dosimetry of 82Rb. *J Nucl Med.* 2010;51:1592–1599.

19. International Commission on Radiological Protection. Radiation dose to patients from radiopharmaceuticals: A compendium of current information related to frequently used substances. *ICRP Publication*. 2015;128:Ann. ICRP 44(2S).
20. Hunter CR, Hill J, Ziadi MC, Beanlands RS, deKemp RA. Biodistribution and radiation dosimetry of (82)Rb at rest and during peak pharmacological stress in patients referred for myocardial perfusion imaging. *Eur J Nucl Med Mol Imaging*. 2015;42:1032–1042.
21. Schelbert HR, Phelps ME, Hoffman EJ, Huang SC, Selin CE, Kuhl DE. Regional myocardial perfusion assessed with N-13 labeled ammonia and positron emission computerized axial tomography. *Am J Cardiol*. 1979;43:209–218.
22. Som P, Atkins HL, Bandoypadhyay D, et al. A fluorinated glucose analog, 2-fluoro-2-deoxy-D-glucose (F-18): nontoxic tracer for rapid tumor detection. *J Nucl Med*. 1980;21(7): 670–675.
23. Maddahi J, Czernin J, Lazewatsky J, et al. Phase I, first-in-human study of BMS747158, a novel 18F-labeled tracer for myocardial perfusion PET: dosimetry, biodistribution, safety, and imaging characteristics after a single injection at rest. *J Nucl Med*. 2011;52:1490–1498.
24. Berman DS, Maddahi J, Tamarappoo BK, et al. Phase II safety and clinical comparison with single-photon emission computed tomography myocardial perfusion imaging for detection of coronary artery disease: flurpiridaz F 18 positron emission tomography. *J Am Coll Cardiol*. 2013 Jan 29;61(4):469–477.
25. Carroll LR, Kertz P, Orcut O. The orbiting rod source: improving performance in PET transmission correction scans. In: *Emission Computed Tomography: Current Trends*. New York, NY: The Society of Nuclear Medicine; 1983:235–247.
26. Hsu BL, Case JA, Moser KW, Bateman TM, Cullom SJ. Reconstruction of rapidly acquired germanium-68 transmission scans for cardiac PET attenuation correction. *J Nucl Cardiol*. 2007;14:706–714.
27. Padole A, Ali Khawaja RD, Kalra M, Singh S. CT radiation dose and iterative reconstruction techniques. *AJR Am J Roentgenol*. 2015;204:W384-W392.
28. de Juan R, Seifert B, Berthold T, von Schulthess GK, Goerres GW. Clinical evaluation of a breathing protocol for PET/CT. *Eur Radiol*. 2004;14:1118–1123.
29. Alessio AM, Kohlmyer S, Branch K, Chen G, Caldwell J, Kinahan P. Cine CT for attenuation correction in cardiac PET/CT. *J Nucl Med*. 2007;48:794–801.
30. Goerres GW, Kamel E, Heidelberg TN, Schwitter MR, Burger C, von Schulthess GK. PET-CT image co-registration in the thorax: influence of respiration. *Eur J Nucl Med Mol Imaging*. 2002;29:351–360.
31. Xia T, Alessio AM, De Man B, Manjeshwar R, Asma E, Kinahan PE. Ultra-low dose CT attenuation correction for PET/CT. *Phys Med Biol*. 2012;57:309–328.
32. Abdoli M, Dierckx RAJO, Zaidi H. Metal artifact reduction strategies for improved attenuation correction in hybrid PET/CT imaging. *Med. Phys*. 2012;39:3343–3361.
33. Gould L, Pan T-S, Laghin C, Johnson NP, Guha A, Sdringola S. Frequent diagnostic errors in cardiac PET/CT due to misregistration of CT attenuation and emission PET images: a definite analysis of causes, consequences and corrections. *J Nucl Med*. 2007;48:1112–1121.
34. Chang S, Nabi F, Xu J, et al. The coronary artery calcium score and stress myocardial perfusion imaging provide independent and complementary prediction of cardiac risk. *J Am Coll Cardiol*. 2009;54:1872–1882.
35. Einstein AJ, Johnson LL, Bokhari S, et al. Agreement of visual estimation of coronary artery calcium from low-dose CT attenuation correction scans in hybrid PET/CT and SPECT/CT with standard Agatston Score. *J Am Coll Cardiol*. 2010;56:1914–1921.
36. Cherry SR, Dahlborn M, Hoffman EJ. 3D PET using a conventional multislice tomography without septa. *J Comput Assist Tomogr*. 1991;15:655–668.
37. Dilsizian V, Bacharach SL, Beanlands SR, et al. ASNC imaging guidelines/SNMMI procedure standard for positron emission tomography (PET) nuclear cardiology procedures. *J Nucl Cardiol*. 2016;23:1187–1226.
38. Lekx KS, deKemp RA, Beanlands RS, et al. 3D versus 2D dynamic 82Rb myocardial blood

flow imaging in a canine model of stunned and infarcted myocardium. *Nucl Med Commun.* 2010;31:75–81.

39. El Fakhri G, Surti S, Trott CM, Scheuermann J, Karp JS. Improvement in lesion detection with whole-body oncologic time-of-flight PET. *J Nucl Med.* 2011 Mar;52(3):347–353.
40. Hudson HM1, Larkin RS. Accelerated image reconstruction using ordered subsets of projection data. *IEEE Trans Med Imaging.* 1994;13(4):601–609.
41. Akamatsu G, Ishikawa K, Mitsumoto K, et al. Improvement in PET/CT image quality with a combination of point-spread function and time-of-flight in relation to reconstruction parameters. *J Nucl Med.* 2012;53:1716–1722.
42. Teoh EJ, McGowan DR, Macpherson RE, Bradley KM, Gleeson FV. Phantom and clinical evaluation of the bayesian penalized likelihood reconstruction algorithm q.Clear on an LYSO PET/CT system. *J Nucl Med.*2015;56: 1447–1452.

EDITOR'S PERSPECTIVE

Gary V. Heller

Radiation exposure through medical imaging procedures has been a concern for patients, society, and healthcare providers for several decades. This is of particular concern for patients with known or suspected CAD who often undergo more than one imaging procedure with a radiation source. The American Society of Nuclear Cardiology has recommended reducing radiation exposure in myocardial perfusion stress testing below current levels, proposing that cardiac PET would be a reasonable means of accomplishing this.[1] This current chapter on cardiac PET radiation exposure is excellent in its inclusive description of current data as well as listing methods to further reduce PET radiation for patients. The conclusion is that cardiac PET procedures are already below ASNC recommendations and the author describes methods available to further reduce PET radiation exposure.

A very important conclusion from this chapter and the data are that radiation exposure from either of the two PET myocardial perfusion agents is low, substantially lower than current SPECT practices and much lower than ASNC recommendations.[2] This is in no small part due to the very short half-lives of both agents, but even FDG imaging—which has a 2-hour half-life—the radiation exposure of approximately 6 mSv is well below those recommendations.

Radiation exposure to the patient should be part of the decision-making process for the referring healthcare provider. For example, in considering positive attributes in comparison to other modalities, especially current SPECT, the ASNC/SNMMI Position Statement lists low radiation exposure of a PET study as one of the compelling reasons to choose cardiac PET over other imaging modalities.[3] In this article, it specifically recommended this approach to young patients, particularly those with known CAD, on the assumption that such patients over their lifetime are very likely to undergo many imaging procedures with radiation exposure due to numerous future clinical scenarios requiring testing.

Lowering radiation exposure has been on the minds of practicing healthcare providers for a number of years, and society has responded by recommending lower exposure tests and encouraging development of methods to further lower exposure. As stated previously, while currently cardiac PET radiation exposure is low, the author presents several practical and technical methods to further reduce already low radiation. This will be an important consideration for any laboratory with an established PET program. Several of the methods are within reach, such as moving from 2D- to 3D-imaging, as well as eliminating a second attenuation correction study when not necessary (which is often). Does all this really matter? This is much difficult to answer, as it would require a large prospective trial to do so. A recent article demonstrated that DNA damage occurs at doses higher than 3 mSv. However, all cell DNA responses for doses <25 mSv were related to cell death and not cell cycle regulation.[4] The authors concluded that there is little evidence that low-dose radiation causes carcinogenesis at any commonly used dosages in nuclear cardiology. For dosages commonly used in cardiac PET, no detectable DNA changes were produced. This radiation exposure level per patient is achievable with many of the PET studies being performed.

In summary, this chapter reviews data on radiation exposure with cardiac PET procedures and methods aiming to further reduce exposure in selected patients. Low radiation exposure with cardiac PET procedures should be reassuring to referring healthcare providers and patients as well as the nuclear cardiology community. It should also be emphasized that low radiation exposure is only one of many compelling reasons to consider cardiac PET for optimal patient care.

References for Editor's Perspective

1. Cerqueira MD, Allman KC, Ficaro EP, Hansen CL, Nichols KJ, Thompson R C, et al. American Society for Nuclear Cardiology Information Statement: recommendations for reducing radiation exposure in myocardial perfusion imaging. *J Nucl Cardiol.* 2010;17:709-718.
2. Desiderio MC, Lundbye JB, Baker WL, et al. Current Status of Patient Radiation Exposure of Cardiac PET and SPECT Myocardial Perfusion

Imaging: a report from the Intersocietal Accreditation Commission Database. *Circ Cardiovasc Imaging*. 2018. In press.

3. Bateman TM, Dilsizian V, Beanlands RS, DePuey EG, Heller GV, Wolinsky DA. American Society of Nuclear Cardiology and Society of Nuclear Medicine and Molecular Imaging Joint Position Statement on the clinical indications for myocardial perfusion PET. *J Nucl Cardiol.* 2016;23(5):1227-31.
4. Lee WH, Nguyen P, Hu S, et al. Variable activation of the DNA damage response pathways in patients undergoing single-photon emission computed yomography myocardial perfusion imaging. *Circ Cardiovasc Imaging.* 2015;8:e002851.

SECTION

5

MYOCARDIAL VIABILITY ASSESSMENT: THE CURRENT ROLE OF CARDIAC PET

Cardiac PET Myocardial Viability Assessment: Emerging Clinical Data

CHAPTER 9

S. Massalha, Rob S. Beanlands, and Gary R. Small

INTRODUCTION

The utility of myocardial viability imaging hinges on the premise that recovery of left ventricular (LV) function in ischemic heart disease can be achieved through coronary revascularization and results in improved outcomes and quality of life. Rahimtoola first characterized that chronic impaired coronary perfusion resulted in impaired contractility, which he termed hibernation.[1] He suggested that a heart with reduced LVEF from hibernation could be improved by revascularization. The challenge since that time has been for viability imaging to identify those patients whose hearts will recover function and who will subsequently experience improvement in quality of life. It is a challenge that remains valid and alive 30 years after those early descriptions.

Emerging data from ischemic heart failure statistics have highlighted the plight of these patients. Mortality rates remain disconcerting high; all-cause mortality at 10 years is approximately 70% of medically managed and 60% of surgically treated individuals in the younger population and even higher in older patients.[2] Mortality can also be high early in the course of the condition, depending on the treatment chosen. Mortality at surgical revascularization can be as high as 8% within 30 days even with modern operative techniques.[2] The need, therefore, remains to accurately, thoroughly, and thoughtfully evaluate patients with ischemic heart failure to optimize management decisions.

In this chapter, cardiac PET viability assessment is described and five areas of emerging data are covered:

1. The STICH trial and STICH viability substudy
2. PARR-2 and Ottawa Five: has time altered the figures?
4. Quality of life outcomes: cardiac PET viability assessment can help
5. Combination of PET and MRI to refine and redefine viability definition

MECHANISMS OF PET VIABILITY IMAGING

Two types of dysfunctional but viable myocardial segments are described: stunned and hibernating. Stunned myocardium is the result of short episodes of ischemic insults that cause a temporarily depressed contractility in the corresponding area with no infarction. This phenomenon is generally associated with normal resting coronary blood flow. In contrast, hibernating myocardium reflects reduced resting perfusion and down regulation of coronary blood flow that is thought to be the result of repetitive ischemia with retained glucose metabolic activity.[3] The net result in terms of a reduction in LV contractility is observed with both stunning and hibernation. Stunning may recover spontaneously, while the persistent dysfunction of hibernating myocardium has the potential for LV functional recovery following adequate revascularization. These pathways are described in Figure 9-1.

Scarred myocardium from previous myocardial infarction or chronic ischemia is to be distinguished from viable (stunned or hibernating) areas. Some myocardial segments may contain both scar and viable proportions, typically referred to as nontransmural scar. At a segmental level, the ratio of scar to viable myocardium will determine whether revascularization of that area may restore normal contractile function. The net balance of scarred versus viable myocardium from each LV segment determines whether global improvement in LV ejection fraction is likely to be observed following revascularization.

CARDIAC PET METABOLIC EVALUATION OF MYOCARDIAL VIABILITY

Generally the assessment of viability is reserved for patients with low-ejection fraction, often considered as 35% LVEF or less. The evaluation of myocardial viability can begin by an assessment of perfusion, either with SPECT or PET. Ischemia detected on stress/rest imaging in an area of hypokinesis indicates viable myocardium. Impaired resting perfusion may also be detected on perfusion imaging. Characteristically this is described as reduced tracer uptake on resting perfusion imaging, which does not deteriorate on stress imaging. Such abnormalities may represent transmural scar, nontransmural scar, or viable myocardium.

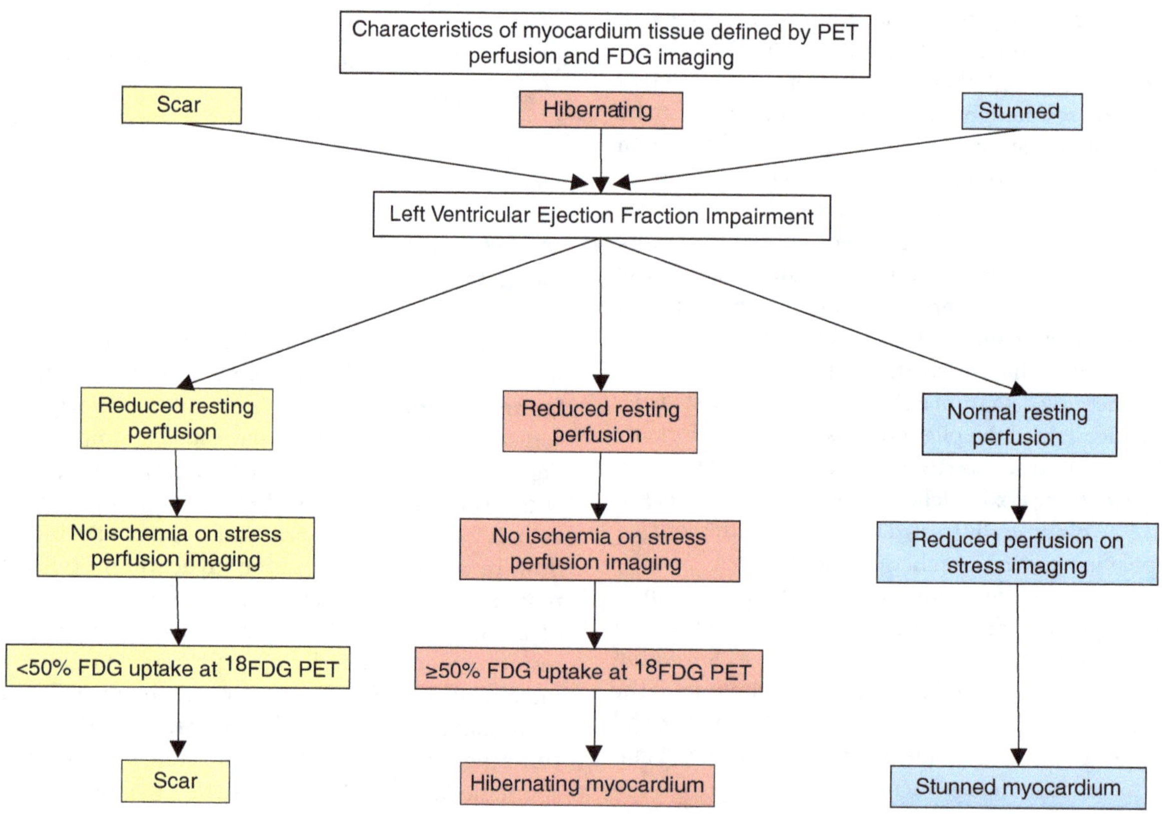

FIGURE 9-1 Characterization of Dysfunctional Myocardium in Ischemic Heart Failure. A schematic representation of the different types of tissue present in dysfunctional myocardium: scar tissue, hibernating or stunned myocardium.

In order to differentiate between scar (nonviable) or viable myocardium, cardiac PET utilizes the metabolic adaptation of cardiomyocytes that have been exposed to chronic poor perfusion. Chronically ischemic cardiomyocytes shift from using free fatty acids (FFA) to glucose as their primary energy substrate.[4] The change in energy substrate can be detected by an F-18 tracer labeled with glucose, F-18 fluorodeoxyglucose PET imaging (^{18}FDG). Myocardial segments with preserved FDG uptake and markedly reduced perfusion is considered hibernating and viable while those with absent FDG uptake and reduced perfusion tracer uptake are considered nonviable scar.

Figure 9-2 demonstrates a cardiac PET viability study of a 66-year-old female patient with progressive dyspnea and a severely reduced LV systolic function with an LVEF of 25%. In this figure the N-13 ammonia ($^{13}NH_3$) perfusion and the corresponding ^{18}FDG uptake images are in Panel A. On the perfusion images there is a moderate reduction in tracer uptake in the entire lateral inferior-lateral, anterior-lateral segments, and apex. In contrast there is >50% uptake of ^{18}FDG in these areas.

These regions of *mismatch* between resting $^{13}NH_3$ uptake and ^{18}FDG uptake are considered to represent areas of viable myocardium. In contrast *matched* defects with reduced $^{13}NH_3$ and ^{18}FDG uptake would be representative of scar. In a case such as Figure 9-2, with a relatively large amount of viable myocardium and minimal scar volume the patient may well benefit from revascularization, and a recommendation was made for further evaluation of the coronary anatomy. Coronary angiography in this patient demonstrated 2-vessel coronary disease with a mid-LAD 90% stenosis and an occluded RCA with left-sided collaterals to the distal branches. Two 2-vessel CABG was performed to the distal RCA and LAD and postsurgical revascularization the LVEF improved to 55%.

ADDRESSING THE FINDINGS OF STICH IN RELATION TO CONTEMPORARY VIABILITY ASSESSMENT

The utility of identifying viable myocardium in an era of contemporary surgical and medical practice was recently considered in the STICH and PARR 2 studies.[5,6] In 2011, the STICH trial (surgical treatment for ischemic heart failure) was published.[5] The trial determined to identify the role of surgical revascularization versus medical management in patients with ischemic heart disease, impaired LV ejection fraction (</=35%), and suitable coronary artery surgical targets. The trial recruited 1212 patients and randomized them to optimal medical care versus optimal medical care plus coronary artery bypass surgery (CABG). A trend was seen at 12 months for an improvement in cardiovascular mortality with CABG versus medical therapy ($P = 0.05$).

An investigator-selected nonrandomized subpopulation (601 patients) of the trial underwent viability imaging.[7] Viability in these individuals was defined as 5 or more segments of abnormal resting segments but manifesting contractile reserve during dobutamine stress echo or having 11 or more viable segments on the basis of relative tracer uptake at SPECT imaging. In this nonrandomized population of patients the substudy determined that preoperative viability assessment did not predict cardiovascular or total mortality.

Unfortunately, this substudy inadvertently gave rise to the controversial notion that viability assessment was not useful in the evaluation of patients with ischemic heart failure. This conclusion, however, does not reflect the many limitations and details of the STICH substudy.

Of considerable importance, viability assessment in the STICH trial was not randomly allocated. While randomization may have afforded some balance this would have been complicated and impractical. Nevertheless, without randomization it is possible that selection bias may have impacted the use of viability imaging. An additional important limitation to the substudy was that only a small percentage of patients that underwent CABG (19%) were deemed negative for myocardial viability. This limited the power of the analysis, and rendered a nonsignificant difference likely. Other limitations of the study included the fact that sensitive standard viability assessment with ^{18}FDG PET was not performed nor were there any management recommendations made following viability assessment that might have optimized outcomes in the study.

The STICH viability paper should be acknowledged as an observational study imbedded in a randomized trial. It observed that nonrandomized

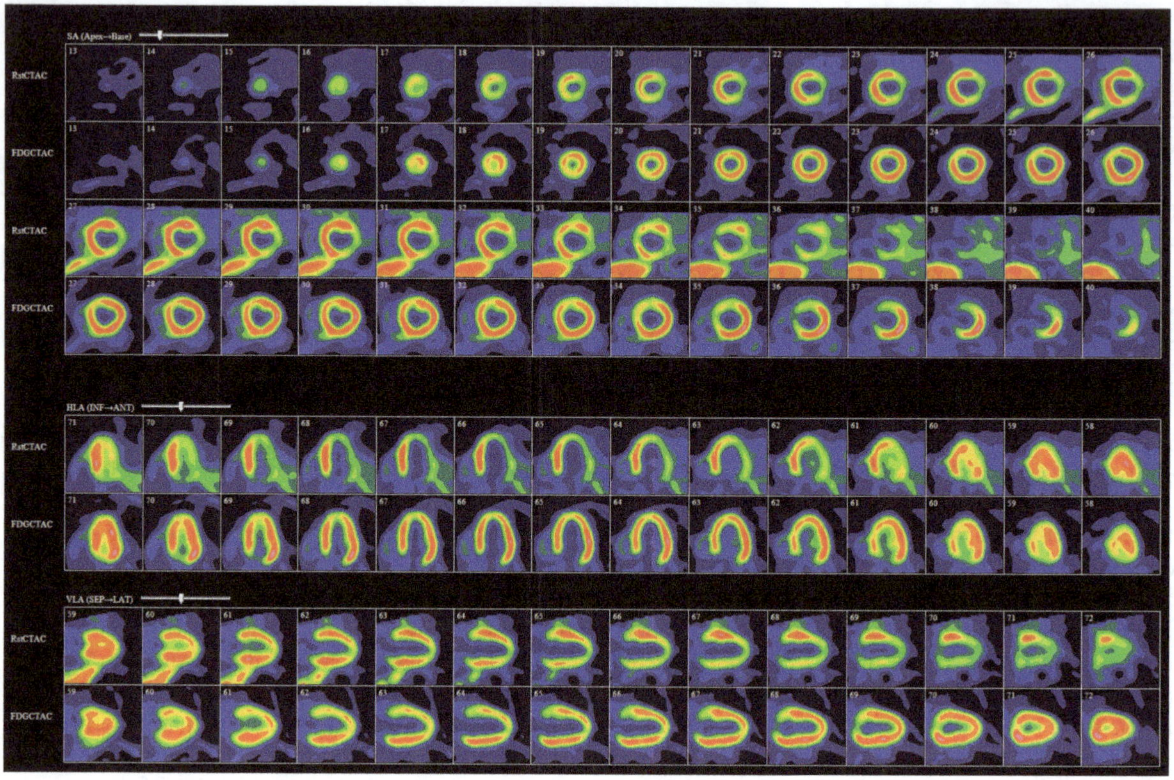

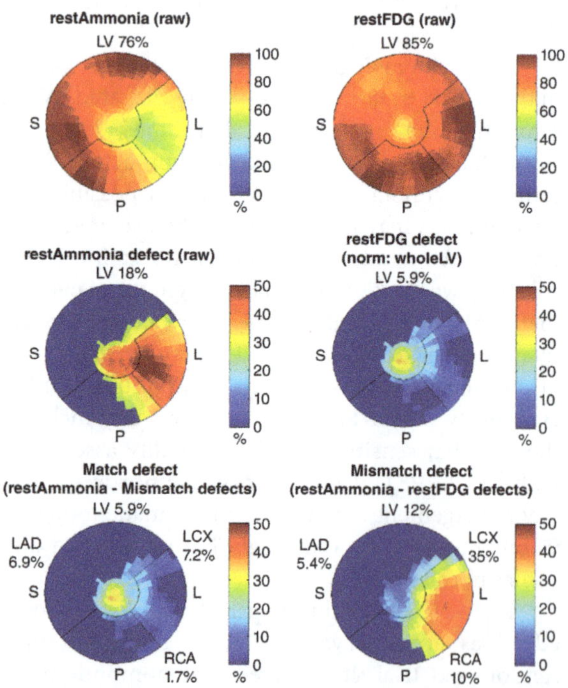

FIGURE 9-2 An Example of PET Imaging in Viability Assessment. (A): Relative metabolic and perfusion imaging using FDG and 13-ammonia ($^{13}NH_3$). Resting perfusion: moderate tracer uptake reduction in lateral, basal to mid-infero-lateral, and antero-lateral segments. Metabolic imaging: FDG in all areas of reduced perfusion. (B): Quantitative metabolic/perfusion imaging using ^{18}FDG and 13-ammonia ($^{13}NH_3$) in the same patient as (A). Quantitative resting perfusion imaging confirms a moderate reduction in tracer uptake in the lateral, infero-lateral, and antero-lateral segments. FDG uptake remains preserved (>50%) in these areas. Area of mismatch (resting FDG uptake but reduced perfusion) by quantitative analysis was 5.9%. Scar volume (reduced perfusion and reduced FDG uptake) is minimal, <1%. The LV is therefore almost entirely viable.

stress/rest SPECT imaging or stress echocardiography assessment was not useful in determining cardiovascular outcomes in a population of patients with ischemic heart failure. It helped to generate a hypothesis that stress/echo or SPECT imaging may not be superior to physician gestalt, but in the setting of extreme study-design limitations. In future studies it is hoped that, if possible and practical, the limitations of STICH viability paper can be avoided.

The 10-year follow-up data from STICH were published in 2016.[2] An absolute 10% improvement in total mortality with surgical revascularization in comparison to medical management was seen (79% versus 68% for patients >67 years of age and 60% versus 48% for those <54 years of age for medical versus surgical management respectively $P < 0.005$) (Figure 9-3). The long-term data also established the high incidence of postoperative mortality in patients with ischemic heart failure (2%-8% at 30 days, depending on the patient's age). The STICH study has, therefore, taught much in terms of outcomes in ischemic heart failure. It has highlighted the difficulties clinicians and their patients face in weighing up whether the risks of adverse perioperative events can be mitigated by potential long-term survival benefits. Whether the STICH viability paper helped clinicians formulate decisions in ischemic heart failure patients is worth considering. Firm conclusions as to the utility of stress echo or SPECT imaging to guide management strategy cannot be gleaned from these data and it remains to be determined whether evaluation with other imaging modalities might have been more useful. In leaving these questions unanswered, the STICH viability paper has perhaps highlighted, paradoxically, the critical importance of a thorough and systematic evaluation of these complex cases by accurate imaging methods. At the outset, the primary objective of STICH was to investigate the benefit of CABG versus medical therapy and the results of STICH point out that this assessment remains important for decision making.

SUPPORTIVE PROSPECTIVE DATA FOR A PET IMAGING STRATEGY: THE PARR-2 STUDY AND 5-YEAR OUTCOMES

To date, the largest randomized study to evaluate viability imaging in patients with severe LV dysfunction and the only study to investigate whether ^{18}FDG PET-assisted management has a beneficial effect on clinical outcomes is the PARR-2 (PET and recovery following revascularization-2) study.[6] In PARR-2, 430 patients were recruited with suspected or confirmed

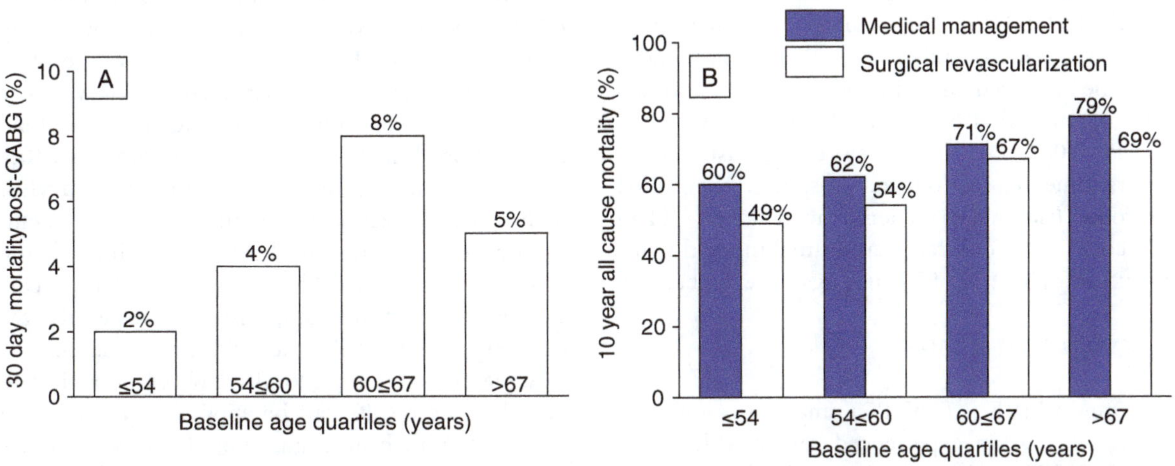

FIGURE 9.3 Mortality in Ischemic Heart Failure. Figures adapted from the 10-year follow-up data from STICH (2). Early, 30-day mortality postcoronary artery bypass surgery is demonstrated in (A). In (B) 10-year total mortality for patients with ischemic heart failure is shown in solid blue for medically managed patients and in solid white for those managed with surgical intervention (P= 0.004). (Data from Velazquez EJ, Lee KL, Jones RH, et al: Coronary-Artery Bypass Surgery in Patients with Ischemic Cardiomyopathy, N Engl J Med. 2016 Apr 21;374(16):1511-1520)

coronary artery disease and an EF of <35% and were randomized to a standard care versus PET imaging-assisted care.[6] Those that were randomized to the PET-assisted arm were assessed using FDG and perfusion PET. Following PET assessment a report of the viability data was issued along with a guidance statement indicating the likely benefit or otherwise of revascularization.

At 12-month follow-up both management arms of the study were seen to share similar event rates in the composite end-point (cardiac death, myocardial infarction, or recurrent hospital admission for cardiac causes). The primary composite end-point occurred in 30% of the PET group versus 36% exposed to standard care (HR 0.78 for PET versus standard care, 95% CI 0.58-1.1; $P = 0.15$). PARR-2 was also a test of the tendency of clinicians to adhere to the advice from imaging studies. In 25% of cases in fact clinicians chose to ignore the PET imaging advice. Furthermore post hoc analyses of the data revealed that when PET recommendations were adhered to, a reduction in adverse events was observed in the FDG PET-assisted patients (HR = 0.62 (95% CI 0.42-0.93; $P = 0.019$).

Five-year outcomes from PARR-2 were published in 2016.[8] Similar event rates were again seen in the primary composite event rates between PET guided versus standard care. Fifty-three percent of patients in the PET-guided care arm suffered a primary end-point versus 57% in the standard care arm (HR 0.82 95% CI 0.62-1.07 $P = 0.15$). In patients where physicians and patients adhered to PET recommendations, the improved outcomes observed at 12 months were maintained at 5 years (HR 0.73 95% CI 0.54-0.99, $P = 0.042$). PARR-2, therefore, demonstrated for the first time in a randomized prospectively enrolled controlled trial that in ischemic heart failure ^{18}FDG PET could assist clinical decision making and clinical outcomes if ^{18}FDG PET findings were adhered to.

OTTAWA FIVE STUDY

The Ottawa FIVE (^{18}FDG PET imaging of myocardial viability in an experienced center with access to ^{18}FDG PET and integration with clinical management teams) study considered PARR-2 patients recruited and managed at a single center.[9] At this center, cardiologists, cardiac surgeons, and heart failure specialists worked closely with experienced nuclear cardiologists with expertise in PET viability imaging. In the Ottawa FIVE cohort there was a >50% reduction in the primary end-point in the PET group in comparison to standard care (19% vs 41% for the primary end-point in PET vs standard care respectively, hazard ratio, 0.34; 95% confidence interval, 0.16-0.72; $P = 0.005$) (Figure 9-4). This substudy highlights that when PET imaging is integrated into clinical care, prognosis in ischemic heart failure can be improved.

CONCLUSIONS FROM STICH AND PARR-2

The emergent long-term follow-up data from STICH and PPAR-2 are a reminder of the need for better treatments, better assessment and clearer management pathways in these complex patients. STICH highlighted the need for accurate assessment. PARR-2 determined that viability imaging results could be relied on to assist clinical decision making. Ottawa FIVE suggests closer collaboration with experience across subspecialties in cardiology might also help improve the impact from ^{18}FDG imaging in these patients. The mortality rates in STICH at 10 years indicate that this condition should continue to remain a high priority for clinicians and researchers alike.

Corroborative data to support Ottawa FIVE and PPAR-2 results is available from a single center study examining ^{18}FDG PET imaging in 648 consecutive patients with known or suspected coronary artery disease and either regional or global LV systolic dysfunction.[10] In this study, patients who had >10% hibernating myocardium had improved survival with revascularization versus medical management. In contrast, in patients who had <5% hibernating myocardium a survival benefit was seen with medical management in comparison to revascularization (Figure 9-5). This study did have limitations as a single center nonrandomized observational trial. Whether the results can be applied more generally to the ischemic heart failure population will require further study. Nevertheless, the approach of the study investigators goes some way to help clinicians determine whether revascularization might be of benefit in this high-risk population and is consistent with the findings from Ottawa FIVE and PPAR-2 studies.

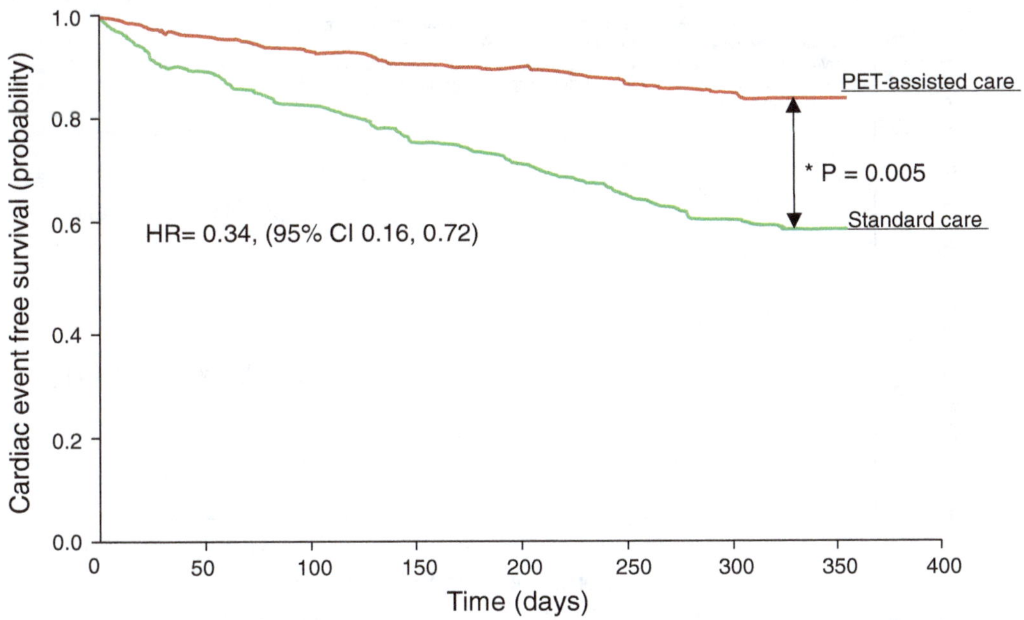

FIGURE 9-4 Impact of PET Assisted Care When PET Recommendations Were Adhered To. Adapted figure from the Ottawa Five cohort of PARR2 (111 patients).[9] When PET-assisted care is adhered to at an experience center a reduction of cardiovascular end points (death, myocardial infarction, or nonelective hospitalization for cardiac cause) is seen and the impact of PET in viability assessment is appreciated ($P = 0.005$). (Reproduced from Abraham A, Nichol G, Williams KA, et al: 18F-FDG PET imaging of myocardial viability in an experienced center with access to 18F-FDG and integration with clinical management teams: the Ottawa-FIVE substudy of the PARR 2 trial, J Nucl Med. 2010 Apr;51(4):567-574)

ARRHYTHMIA RISK ASSESSMENT: AN IMPORTANT PART OF CARDIAC PET VIABILITY IMAGING?

Patients with ischemic heart failure may be at risk of fatal ventricular arrhythmias. Guidelines for implantable cardiac defibrillators (ICDs) exist for both primary and secondary prevention. The PAREPET (Prediction of ARrhythmic Events with Positron Emission Tomography) study considered whether PET assessment of sympathetic denervation could predict cardiac events in patients suitable for primary prevention ICDs.[11]

Disruption of balanced ventricular sympathetic innervation may contribute to the development of malignant ventricular arrhythmias in ischemic heart failure. Chronic ischemia or prior myocardial infarction induces myocardial scar formation and sympathetic denervation to affected areas. It is the inhomogeneity of sympathetic innervation that appears to produce an arrhythmic substrate.[11] C11 meta-hydroxyephedrine (^{11}CHED) was used in PAREPET as a PET-radiolabeled catecholamine analog for imaging the autonomic nervous system. This tracer characterizes the norepinephrine presynaptic uptake and storage capacity and provides quantitative indication of the integrity of sympathetic function.[12]

In PAREPET ^{11}CHED uptake was assessed in 204 patients with ischemic heart failure (LVEF </=35%), unsuitable for coronary revascularization; PET perfusion imaging and viability assessment with ^{18}FDG was also performed. Patients were followed for a median of 4.1 years; the primary end-point was sudden cardiac arrest (SCA) as documented by arrhythmic death or appropriate ICD discharge.[11]

The amount of denervated LV was seen to be associated with SCA ($P = 0.001$). For each 1% increase in denervated myocardium there was a 5.7% increase in risk of SCA. Patients with the highest tertile of

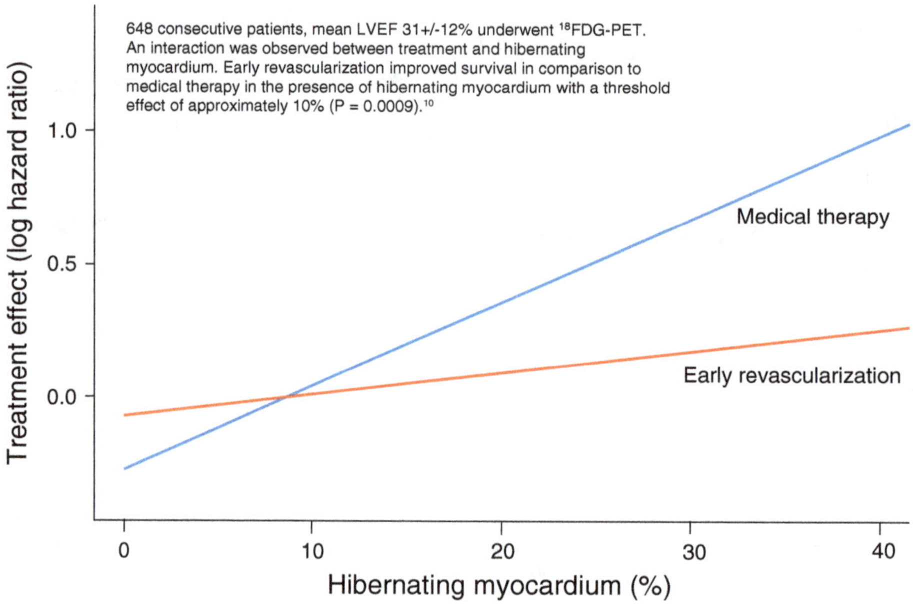

FIGURE 9-5 Relationship Between Percentage Hibernating Myocardium and Hazard Ratio (All-Cause Mortality). Increasing percentage of hibernating myocardium was associated with improved survival in patients undergoing revascularization (solid red line) comparison to medical management (solid blue line) (*P* = 0.0009). A threshold effect for this interaction was seen from percentage hibernating myocardium >10%.[10] (Reproduced from Ling LF, Marwick TH, Flores DR, et al: Identification of therapeutic benefit from revascularization in patients with left ventricular systolic dysfunction: inducible ischemia versus hibernating myocardium, Circ Cardiovasc Imaging. 2013 May 1;6(3):363-372)

sympathetic denervation had an annual SCA event rate of 6.7% whereas the intermediate and lowest tertile had annual SCA event rates of 2.2% and 1.2%, respectively (Figure 9-6).

PAREPET extends the potential utility of PET imaging in ischemic heart failure beyond quantification of LV scar and viability. ^{11}CHED imaging might help to confirm which patients are at highest risk of SCA and could be used to expedite ICD implantation in those patients at highest risk. PAREPET did not recruit those patients with ischemic heart failure who could be managed by revascularization. Whether patients with coronary anatomy suitable for revascularization might also be at risk of arrhythmic death from denervation will require further study. The PAREPET studies suggest that in the future, it could be considered reasonable to perform ^{11}CHED imaging in patients with ischemic heart failure who were unsuitable for revascularization but in whom further risk stratification for primary prevention ICD implantation was desirable. Further studies are needed to support this concept.

QUALITY OF LIFE OUTCOMES: CARDIAC PET VIABILITY ASSESSMENT CAN HELP

A very important aspect of the long-term success of revascularization in patients with heart failure is how the patients feel and their quality of life. Few studies have considered the potential that PET viability-assisted management could have on the quality of life in patients with ischemic heart failure.[13,14] DiCarli et al considered symptom improvement in 36 patients with ischemic heart failure undergoing surgical revascularization.[13] Percentage improvement in functional status post CABG correlated linearly with the amount of hibernating myocardium as assessed by ^{18}FDG PET.[13] Quality of life improvement would be expected to follow symptom improvement, yet quality of life might also be improved through the reassurance of

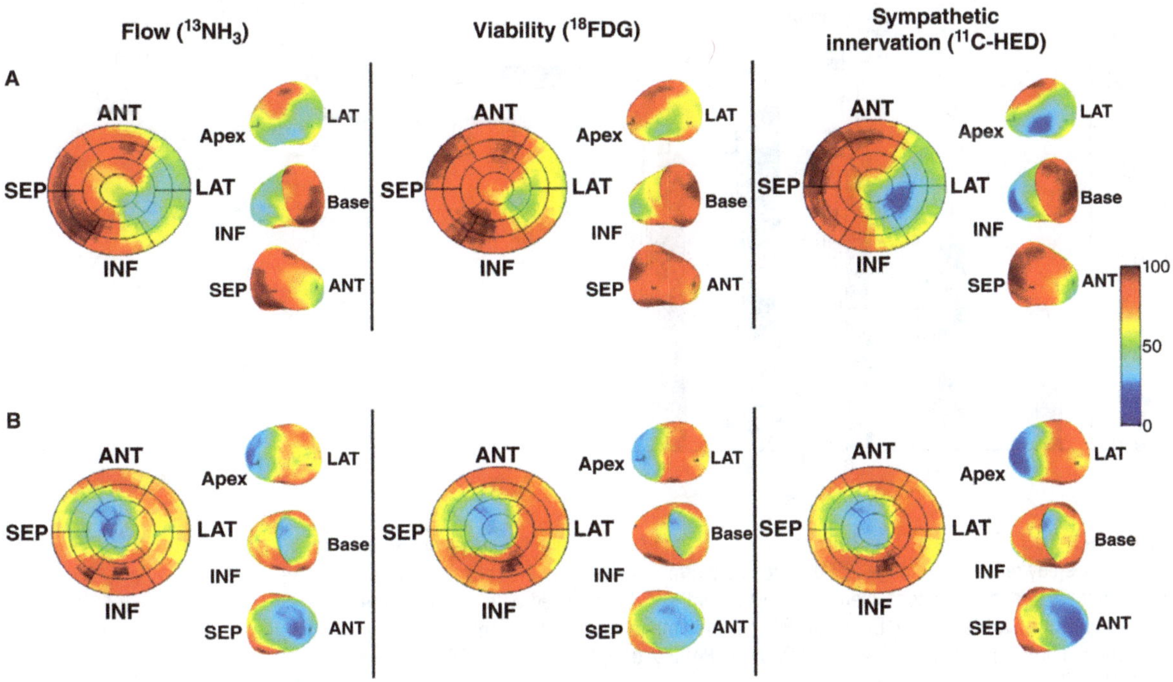

FIGURE 9-6 An Example of PET Imaging of Flow, Viability, and Sympathetic Innervation. Adapted figure from PAREPET (Prediction of ARrhythmic Events with Positron Emission Tomography) study.[11] (A): Patient who experienced a sudden cardiac arrest. The images demonstrate a larger volume of myocardium with sympathetic denervation (^{11}C-HED defect) than the infarct size (matched $^{13}NH_3$ and ^{18}FDG defect). (B): Patient with matched reductions in flow, infarct volume, and sympathetic denervation. (Reproduced from Fallavollita JA, Heavey BM, Luisi AJ, et al: Regional myocardial sympathetic denervation predicts the risk of sudden cardiac arrest in ischemic cardiomyopathy, J Am Coll Cardiol. 2014 Jan 21;63(2):141-149)

thorough evaluation in ischemic heart failure as per the findings of the quality of life arm of PARR-2.[14]

In this analysis of PARR-2 data the EQD-5 (European Quality of Life-5 dimensions) questionnaire was used to assess 5 dimensions associated with quality of life: mobility, self-care, usual activities, pain/discomfort, and anxiety/depression. EQD-5 was applied to both PPAR-2 groups, the PET-assisted arm and the standard care arm. Quality of life scores improved in the PET-assisted arm at 6 months with a trend to a persistent benefit at 12 months. In PARR-2 PET guidance was not followed in 25% of PET-assisted care patients.

When PET guidance was adhered to, quality of life scores improved whether revascularization was performed or not (Figure 9-7). In this figure, improved quality of life measures were maintained throughout the study. This perhaps speaks to the importance of patient reassurance experienced through careful and thoughtful evaluations even if no further therapeutic options are found to be ultimately available.

The PARR-2 quality of life study is a reminder that in clinical conditions where the prognosis is bleak, the quality of life is tremendously important to patients. These results suggest that patients appreciate the experience of careful and considerate assessment even in the absence of revascularization.

COMBINATION OF PET AND MRI TO REFINE AND REDEFINE VIABILITY DEFINITION

Cardiac magnetic resonance imaging (CMR) with gadolinium has been demonstrated to provide viability information and is commonly perceived as a competitor to ^{18}FDG PET as the imaging modality of choice in viability assessment. CMR is a useful technique for evaluating cardiac function and determining the presence and extent of myocardial scar. The ability of recently developed CMR-PET cameras to combine CMR and PET modalities at one sitting could be a

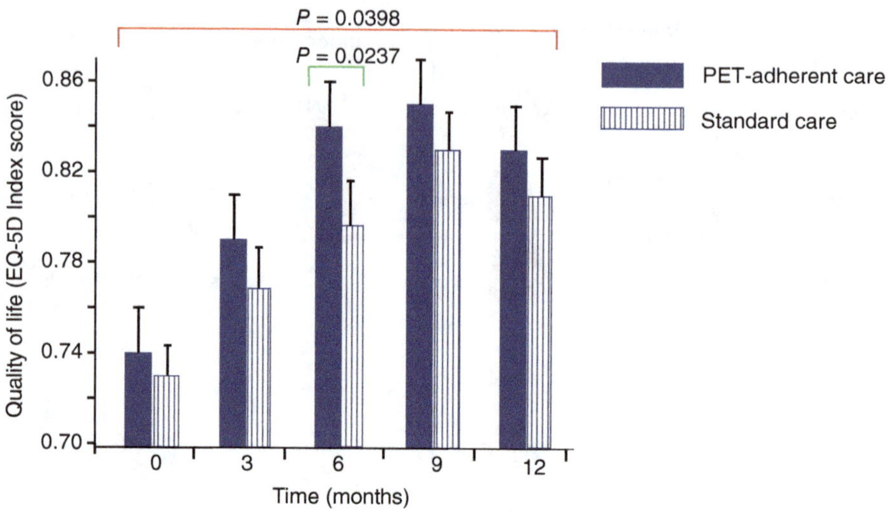

FIGURE 9-7 FDG PET-assisted care can improve quality of life in ischemic heart failure. In patients from PARR2 study randomized to the PET-assisted care arm who were adherent to the PET advice improvement in quality of life was seen at 6 and 12 months.[14] (Reproduced with permission from Shukla T, Nichol G, Wells G, et al: Does FDG PET-assisted management of patients with left ventricular dysfunction improve quality of life? A substudy of the PARR-2 trial, Can J Cardiol. 2012 Jan-Feb;28(1):54-61)

useful tool in ischemic heart failure patients. It would allow the strengths of CMR scar determination to be combined with the sensitivity of ^{18}FDG PET to identify viable hibernating myocardium.

A study of 28 patients 5-7 days postmyocardial infarction used PET-CMR evaluation to predict the recovery of LV segments 6 months postrevascularization.[15] Viability was assessed using standard definitions: at CMR viability was defined by scar of ≤50% transmural width in a myocardial segment. At PET, segments with FDG uptake ≥50% of normal uptake were declared viable. There was substantial intermethod agreement, 82% of dysfunctional segments demonstrated concordant findings (either both techniques agreed a segment was viable or both agreed a segment was nonviable). In only 18% of dysfunctional segments were there discrepant findings. The discrepant findings were all PET nonviable, CMR viable. Functional recovery in these segments at 6 months occurred in only 41% versus 78% when there was intermethod agreement for viability.

No segments were noted to be PET viable/CMR nonviable using the standard definitions. This is perhaps surprising in the context of acute myocardial infarction when myocardial glucose uptake might be expected to be increased as a reflection of inflammation in the healing infarct in addition to areas of stunned and hibernating myocardium.[16] In this setting the recovery of 41% of segments thought to be PET nonviable/MRI viable suggests that the threshold for PET viability might be lower than the 50% definition. A lower threshold of >40%-45% of normal uptake might have led to the detection of some of the viable segments detected by CMR but overlooked by ^{18}FDG-PET.

Combined PET CMR offers the opportunity to marry PET viability assessment with CMR tissue and function evaluation at a single sitting. As a technique it is currently in its infancy but there is already a signal that when combined together the techniques may help to refine and redefine our definitions of viability. Further evaluation will be needed to confirm this early promise.

CONCLUSIONS

This chapter reviews the value of cardiac PET viability assessment using the metabolic tracer FDG. It is a measure of the success of managing acute coronary syndromes and improving medical management of heart failure that patient survival has improved. A consequence to improved longevity is that patients may present in later years with ischemic heart failure with deterioration in LV ejection fraction from progression of their coronary disease. Some may have previously undergone surgical or percutaneous revascularization. This population is often elderly, with multiple co-morbidities, with poor targets for revascularization or with occlusion of prior grafts. It is a challenging cohort to manage but the emergent data from STICH and PARR-2 is that revascularization does improve survival and that viability imaging can help both clinical decision making and patient quality of life. Both studies demonstrated that ischemic heart failure continues to suffer from a poor long-term survival rate. It is hoped that improvements in revascularization techniques, medical management of angina and/or arrhythmia assessment by PET can ameliorate the situation. Ongoing investigations such as AIMI-HF (alternative imaging modalities in ischemic heart failure) may also be informative.[17] AIMI-HF will randomize patients to SPECT, PET, or CMR imaging to determine the optimal imaging strategies in ischemic heart failure. For the foreseeable future, viability assessment with ^{18}FDG PET will continue to form an important aspect of the work up of these cases. This will ensure that those most likely to benefit from revascularization are given this opportunity.

REFERENCES

1. Rahimtoola SH. Myocardial hibernation: clinical manifestations and importance. *Dialogues Cardiovasc Med.* 1997;2(2):57–112.
2. Velazquez EJ, Lee KL, Jones RH, et al. Coronary-artery bypass surgery in patients with ischemic cardiomyopathy. *N Engl J Med.* 2016;374(16):1511–1520. doi:10.1056/NEJMoa1602001.
3. Canty JM, Fallavollita JA. Chronic hibernation and chronic stunning: a continuum. *J Nucl Cardiol.* 2000;7(5):509–527. doi:10.1067/mnc.2000.109683.
4. Anavekar NS, Chareonthaitawee P, Narula J, Gersh BJ. Revascularization in patients with severe left ventricular dysfunction: is the assessment of viability still viable? *J Am Coll Cardiol.* 2016;67(24):2874–2887. doi:10.1016/j.jacc.2016.03.571.
5. Velazquez E, Lee K, Deja M, et al. Coronary-artery bypass surgery in patients with left ventricular dysfunction. *N Engl J Med.* 2011;364:1607–1616.
6. Beanlands RSB, Nichol G, Huszti E, et al. F-18-fluorodeoxyglucose positron emission tomography imaging-assisted management of patients with severe left ventricular dysfunction and suspected coronary disease: a randomized, controlled trial (PARR-2). *J Am Coll Cardiol.* 2007;50(20):2002–2012. doi:10.1016/j.jacc.2007.09.006.
7. Bonow RO, Maurer G, Lee KL, et al. Myocardial viability and survival in ischemic left ventricular dysfunction. *N Engl J Med.* 2011;364(17):1617–1625. doi:10.1056/NEJMoa1100358.
8. McArdle B, Shukla T, Nichol G, et al. Long-term follow-up of outcomes with F-18-fluorodeoxyglucose positron emission tomography imaging-assisted management of patients with severe left ventricular dysfunction secondary to coronary disease. *Circ Cardiovasc Imaging.* 2016;9(9):e004331. doi:10.1161/CIRCIMAGING.115.004331.
9. Abraham A, Nichol G, Williams KA, et al. 18F-FDG PET imaging of myocardial viability in an experienced center with access to 18F-FDG and integration with clinical management teams: the Ottawa-FIVE substudy of the PARR 2 trial. *J Nucl Med.* 2010;51(4):567–574. doi:10.2967/jnumed.109.065938.
10. Ling LF, Marwick TH, Flores DR, et al. Identification of therapeutic benefit from revascularization in patients with left ventricular systolic dysfunction inducible ischemia versus hibernating myocardium. *Circ Cardiovasc Imaging.* 2013;6(3):363–372. doi:10.1161/CIRCIMAGING.112.000138.
11. Fallavollita JA, Heavey BM, Luisi AJ, et al. Regional myocardial sympathetic denervation predicts the risk of sudden cardiac arrest in ischemic cardiomyopathy. *J Am Coll Cardiol.* 2014;63(2):141–149. doi:10.1016/j.jacc.2013.07.096.
12. Ungerer M, Hartmann F, Karoglan M, et al. Regional in vivo and in vitro characterization of autonomic innervation in cardiomyopathic human heart. *Circulation.* 1998 Jan 20;97(2):174–180.

13. Di Carli MF, Asgarzadie F, Schelbert HR, et al. Quantitative relation between myocardial viability and improvement in heart failure symptoms after revascularization in patients with ischemic cardiomyopathy. *Circulation*. 1995;92(12):3436 LP-3444. http://circ.ahajournals.org/content/92/12/3436.abstract.
14. Shukla T, Nichol G, Wells G, et al. Does FDG PET-assisted management of patients with left ventricular dysfunction improve quality of life? A substudy of the PARR-2 trial. *Can J Cardiol.* 2012;28(1):54–61. doi:10.1016/j.cjca.2011.09.012.
15. Rischpler C, Langwieser N, Souvatzoglou M, et al. PET/MRI early aftermyocardial infarction: evaluation of viability with late gadolinium enhancement transmurality vs. ^{18}F-FDG uptake. *Eur Heart J Cardiovasc Imaging*. 2015;16(6):661–669. doi:10.1093/ehjci/jeu317
16. Nonogi H, Miyazaki S, Goto Y, Ishida Y, Uehara T, Nishimura T. Efficacy and limitation of F-18-fluorodeoxyglucose positron emission tomography during fasting to assess myocardial viability in the acute phase of myocardial infarction. *Intern Med.* 1998;37(8):653–661. doi:10.2169/internalmedicine.37.653.
17. O'Meara E, Mielniczuk LM, Wells GA, et al. Alternative imaging modalities in ischemic heart failure (AIMI-HF) IMAGE HF project I-A: study protocol for a randomized controlled trial. *Trials.* 2013;14(1):218. doi:10.1186/1745-6215-14-218.

EDITOR'S PERSPECTIVE

Gary V. Heller

Myocardial viability assessment is an important part of the cardiac PET armamentarium, providing a study of a group of patients who are at high risk if the wrong management decision is made. The determination of viability in a region of myocardial dysfunction can change management to a revascularization procedure, rather than medicines, transplant, or mechanical support such as with left ventricular assist devices. This chapter spells out indications for a cardiac PET viability study and the supportive data for FDG imaging that validates its use in this arena. FDG PET as a metabolic study has important advantages over other imaging studies that rely primarily upon either perfusion or function data. An important aspect of this chapter is a careful discussion and dissection of the STICH Trial, the results of which are frequently misunderstood, and how FDG-PET imaging differs from the modalities represented in that trial. The authors present more recent outcome data for FDG-PET, demonstrating improvements in survival, ventricular function, and quality of life when the results of FDG PET imaging are adhered to in management decisions.

In this editor's experience, patients who are candidates for viability assessment are complex with both CAD and heart failure. Cardiac FDG PET can play a key role in determining whether the patient is a good revascularization candidate. However, this study is often part of a layered approach to viability assessment. It comes into play after an ischemic workup with either rest/stress SPECT or PET leaves uncertainty about viability of dysfunctioning but not clearly ischemic myocardium, and after angiography, has confirmed that revascularization is an option if myocardium is confirmed viable. Its role in decision-making requires an understanding of concepts such as hibernation, stunning, and infarction.

This chapter has superbly described the current literature supporting the value of FDG PET in viability assessment. It also addresses the challenge of demonstrating its value, given that the complexity of the patient population is such that it is often only one of a number of considerations that go into management decisions. When management is based on metabolic considerations only, it can clearly predict outcomes. Subsequent chapters describe patient preparation and interpretation of results to augment the supportive FDG literature.

Patient Preparation for FDG PET Viability Imaging

CHAPTER 10

Hiroshi Ohira, Jennifer Renaud, Robert A. deKemp, May Aung, Terrence D. Ruddy, and Rob Beanlands

INTRODUCTION

The heart consumes more energy than any other organ in order to maintain its contractile performance.[1] The healthy myocardium possesses the superb ability to utilize a wide variety of substrates including: free fatty acids, glucose, lactate, pyruvate, ketone bodies, and amino acids as energy sources, which makes it possible for it to function as a constant pump. In the healthy adult myocardium, free fatty acids are the major energy source; however, under certain conditions, such as the postprandial state when glucose is more available, the heart is capable of switching to a glucose-predominant substrate utilization pattern.[2,3] During ischemia, when there is reduced oxygen available to the tissue, the heart must use anaerobic glycolysis for ATP and energy production. As such, glucose becomes the primary substrate for ischemic myocardium. ^{18}F-fluorodeoxyglucose (FDG) is a glucose analog whose uptake parallels glucose and, therefore, can be used to reflect glucose utilization and the metabolic state of the myocardium. Viable myocardium that is ischemic or hibernating will take up glucose and thus FDG. Likewise normal myocardium (which is, of course, also viable) in the postprandial state will take up glucose and as such FDG.

As a metabolic viability test, cardiac PET imaging with FDG can assess the myocardium in either a fasting or a glucose-loaded state. A fasting protocol is preferred when one wants to suppress FDG uptake in normal tissue, as in the detection of inflammatory or infectious diseases, including: cardiac sarcoidosis, vasculitis, and infection of intravascular devices, pacemakers, and catheters. The fasting protocol is useful to suppress physiological myocardial FDG uptake, making it easier to distinguish between physiological and pathological FDG uptake (see Chapter 14 for discussion of preparation for FDG inflammation imaging).

In contrast, a glucose load protocol is selected for assessing myocardial viability in order to enhance FDG (glucose) uptake in the viable myocardium (both normal and ischemic/hibernating tissue). The most common protocol for glucose loading is with an oral load of 25–100 g. The glucose load induces a rapid increase in insulin secretion from β(beta)-cells of the pancreas, which enhances FDG uptake in the viable myocardium through the glucose transporter 4 (GLUT-4).[4] However, oral glucose loading may not be as effective in patients with impaired glucose tolerance or diabetes because of the impaired response of the cells (including myocardial cells) to insulin stimulation as a result of insulin resistance, as well as a decrease in glucose transporter activity and reduction in transport rates owing to pretranslational suppression of GLUT-4 gene expression[5] or their limited ability to produce endogenous insulin. Thus, the use of insulin along with close monitoring of blood glucose levels is used (routinely in some sites) to improve image quality in patients with diabetes or glucose intolerance.

In this chapter, we focus on FDG PET viability imaging with the glucose load protocol in patients with or without diabetes mellitus.

PATIENT PREPARATION FOR A PET VIABILITY STUDY

It is important to choose the right protocol for the right patient (either oral glucose load, intravenous insulin injections after oral glucose load, or an euglycemic-hyperinsulinemic clamp) in order to obtain optimal cardiac FDG PET images. The presence of diabetes mellitus can substantially affect the assessment of myocardial viability using FDG PET.[6] In patients with diabetes, the myocardium-to-background ratio can be decreased compared with patients who do not have diabetes. This can be explained by lower myocardial glucose (and FDG) uptake and higher plasma glucose (and FDG) levels. Therefore, the status of glucose tolerance should be known prior to the scan, if at all possible. Diabetes can be diagnosed based on hemoglobin A1c (Hb $A1_C$) criteria or plasma glucose criteria; fasting plasma glucose (FPG) or the 2-h plasma glucose (2-h PG) value after a 75-g oral glucose tolerance test (OGTT).[7,8]

The ASNC guidelines and University of Ottawa Heart Institute (UOHI) protocols are shown in Tables 10-1 and 10-2 and Appendices 10-1 through 10-3, respectively.[9]

Patients Without Known Diabetes Mellitus

After at least 6 hours of fasting, an oral load of 25–100 g glucose is given.

At UOHI, the dosage of glucose is based on the baseline blood glucose (BG) level, measured by a glucometer. If BG is <90 mg/dL (5 mmol/L), 50 g of glucose is orally administered (see Appendix 10-1). If BG is 90–125 mg/dL (5.1–6.9 mmol/L), 25 g of glucose is given.

Table 10-1

Patient Preparation for ^{18}F-FDG PET Cardiac Viability Assessment

Procedure	Steps for standardization	Technique
Fasting period	Step 1: Fast patient	
	*6-12 hours	Preferred
	<6 hours	Suboptimal
	Step 2: Check blood glucose (BG) and the glucose load (choose one of the following 3 options)	
Oral glucose load	Option 1: Oral glucose loading	
	IF:fasting BG <~250 mg/dL (13.9 mmol/L) THEN: (1) oral glucose load: typically 25–100 g orally (see Table 10-2) (2) monitor BG (see Table 10-2)	Standard
	IF: fasting BG >~250 mg/dL(13.9 mmol/L) THEN: see Table 10-2	Standard
IV protocol	Option 2: Dextrose IV infusion	Optional
	(see ASNC/SNMMI Guidelines for details)	
Acipimox	Option 3: Acipimox	
	Acipimox, 250 mg orally not available in the United States	
18F-FDG injection	Step 3: Administer ^{18}F-FDG	
	Time: Dependent on which option was selected	
	Standard IV administration of ^{18}F-FDG	
Begin PET imaging	0-90 minutes post ^{18}F-FDG injection (45–60 min postinjection for standard static imaging)	

(Reproduced with permission from Dilsizian V, Bacharach SL, Beanlands RS, et al: ASNC imaging guidelines/SNMMI procedure standard for positron emission tomography (PET) nuclear cardiology procedures, J Nucl Cardiol. 2016 Oct;23(5):1187-1226)

Table 10-2

Guidelines for BG Maintenance (After Glucose Administration) for Optimal 18F-FDG Cardiac Uptake, BG of Approximately 100–140 mg/dL (5.55–7.77 mmol/L) at Time of Injection of 18F-FDG

BG at 45–60 min after administration	Restorative measure	Technique
130–140 mg/dL (7.22–7.78 mmol/L)	1 U regular insulin IV	Standard
140–160 mg/dL (7.78–8.89 mmol/L)	2 U regular insulin IV	
160–180 mg/dL (8.89–10 mmol/L)	3 U regular insulin IV	
180–200 mg/dL (10–11.11 mmol/L)	5 U regular insulin IV	
>200 mg/dL (>11.11 mmol/L)	Notify physician	

BG = blood glucose; FDG = fluorodeoxyglucose; IV = intravenous; mg = milligram; mmol = millimoles; L = liter; dL = deciliter; U = unit

(Reproduced with permission from Dilsizian V, Bacharach SL, Beanlands RS, et al: ASNC imaging guidelines/SNMMI procedure standard for positron emission tomography (PET) nuclear cardiology procedures, J Nucl Cardiol. 2016 Oct;23(5):1187-1226)

When BG is greater than 126 mg/dL (>7 mmol/L), the value is considered to be in the diabetic range of glucose intolerance (although BG measurement by a glucometer cannot be used for the diagnosis of diabetes). In such a situation, 25 g of oral glucose load along with 1–2 U of regular insulin is administered intravenously.

We typically administer 1–2 U of regular insulin when BG is 126–180 mg/dL (7–10 mmol/L). The dose of regular insulin is determined based on the patient's body weight. Lean patients tend to develop hypoglycemia after insulin administration, thus walking is an alternative choice to decrease BG used at some institutions.

Blood glucose is measured 20 minutes after the insulin administration in order to identify hypoglycemia and to determine whether walking or the need for more insulin is necessary. When BG is greater than 181 mg/dL (>10 mmol/L), our team discusses whether administration of a larger dose of regular insulin or a switch to the euglycemic-hyperinsulinemic clamp is the best choice for a given patient. One hour postglucose load and insulin (if applicable), we recheck the BG to determine if this has achieved the optimal range (100–140 mg/dL = 5.55–7.77 mmol/L). When the BG is less than 144 mg/dL (<8 mmol/L), we proceed with FDG injection. When the BG is equal or greater than 144 mg/dL (>8 mmol/L), we use supplemental insulin (see Appendix 10-1). FDG is administered 1 hour postglucose load and insulin (if applicable). FDG can be given at the same time as supplemental insulin, if required. We recheck BG after 30 minutes if supplemental insulin has been given.

At this point, typically, 5–15 mCi of FDG is injected in a peripheral vein after the aforementioned preparation procedure. PET imaging acquisition begins at 45–60 min after FDG injection.

Acipimox, which is a nicotinic acid derivative, may be an alternative method, although this is not available in North America. It is reported that Acipimox inhibits lipolysis in the peripheral tissues, which decreases the plasma level of fatty acids and indirectly stimulates myocardial glucose (and FDG) uptake.[10,11] Niacin may be used for a similar effect but in general is not applied because of associated flushing side effects.[12]

Patients With Diabetes Mellitus

The same fasting period with nondiabetic patients is applied to diabetic patients. The simple fast and oral glucose loading method is often not effective in patients with diabetes because of their limited ability to secrete insulin in the β-cell in the pancreas and/or increased insulin resistance in the insulin target organs. Several protocols are advocated in order to promote myocardial FDG uptake, including oral glucose load with supplemental insulin, euglycemic-hyperinsulinemic clamp, shorter intravenous glucose/insulin-loading procedures, and the administration of nicotinic acid derivatives.

Oral glucose load with supplemental insulin and close monitoring of BG yields satisfactory results in many diabetic patients (Table 10-2). The euglycemic-hyperinsulinemic clamp protocol on the other hand is a more rigorous but time-consuming approach[12]; however, it provides consistently high-quality images in almost all patients with diabetes[12] (see Appendix 10-2). A simplified intravenous glucose/insulin/potassium (GIK) infusion protocol has also been used as an alternative method.[13]

Vitale et al performed a direct comparison among three protocols including the standard protocol, consisting of oral glucose loading and boluses of insulin based on blood glucose; the niacin protocol, consisting of pretreatment with niacin to lower free fatty acids; and the insulin clamp protocol, consisting of euglycemic-hyperinsulinemic clamp in patients with noninsulin-dependent diabetes, coronary artery disease and severe left ventricular dysfunction. Of the three protocols, the insulin clamp method yielded the highest FDG PET image quality.[14] While the other approaches are acceptable,[13] for sites that are able to perform the technique, the euglycemic-hyperinsulinemic clamp is considered to be a preferred method in this population.

Tables 10-1 and 10-2 are advocated protocols from ASNC guidelines.[9] The protocols at our institute are noted in Appendices 10-1, 10-2, and 10-3.

REFERENCES

1. Neubauer S. The failing heart: an engine out of fuel. *N Engl J Med.* 2007;356:1140–1151.
2. Neely JR, Rovetto MJ, Oram JF. Myocardial utilization of carbohydrate and lipids. *Prog Cardiovasc Dis.* 1972;15:289–329.
3. Neely JR, Morgan HE. Relationship between carbohydrate and lipid metabolism and the energy balance of heart muscle. *Annu Rev Physiol.* 1974;36:413–459.
4. Shepherd PR, Kahn BB. Glucose transporters and insulin action: implications for insulin resistance and diabetes mellitus. *N Engl J Med.* 1999;341:248–257.
5. Garvey WT, Hardin D, Juhaszova M, Dominguez JH. Effects of diabetes on myocardial glucose transport system in rats: implications for diabetic cardiomyopathy. *Am J Physiol.* 1993;264:H837-H844.
6. Ohtake T, Yokoyama I, Watanabe T, et al. Myocardial glucose metabolism in noninsulin-dependent diabetes mellitus patients evaluated by FDG-PET. *J Nucl Med.* 1995;36:456–463.
7. International Expert Committee report on the role of the A1C assay in the diagnosis of diabetes. *Diabetes Care.* 2009;32:1327–1334.
8. Diagnosis and classification of diabetes mellitus. *Diabetes Care.* 2014;37 Suppl 1:S81-S90.
9. Dilsizian V, Bacharach SL, Beanlands RS, et al. ASNC imaging guidelines/SNMMI procedure standard for positron emission tomography (PET) nuclear cardiology procedures. *J Nucl Cardiol.* 2016;23:1187–1226.
10. Musatti L, Maggi E, Moro E, Valzelli G, Tamassia V. Bioavailability and pharmacokinetics in man of acipimox, a new antilipolytic and hypolipemic agent. *J Int Med Res.* 1981;9:381–386.
11. Knuuti MJ, Yki-Jarvinen H, Voipio-Pulkki LM, et al. Enhancement of myocardial [fluorine-18] fluorodeoxyglucose uptake by a nicotinic acid derivative. *J Nucl Med.* 1994;35:989–998.
12. Knuuti MJ, Nuutila P, Ruotsalainen U, et al. Euglycemic hyperinsulinemic clamp and oral glucose load in stimulating myocardial glucose utilization during positron emission tomography. *J Nucl Med.* 1992;33:1255–1262.
13. Martin WH, Jones RC, Delbeke D, Sandler MP. A simplified intravenous glucose loading protocol for fluorine-18 fluorodeoxyglucose cardiac single-photon emission tomography. *Eur J Nucl Med.* 1997;24:1291–1297.
14. Vitale GD, deKemp RA, Ruddy TD, Williams K, Beanlands RS. Myocardial glucose utilization and optimization of (18)F-FDG PET imaging in patients with non-insulin-dependent diabetes mellitus, coronary artery disease, and left ventricular dysfunction. *J Nucl Med.* 2001;42:1730–1736.

APPENDIX 10-1

Ottawa (UOHI) Protocol for Blood Glucose Management in Patients Not Known to Have Diabetes Undergoing Myocardial Tissue Viability Studies With FDG PET

Procedure

- Patients are to be fasting 6–12 hours (preferred) or a minimum of 6 hours (see Table 1 from ASNC guidelines 2016).
- Hold diuretics (easier for patient to tolerate time in scanner; resume after scanning).
- Resting perfusion scan must be performed prior to FDG imaging if scan is on the same day as FDG. If scan is performed on separate day, it must be within 2 weeks of FDG scan (if patient stable), (unstable patients resting scan must be on same day (or within 1 day of FDG imaging).
- Check Blood Glucose Level (BG) on glucometer (when drawing blood from IV use 1 cc TB syringe and discard 0.3 cc blood before checking the BG. Remember to flush lock afterwards). Baseline potassium, glucose, creatinine blood tube drawn (needed if supplemental insulin given).
- If BG is <90 mg/dL (5 mmol/L) **give 50 g of an oral glucose load**
- If BG is 91–125 mg/dL (5.1–6.9 mmol/L) **give 25 g oral glucose load**
- If BG is 126–180 mg/dL (7-10 mmol/L) **give 25 g of oral glucose load and regular insulin (at UOHI: give 1–2U of insulin IV, with 5U insulin patients became hypoglycemic) OR (have patients walk [if able] to help decrease blood glucose levels). Check BG in 20 minutes.**
- If BG is >180 mg/dL (10 mmol/L) **notify MD to decide re larger dose of insulin or switch to insulin/glucose clamp protocol.**
- 1 hour after Glucose load and insulin (if required) check BG.
- If BG is <144 mg/dL (8 mmol/L) **proceed with FDG injection.**
- If BG is 144–159 mg/dL (8-8.8 mmol/L) **give 1U-2U of regular insulin.**
- If BG is 160–180 mg/dL (8.9–10 mmol/L) **give 3U of regular insulin.**
- If BG is 181–200 mg/dL (10.1–11.1 mmol/L) **give 5U of regular insulin.**
- If BG >200 mg/dL (11.1 mmol/L) **give up to 10U of regular insulin. Notify MD for insulin orders.**
- If BG slightly >144 mg/dL (8 mmol/L) **have patient walk (if able) to help reduce blood glucose levels.**
- Injection of FDG 1 hour postglucose load (can be given at the same time as supplemental insulin, if required). ***(ASNC: optimal BG should be between 100 and 140 mg/dL = 5.55 - 7.77 mmol/L to inject FDG [see Table 2]).***
- Recheck BG after 30 minutes if insulin was given.
- FDG imaging 45–60 minutes post-FDG injection (refer to FDG imaging protocol).
- Patients receive nourishment after the procedure due to their fasting state. Normal BG is 63–104 mg/dL (3.5–5.8 mmol/L). If the patient's BG is lower than 63 mg/dL (3.5 mmol/L) or patient exhibits symptoms of hypoglycemia, a glucose-loaded drink may be required to raise the BG to within the acceptable range.
- Assess posttest blood pressure, heart rate, and final BG. Refer to potassium protocol if supplemental insulin given.
- Diabetic patients may require closer monitoring of BG and higher doses of insulin or additional doses of insulin if BG does not stabilize/decrease. The euglycemic-hyperinsulinemic clamp protocol is an alternative method to be used for diabetic patients (preferred). **UOHI only uses the clamp protocol for patients with known diabetes mellitus.**

APPENDIX 10-2

Ottawa (UOHI) Protocol for Blood Glucose Management in Patients With Known Diabetes Mellitus Undergoing Myocardial Tissue Viability Studies With FDG PET

1. **Glucose Insulin Clamp Protocol:**
   - Patients with known diabetes mellitus.
   - Hold diuretics (easier for patient to tolerate time in scanner; resume after scanning).
   - Patients must fast 6–12 hours. If fasting overnight, hold oral diabetic medications/insulin.
   - Schedule diabetic patients in the morning (preferred). If diabetic patient is scheduled for afternoon, patient may have light breakfast and medications as required.
2. **Patient Preparation:**
   - Two saline locks are required. One for insulin/glucose infusion and the other to check Blood Glucose Level (BG), this should be distal to any infusion lock or in the opposite arm. Finger pricks are an alternative to using the saline lock for checking BG if unable to access second IV site.
   - Check BG on glucometer (when drawing blood from IV use 1 cc TB syringe and discard 0.3 cc blood before checking the BG. Remember to flush lock afterward). Baseline potassium, glucose, creatinine blood tube drawn.
   - If BG is >10 mmol/L, notify MD and obtain orders for insulin bolus prior to starting infusion. (ie, MD may order: if BG is 180-270 mg/dL (10-15 mmol/L) **5U regular insulin,** if BG is >270 mg/dL (15 mmol/L) **10U regular insulin.**
   - Calculate amount of insulin to be used for clamp. **Insulin dose:** pt's weight (kg) × 0.25 = # of IU of regular insulin to be added per NaCl 50 cc bag, that is **UOHI–double the amount of insulin to be added to 100 cc volume NaCl bag (used at UOHI).**
   - Resting perfusion scan must be performed prior to FDG imaging if scan is on the same day as FDG. If scan is performed on separate day, it must be within 2 weeks of FDG scan (if patient stable). Unstable patients resting scan must be on same day or within 1 day of FDG imaging.
3. **Insulin Infusion:**
   - Run IV insulin infusion as per Glucose Insulin Clamp Data sheet. (originally adapted from Munich protocol)
   - 48 cc/hour × 4 minutes.
   - 24 cc/hour × 3 minutes.
   - 12 cc/hour for remainder of infusion.
   - **Check BG every 5 minutes.** If patient exhibits symptoms of hypoglycemia, check BG sooner.
   - Best images are obtained when BG is approximately 90 mg/dL (5 mmol/L). **NOTE:** BG is patient specific, therefore adjust as tolerated. Goal is to see a decrease in BG or keep at approximately90 mg/dL (5 mmol/L).
   - If after initial load patient BG is not dropping, patient may need additional regular insulin bolus (2U at a time).
4. **Glucose Infusion:**
   - An exogenous 20% glucose infusion is started (if required) at a rate of 1–5 cc/hour and adjusted until a steady state is achieved. The glucose infusion is adjusted according to the BG over the preceding 5 minutes. Glucose infusion is usually started after insulin infusion. Glucose infusion start time varies depending on the patients BG. For example, in a case where the patients fasting blood glucose is low (ie, took insulin, but did not eat) then the glucose infusion will be started prior to the insulin infusion.
   - FDG injection (BG is stable and beginning to decrease). FDG imaging see FDG imaging protocol.
   - Turn off insulin approximately 30 minutes post-FDG injection. Do not turn off the glucose infusion (if running). Continue to check BG for another 20–30 minutes depending on BG and turn off the glucose infusion when the BG has returned to baseline.
   - Patients receive nourishment after the procedure due to their fasting state. Normal BG is 63-104 mg/dL 63 mg/dL (3.5 mmol/L). If the patient's BG is lower than 3.5 mmol/L or he/she exhibits symptoms of hypoglycemia, a glucose load drink may be required to raise the BG to within the acceptable range.
   - Assess post–blood pressure, heart rate, and final BG.
   - Slow K+: document if given or not required. See potassium protocol.

APPENDIX 10-3

Ottawa (UOHI) Protocol for Blood Glucose Management in Patients Undergoing Myocardial Tissue Viability Studies With FDG PET

Potassium Protocol

All diabetic patients booked for a FDG viability scan will have potassium (K+), glucose, and creatinine levels drawn on the day of the study. This protocol is also used for any patient that has received insulin during the viability scan; therefore, it may be relevant to nondiabetic patients as well.

If K+ level is >4.0 mEq/L (mmol/L)	▶ **No supplement is required.**
If K+ level is 3.5–3.9 mEq/L (mmol/L)	▶ **Give potassium chloride tablets (Slow K 3 tablets equivalent to 24 mEq) at the end of the scan.**
If K+ level is <3.5 mEq/L (mmol/L)	▶ **Give potassium chloride tablets (Slow K 3 tablets equivalent to 24 mEq) as soon as possible.** **Draw a stat K+ level at the end of the scan.** **Follow up with a K+ level the next morning.**
If K+ level is <3.0 mEq/L (mmol/L) OR an abnormal creatinine level	▶ **Individual patient orders are received from the physician.**

EDITOR'S PERSPECTIVE

Gary V. Heller

Patient preparation for FDG PET viability studies is a critical aspect to the success of the resulting images and, ultimately clinical value. The authors of this chapter have elucidated the various protocols that are practical and important for successful and useful imaging. The patient preparation for viability generally requires a nurse to assist in the blood draw and administration of medications. It is also important to monitor the patient during this phase, especially during glucose stabilization. For clinical laboratories primarily performing cardiac PET MPI studies, a decision needs to be made regarding where the patient stays after the injection of FDG, as there is a wait time of 45 minutes before acquisition. Generally, for centers also performing FDG oncology studies, there is an already constructed holding room for such purpose. For those facilities in which this is not available, clinical labs tend to perform this test at the end of the day, and once FDG is injected, keep the patient in the lead-shielded imaging room.

The authors have emphasized that there are differences in the preparation of non-diabetic and diabetic patients, as well as the importance of identifying the presence of diabetes prior to testing. In those patients in which careful preparation is not performed, image quality can suffer. This is particularly true in diabetic patients. The authors describe the importance of accurate assessment and the decision, at times, to use the Euglycemic-hyperinsulinemic clamp protocol as an alternative to a higher dose of insulin. This procedure may not be available in clinical laboratories, but its use is now being suggested and is included in this chapter for consideration for potential future use, as more data emerge.

Unfortunately, an FDG PET viability study can be time-consuming, at times confusing for staff, and frustrating for patients. Considerations include glucose loading (oral, intravenous, and how much), insulin injection protocols, when after insulin and how often to check blood glucose levels, and when to inject FDG. Often this study requires physician availability to address questions that arise. If the performing team is not reasonably experienced and does not have clear guidance, the protocol can last hours. Finally, patient safety is paramount. These patients need to be constantly observed, as severe hypoglycemia can develop quickly.

This thoughtful chapter on patient preparation describes the importance of proper procedures. It emphasizes differences in management between diabetic and non-diabetic patients. It provides guidance about what can be a challenging study from a team of experts in this field.

Interpretation of Cardiac PET Myocardial Viability Studies

CHAPTER 11

Fernanda Erthal, Ali Alenazy, and Terrence D. Ruddy

ABBREVIATIONS

^{18}FDG	^{18}F-fluorodeoxyglucose
CAD	coronary artery disease
EF	ejection fraction
LAD	left anterior descending
LCX	left circumflex
LV	left ventricular
PET	positron emission tomography
RCA	right coronary artery

INTRODUCTION

Heart failure is a common cardiac diagnosis and the prevalence is increasing, with a prediction of more than 8 million affected adults in the United States by 2030.[1] Despite recent improvement in survival, prognosis remains poor with a 5-year mortality of 50% following diagnosis.[2] The most frequent etiology continues to be coronary artery disease (CAD) in the developed countries.[3] Evidence supports the idea that viability imaging to guide revascularization therapy may be the best strategy for patients with multiple comorbidities and severe left ventricular (LV) dysfunction.[4–12] Several studies have demonstrated that revascularization in appropriate patients with CAD improves outcomes in these high-risk patients.[6] Viable but dysfunctional myocardium caused by abnormal coronary flow may restore its function with normalization of coronary blood flow. In this chapter, we review the approach to the interpretation of viability scans acquired with ^{18}F-fluorodeoxyglucose (^{18}FDG) and positron emission tomography (PET) and reporting with recommendations for clinical management. This topic has been reviewed in the recent PET imaging guidelines cosponsored by the American Society of Nuclear Cardiology and the Society of Nuclear Medicine and Molecular Imaging.[13]

VIABLE, STUNNED, AND HIBERNATING MYOCARDIUM

Viable, stunned, and hibernating myocardium are important concepts that need to be understood for appropriate interpretation of PET viability scans. Viable versus nonviable dysfunctional myocardium is a simple binary classification that refers to dysfunctional myocardium that may recover (viable or stunned/hibernating) or not (nonviable or scar) with revascularization.

Dysfunctional viable myocardium may have a spectrum of different levels of metabolism and flow caused by repeated transient or persistent ischemia.[14] Stunned myocardium may occur after ischemia and is characterized by normal rest flow and transiently impaired contractility caused by previous ischemia.[15–17] Microscopically, stunned myocardium has minimal structural injury but complex metabolic changes.[18–20] The severity of impaired metabolism will depend on the number, extent, and duration of the ischemic episodes.[21] Stunned myocardium may completely recover normal function or progress to a hibernation (still viable) or irreversible fibrosis (nonviable). Hibernating myocardium is dysfunctional myocardium with reduced rest flow and function that occurs after chronic repeated episodes of reduced blood supply.[21] By definition, hibernating myocardium is considered viable and has the capacity to recover function if adequate revascularization is performed in a timely fashion.[22,23] Glucose metabolism is preserved or even enhanced in hibernating myocardium because of preferential use of glucose by ischemic myocardium.[24–31] ^{18}FDG is a glucose analogue taken up by the myocyte-like glucose using sarcolemmal transporters and phosphorylated by hexokinase to ^{18}FDG-phosphate.[32] ^{18}FDG-phosphate is "trapped" in the myocyte because it cannot be further metabolized and is used as a marker of glucose transport by viable ischemic (hibernating) or nonischemic myocardium with viability imaging. Thus, preservation of ^{18}FDG uptake in areas of reduced perfusion is consistent with viability (perfusion-metabolism mismatch) and indicates hibernation. Conversely, reduced ^{18}FDG uptake in a region of reduced perfusion and of similar or greater degree indicates nonviability (perfusion-metabolism match) and indicates scar. Of note, regions with normal perfusion are viable, even with reduced ^{18}FDG, and may represent stunned myocardium.

IMAGE INTERPRETATION OF FDG PET

The standard interpretation of metabolic FDG studies is in comparison to rest myocardial perfusion. It is virtually impossible to interpret a metabolic FDG study without such comparison. ^{18}FDG PET images are best interpreted with rest PET perfusion images. Rest PET perfusion images are typically acquired with either ^{13}N-ammonia or ^{82}Rb. Although SPECT perfusion images can be used for comparison, interpretation can be difficult because attenuation artifacts in nonattenuation-corrected SPECT images or possible suboptimal correction when attenuation-correction is available.[13]

Image interpretation begins with examination of the coregistration of the fused emission and transmission images using the transaxial, coronal, and sagittal slices.[13] Misalignment may result in attenuation correction artifacts with undercorrection possibly resulting in anterior or anterolateral perfusion defects or overcorrection resulting in inferior wall "hot spots" on ^{18}FDG imaging and errors in interpretation if not recognized.[33] ^{18}FDG and perfusion images are reoriented and displayed as short-axis view (SAO), horizontal long axis (HLA), and vertical long axis (VLA) slices.[13] All slices need to be aligned and displayed adjacent to each other and interpreted according to the ASNC 17-segment model.[13]

Generally, the format is that the rest perfusion study (the same position as a "stress/rest" study) be above the ^{18}FDG study. The ^{18}FDG and perfusion images need to be normalized to the same normal myocardial region, which is usually the region on the perfusion image with the highest counts.[13] This normal region could also be identified or confirmed as normal from stress perfusion images or angiographic data if available. The electrocardiogram should also be reviewed at this time, because the left bundle branch block may lead to reduced ^{18}FDG uptake in the septum.[34] The septal region should not be used for normalization in patients with left bundle branch block (LBBB).[13] Persistent blood pool activity may alter myocardial activity and decrease defect severity on perfusion imaging or increase apparent ^{18}FDG uptake on metabolic imaging. Impaired LV systolic function may result in slower blood pool clearance. Blood pool activity should be minimized by optimal timing of the image acquisition or frame selection for the static images using later frames. Alternatively, the display settings for the lower limits of the color or grayscale can be adjusted to correct for blood pool differences.

Regional perfusion and ^{18}FDG metabolic images are evaluated together. Dysfunctional regions can be identified from gated perfusion images or from other clinical data and are the focus of attention. In a given region, perfusion is assessed as reduced or preserved. Four patterns of perfusion-metabolism can be seen (Figures 11-1 to 11-4) and are useful to separate viable from nonviable myocardium[13]: (1) reduced perfusion and preserved ^{18}FDG (perfusion-metabolism mismatch) identifying hibernating myocardium (viable). (2) Reduced perfusion and ^{18}FDG (perfusion-metabolism match) indicating scar (nonviable). (3) Preserved perfusion and ^{18}FDG showing normal myocardium (viable). (4) Preserved perfusion and reduced ^{18}FDG (reversed perfusion-metabolism mismatch) can be seen in patients with repetitive stunning, in the septum with LBBB,[35] with acute coronary syndrome and early following revascularization[20] and with diabetes[35] (viable). These patterns may coexist in a region or coronary territory. The severity of perfusion reduction can be used to define scar as nontransmural (<50%) or transmural (>50%). The extent of hibernating myocardium or scar (% of LV) can be described using qualitative or semiquantitative approaches as small (<10%), moderate (10% to 20%) or large (>20%). In patients with severe LV dysfunction caused by CAD, moderate or larger extents of hibernating myocardium are associated with improved outcomes with revascularization[9] and large amounts of scar predict less recovery of LV function.[7] Management recommendations can be suggested on the basis of the extent of hibernating myocardium and scar.

REPORT

The viability clinical report needs to be descriptive but at the same time concise. The clinical question needs to be answered in a clear way. An example of a report is as follows:

Viability PET Imaging with ^{18}FDG and ^{82}Rb/13N and Rest Gated Imaging

- Indication and clinical history: describe patient comorbidities, coronary anatomy, result of previous studies, previous cardiac procedures, and currents symptomatology
- Protocol: describe the used protocol and if patient had followed the diet instructions
- Rest ECG: presence/absence of LBBB/pacemaker, cardiac rhythm
- Study quality and presence of artifacts
- Imaging interpretation
  - Rest perfusion images: describe the tracer uptake distribution
  - FDG images: describe the tracer uptake distribution
  - Gated images: describe both perfusion and FDG, providing left ventricle end systolic and end diastolic volumes and left ventricle ejection fraction
- Conclusion: summarize the findings clearly stating the areas of viability and scar in accordance with coronary distribution. We recommend reporting the total percentage of scar and viability.
- Recommendation: This is optional, although communication with the referring healthcare provider is very important and usually appreciated.

CLINICAL CASES

Case 1 (Figure 11-1)

A 72-year-old female presented with dyspnea (NYHA III) and congestive heart failure. Past history

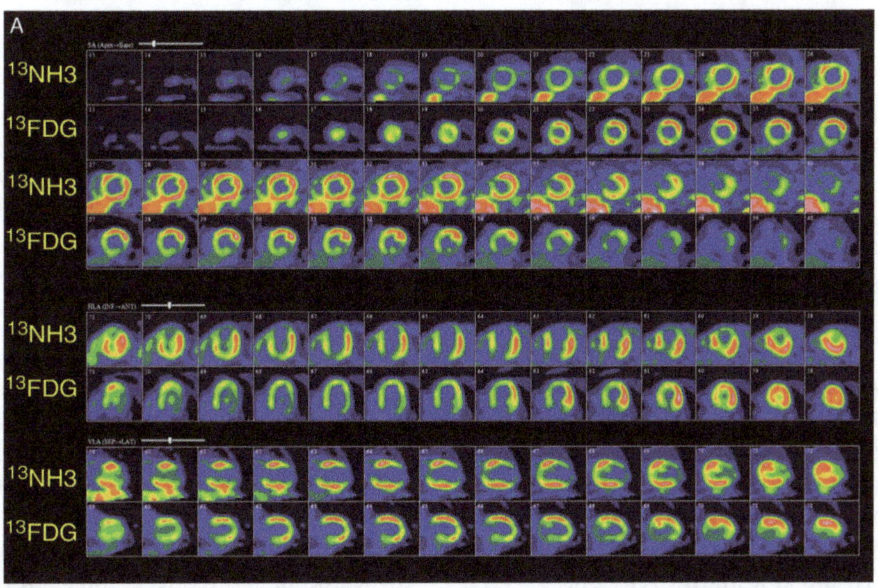

FIGURE 11-1 *(Continue)*

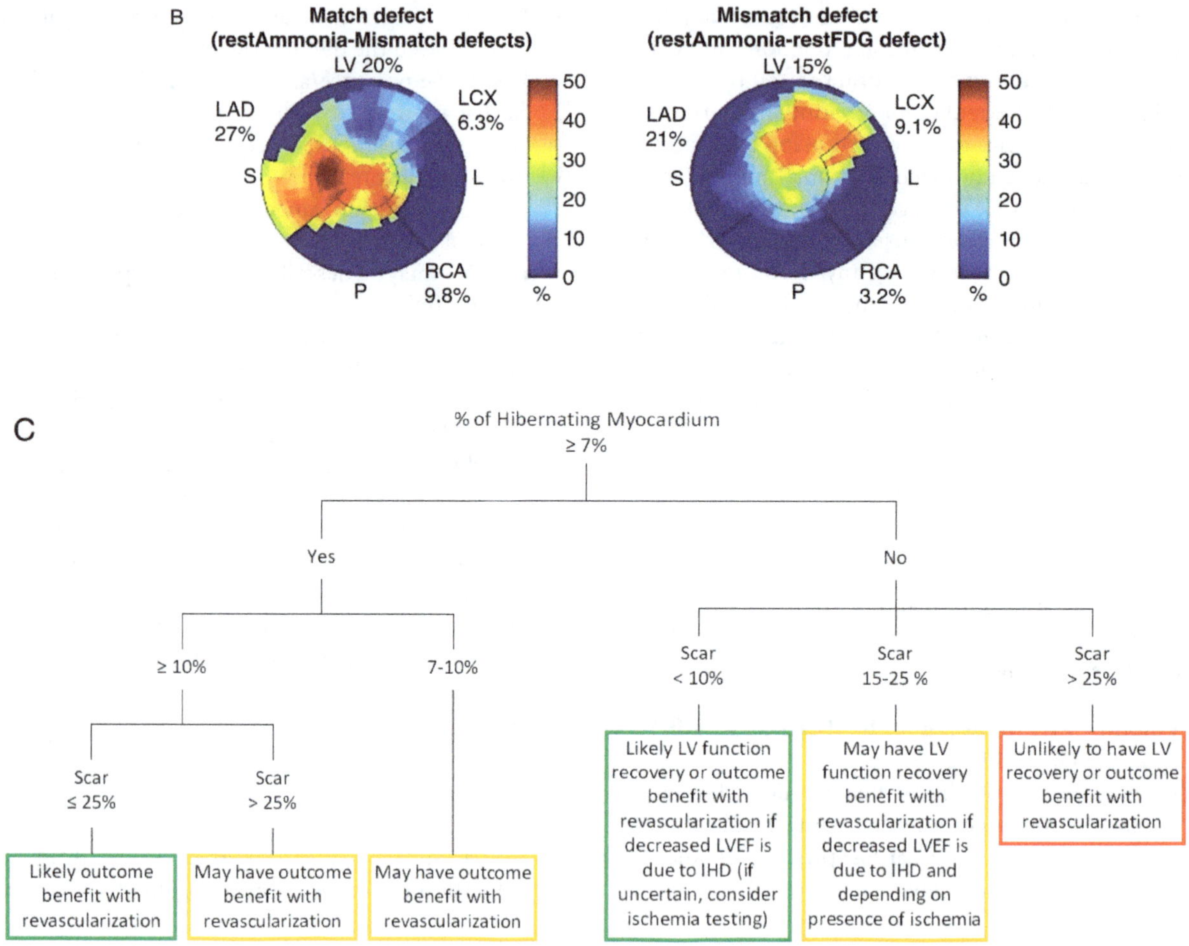

FIGURE 11-1 Hibernating Myocardium and Scar.The PET $^{13}NH3$ perfusion images show reduced perfusion in the septal, mid- and apical anterior and mid- and apical anterolateral regions and apex (A). The ^{18}FDG images show preserved uptake in the mid- and apical anterior and mid- and apical anterolateral regions consistent with hibernating myocardium and reduced uptake in the septum and apex indicating scar (A). Quantitative analysis (B) determined scar (match defect) as 20% LV and hibernating myocardium (mismatch) as 15% LV. The University of Ottawa Heart Institute decision-guiding flow map (C) is used to guide recommendations for management based on the extents of scar and hibernating myocardium and assuming decreased left ventricular ejection fraction (LVEF) is caused by extensive ischemic heart disease (IHD).

included previous myocardial infarctions, paroxysmal atrial fibrillation, chronic obstructive pulmonary disease, diabetes mellitus type II, and dyslipidemia. Echocardiography showed LV EF of 20% and severe hypokinesia of the anterior wall and septum. Coronary angiography showed 100% proximal LAD, 100% mid-RCA, and 70% mid-LCX lesions.

The PET $^{13}NH3$ perfusion images show reduced perfusion in the septal, mid-, and apical anterior and mid- and apical anterolateral regions and apex (Panel A). The ^{18}FDG images show preserved uptake in the mid- and apical anterior and mid- and apical anterolateral regions consistent with hibernating myocardium and reduced uptake in the septum and apex, indicating scar (Panel A). Quantitative analysis (Panel B) determined scar (match defect) as 20% LV and hibernating myocardium (mismatch) as 15% LV. Patient underwent surgical revascularization (3 grafts) owing to the moderate amount of hibernating myocardium. The recommendation in the report was "Likely outcome benefit with revascularization." At 18-month follow-up, echocardiography showed improved LV EF of 25% and less dyspnea (NYHA II).

Case 2 (Figure 11-2)

A 75-year-old male presented with dyspnea (NYHA 3) and known CAD with remote RCA stenting about 7 years ago. Dipyridamole ^{99m}tetrofosmin SPECT rest and dipyridamole stress imaging large transmural scar in the inferior regions and LV EF of 21%.

The PET ^{13}NH3 perfusion images show severely reduced perfusion in the inferior regions (Panel A).

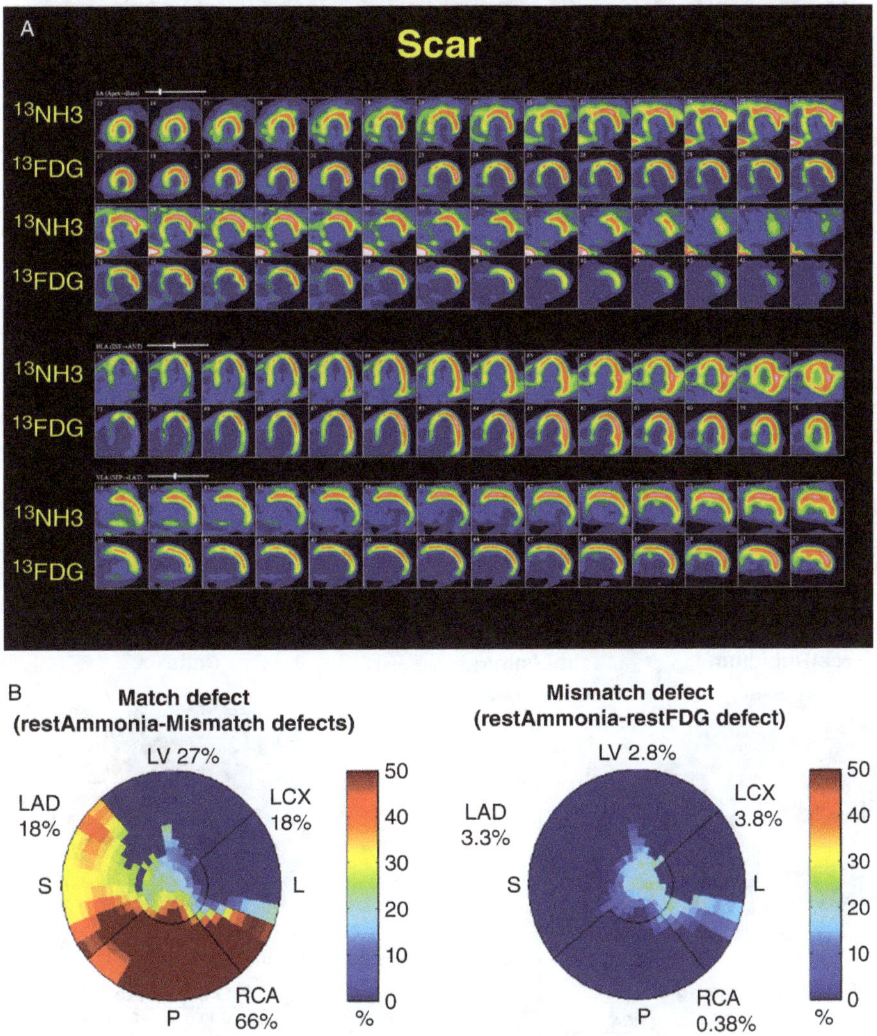

FIGURE 11-2 ScarPET ^{13}NH3 perfusion images show severely reduced perfusion in the inferior regions (A). The ^{18}FDG images show severely reduced uptake in inferior regions indicating scar (A). Quantitative analysis (B) determined scar (match defect) as 27% LV and hibernating myocardium (mismatch) as 2.8% LV.

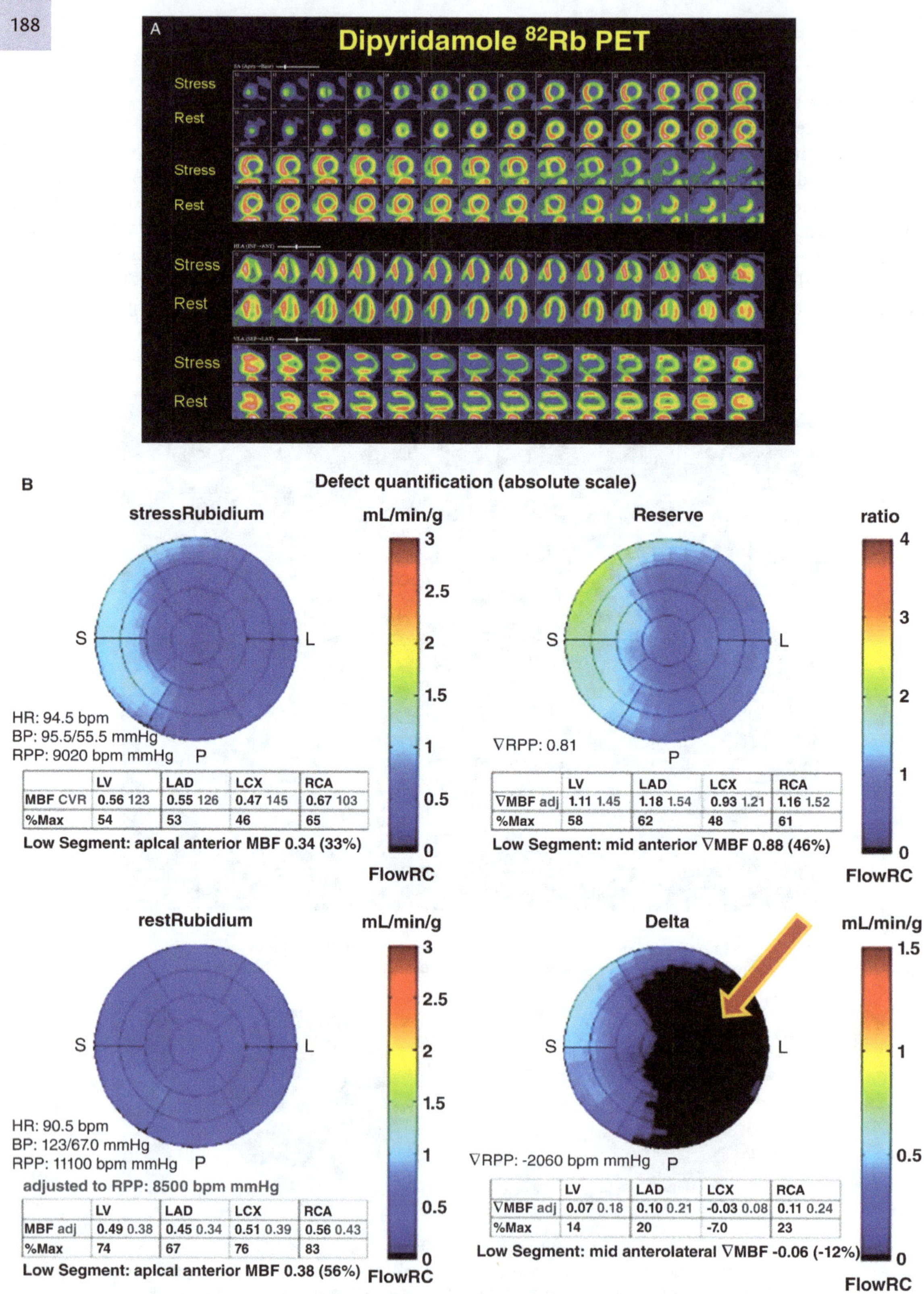

FIGURE 11-3 (*Continue*)

The ^{18}FDG images show severely reduced uptake in inferior regions indicating scar (Panel A). Quantitative analysis (Panel B) determined scar (match defect) as 27% LV and hibernating myocardium (mismatch) as 2.8% LV. The recommendation in the report was "Unlikely to have LV recovery or outcome benefit with revascularization." Patient continued with medical therapy and was stable 2 years later.

Case 3 (Figure 11-3)

A 77-year-old male presented with dyspnea (NYHA III). Echocardiography showed LV EF of 21% and global hypokinesia. Past history included peripheral vascular disease, chronic obstructive pulmonary disease, smoking for 50 pack-years, diabetes mellitus type II, hypertension, and dyslipidemia. Dipyridamole ^{82}Rb PET showed 3 vessel moderate ischemia and nontransmural scar (Panel A). Quantitative myocardial flow analysis (Panel B) showed severely reduced stress flow and flow reserve as well as coronary steal in the lateral regions (red arrow). Coronary angiography 70% proximal and 70% distal LAD, 80% mid LCX, 90% second marginal, 95% proximal, and 99% distal RCA lesions (all with poor distal vessels). Patient was considered for coronary stenting and PET viability imaging was carried out to select target vessels.

The PET ^{13}NH3 perfusion images show moderately reduced perfusion in the anterior, lateral, and inferior regions (Panel C). The ^{18}FDG images show increased uptake in the lateral wall indicating hibernating myocardium (Panel C). The recommendation in the report was "Likely regional LV recovery with revascularization." Patient underwent stenting of LCX lesions and optimal medical therapy. At follow-up 1 year later, LV EF had improved to 26% on echocardiography and patient had less dyspnea (NYHA II).

Case 4 (Figure 11-4)

A 57-year-old male presented with heart failure and severe LV dysfunction with LV EF of 21% by echocardiography. Past history included previous myocardial infarction 2 years earlier and coronary angiography showing severe and diffuse CAD not suitable for stenting and suboptimal for coronary bypass surgery

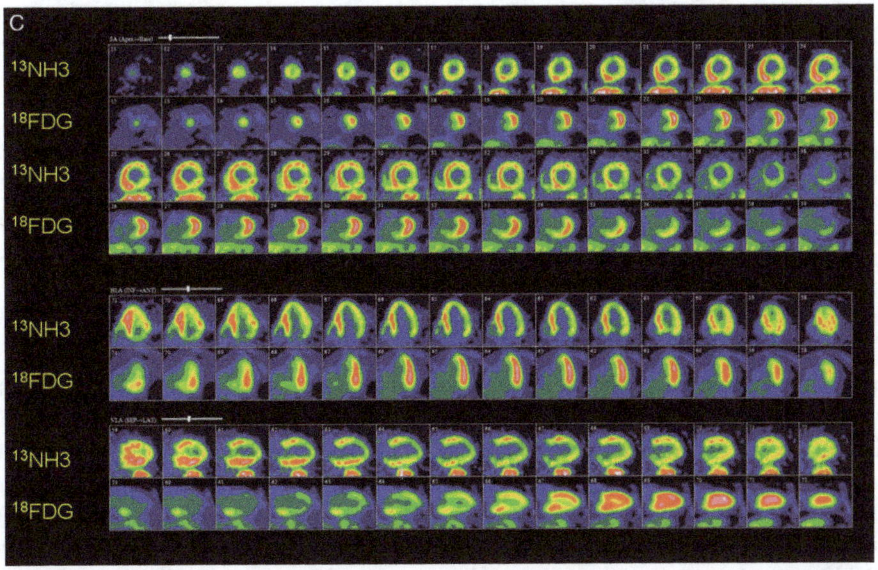

FIGURE 11-3 Hibernating Myocardium. Dipyridamole ^{82}Rb PET showed 3-vessel moderate ischemia and nontransmural scar (A). Quantitative myocardial flow analysis (B) showed severely reduced stress flow and flow reserve as well as coronary steal in the lateral regions (red arrow). PET ^{13}NH3 perfusion images show moderately reduced perfusion in the anterior, lateral, and inferior regions (C). The ^{18}FDG images show increased uptake in the lateral wall indicating hibernating myocardium (C).

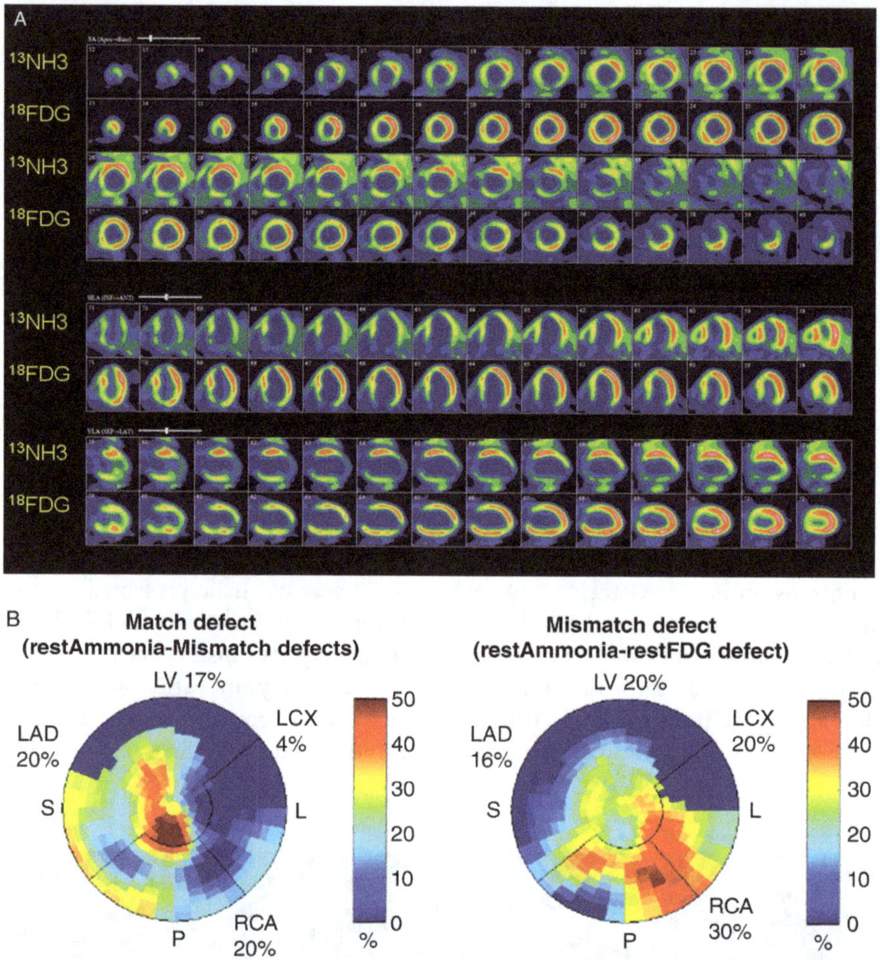

FIGURE 11-4 Hibernating Myocardium and Scar. The PET $^{13}NH3$ perfusion images show reduced perfusion in the mid- to apical anterior and anteroseptal regions, inferior and inferolateral regions and apex (A). The ^{18}FDG images show preserved uptake in the mid- to apical anterior regions, the inferior and inferolateral regions indicating hibernating myocardium and reduced uptake in the mid- to apical anteroseptal regions and apex consistent with scar (A). Quantitative analysis (B) determined scar (match defect) as 17% LV and hibernating myocardium (mismatch) as 20% LV.

caused by poor target vessels and very distal disease, paroxysmal atrial fibrillation, diabetes mellitus type II, and peripheral vascular disease. Repeat angiography showed similar CAD with minimal interval change. Viability imaging was carried out to determine potential benefit of surgery.

The PET $^{13}NH3$ perfusion images show reduced perfusion in the mid- to apical anterior and anteroseptal regions, inferior and inferolateral regions, and apex (Panel A). The ^{18}FDG images show preserved uptake in the mid- to apical anterior regions, the inferior and inferolateral regions indicating hibernating myocardium, and reduced uptake in the mid- to apical anteroseptal regions and apex consistent with scar (Panel A). Quantitative analysis (Panel B) determined scar (match defect) as 17% LV and hibernating myocardium (mismatch) as 20% LV. The recommendation in the report was "Likely outcome benefit with revascularization." Patient underwent surgical revascularization (3 grafts) owing to the moderate amount of hibernating myocardium. At 12-month follow-up, echocardiography showed stable LV EF of 24% on echocardiography and less dyspnea (NYHA II).

CONCLUSIONS

PET viability images should be analyzed with full consideration of the clinical context. All available data should be reviewed and include information from invasive or computed tomographic coronary angiography, stress perfusion imaging, echocardiography, and cardiac magnetic resonance imaging. The clinical question needs to be defined and preferably with the attending staff or team with the goal of a better understanding of the clinical scenario and formulating the best patient-based recommendation. *The report should describe the imaging findings, clinical interpretation, and management recommendations.*

ACKNOWLEDGMENTS

FE is Cardiac Imaging Fellow at the University of Ottawa Heart Institute supported by the UOHI Associates in Cardiology.

DISCLOSURES

TDR receives grant funding from GE Healthcare and Advanced Accelerator Applications International Inc.

REFERENCES

1. Mozaffarian D, Benjamin EJ, Go AS, et al. Heart disease and stroke statistics—2015 update: a report from the American Heart Association. *Circulation* 2015;131:e29–e322.
2. Levy D, Kenchaiah S, Larson MG, et al. Long-term trends in the incidence of and survival with heart failure. *N Engl J Med.* 2002;347:1397–1402.
3. He J, Ogden LJ, Bazzano LA, Vupputuri S, Loria C, Whelton PK. Risk factors for congestive heart failure in US men and women: NHANES I epidemiologic follow-up study. *Arch Intern Med.* 2001;161:996–1002.
4. Lee KS, Marwick TH, Cook SA, et al. Prognosis of patients with left ventricular dysfunction, with and without viable myocardium after myocardial infarction. Relative efficacy of medical therapy and revascularization. *Circulation.* 1994;90:2687–2694.
5. Di Carli MF, Asgarzadie F, Schelbert HR, et al. Quantitative relation between myocardial viability and improvement in heart failure symptoms after revascularization in patients with ischemic cardiomyopathy. *Circulation.* 1995;92:3436–3444.
6. Allman KC, Shaw LJ, Hachamovitch R, Udelson JE. Myocardial viability testing and impact of revascularization on prognosis in patients with coronary artery disease and left ventricular dysfunction: a meta-analysis. *J Am Coll Cardiol.* 2002;39:1151–1158.
7. Beanlands RS, Ruddy TD, deKemp RA, et al. Positron emission tomography and recovery following revascularization (PARR-1): the importance of scar and the development of a prediction rule for the degree of recovery of left ventricular function. *J Am Coll Cardiol.* 2002;40:1735–1743.
8. Beanlands RS, Nichol G, Huszti E, et al. F-18-fluorodeoxyglucose positron emission tomography imaging-assisted management of patients with severe left ventricular dysfunction and suspected coronary disease (PARR-2). *J Am Coll Cardiol.* 2007;50:2002–2012.
9. D'Egidio G, Nichol G, Williams KA, et al. Increasing benefit from revascularization is associated with increasing amounts of myocardial hibernation: a substudy of the PARR-2 trial. *J Am Coll Cardiol Imaging.* 2009;2:1060–1068.
10. Abraham A, Nichol G, Williams KA, et al. 18F-FDG PET imaging of myocardial viability in an experienced center with access to 18F-FDG and integration with clinical management teams: the Ottawa-FIVE substudy of the PARR 2 trial. *J Nucl Med.* 2010;51(4):567–574.
11. Ling LF, Marwick TH, Flores DR, et al. Identification of therapeutic benefit from revascularization in patients with left ventricular systolic dysfunction: inducible ischemia versus hibernating myocardium. *Circ Cardiovasc Imaging.* 2013;6(3):363–372.

12. McArdle B, Shukla T, Nichol G, et al. Long-term follow-up of outcomes with F-18-fluorodeoxyglucose positron emission tomography imaging–assisted management of patients with severe left ventricular dysfunction secondary to coronary disease. *Circ Cardiovasc Imaging.* 2016;9:e004331.
13. Dilsizian V, Bacharach SL, Beanlands RS, et al. ASNC imaging guidelines/SNMMI procedure standard for positron emission tomography (PET) nuclear cardiology procedures. *J Nucl Cardiol.* 2016;23:1187–1226.
14. Lim SP, McArdle BA, Beanlands RS, Hessian RC. Myocardial viability: it is still alive. *Semin Nucl Med.* 2014;44(5):358–374.
15. Braunwald E, Kloner RA. The stunned myocardium: prolonged, postischemic ventricular dysfunction. *Circulation.* 1982;66(6):1146–1149.
16. Ambrosio G, Betocchi S, Pace L, et al. Prolonged impairment of regional contractile function after resolution of exercise-induced angina. Evidence of myocardial stunning in patients with coronary artery disease. *Circulation.* 1996;94(10): 2455–2464.
17. Barnes E, Hall RJC, Dutka DP, Camici PG. Absolute blood flow and oxygen consumption in stunned myocardium in patients with coronary artery disease. *J Am Coll Cardiol.* 2002;39(3):420–427.
18. Bax JJ, Veening MA, Visser FC, et al. Optimal metabolic conditions during fluorine-18 fluorodeoxyglucose imaging; a comparative study using different protocols. *Eur J Nucl Med.* 1997;24(1):35–41.
19. Hashimoto K, Nishimura T, Ishikawa M, et al. Enhancement of glucose uptake in stunned myocardium: role of glucose transporter. *Am J Physiol.* 1997;272(3):H1122-H1130.
20. Anselm DD, Anselm AH, Renaud J, et al. Altered myocardial glucose utilization and the reverse mismatch pattern on rubidium-82 perfusion/F-18-FDG PET during the sub-acute phase following reperfusion of acute anterior myocardial infarction. *J Nucl Cardiol.* 2011;18(4):657–667.
21. Canty JM, Fallavollita JA. Hibernating myocardium. *J Nucl Cardiol.* 2005;12(1):104–119.
22. Fallavollita JA, Malm BJ, Canty JM. Hibernating myocardium retains metabolic and contractile reserve despite regional reductions in flow, function, and oxygen consumption at rest. *Circ Res.* 2003;92(1):48–55.
23. Tillisch J, Brunken R, Marshall R, et al. Reversibility of cardiac wall-motion abnormalities predicted by positron tomography. *N Engl J Med.* 1986;314(14):884–888.
24. Camici P, Ferrannini E, Opie LH. Myocardial metabolism in ischemic heart disease: basic principles and application to imaging by positron emission tomography. *Prog Cardiovasc Dis.* 1989;32(3):217–238.
25. Camici PG, Dutka DP. Repetitive stunning, hibernation, and heart failure: contribution of PET to establishing a link. *Am J Physiol Heart Circ Physiol.* 2001;280(3):H929-H936.
26. Depre C, Vanoverschelde JL, Taegtmeyer H. Glucose for the heart. *Circulation.* 1999;99(4):578–588.
27. Neely JR, Morgan HE. Relationship between carbohydrate and lipid metabolism and the energy balance of heart muscle. *Annu Rev Physiol.* 1974;36:413–459.
28. Liedtke AJ. Alterations of carbohydrate and lipid metabolism in the acutely ischemic heart. *Prog Cardiovasc Dis.* 1981;23(5):321–336.
29. Stanley WC, Lopaschuk GD, Hall JL, McCormack JG. Regulation of myocardial carbohydrate metabolism under normal and ischaemic conditions: potential for pharmacological interventions. *Cardiovasc Res.* 1997;33(2): 243–257.
30. Goodwin GW, Ahmad F, Doenst T, Taegtmeyer H. Energy provision from glycogen, glucose, and fatty acids on adrenergic stimulation of isolated working rat hearts. *Am J Physiol.* 1998;274(4 Pt 2):H1239-H1247.
31. Choi SM, Tucker DF, Gross DN, et al. Insulin regulates adipocyte lipolysis via an akt-independent signaling pathway. *Mol Cell Biol.* 2010;30:5009–5020.
32. Zaret BL, Beller GA. *Clinical Nuclear Cardiology: State of the Art and Future Directions.* 4th ed. New York, NY: Elsevier; 2010.

33. Gould KL, Pan T, Loghin C, Johnson NP, Guha A, Sdringola S. Frequent diagnostic errors in cardiac PET/CT due to misregistration of CT attenuation and emission PET images: a definitive analysis of causes, consequences, and corrections. *J Nucl Med.* 2007;48:1112–1121.
34. Thompson K, Saab G, Birnie D, et al. Is septal glucose metabolism altered in patients with left bundle branch block and ischemic cardiomyopathy? *J Nucl Med.* 2006;47:1763–1768.
35. Paternostro G, Camici PG, Lammerstma AA, et al. Cardiac and skeletal muscle insulin resistance in patients with coronary heart disease: a study with positron emission tomography. *J Clin Invest.* 1996;98:2094–2099.

EDITOR'S PERSPECTIVE

Gary V. Heller

The interpretation and reporting of FDG viability studies is the final result of ordering the right test for the right patient, having performed appropriate patient preparation and imaging, and finally, conveying the information to the referring healthcare provider. Viability studies are more difficult to interpret and convey more useful information to the healthcare provider than standard rest/stress myocardial perfusion imaging studies—notably because of the complexity of the patient as well as of the images. The study is not diagnostic for CAD, but rather to assist in clinical decisions in patients with CAD. The challenge is also to interpret a perfusion study, which is essentially an absence of activity in affected places, in comparison to FDG—in which the only uptake of importance is in the area of the perfusion abnormality. There is often FDG uptake in "normal" tissue, which can be misinterpreted.

This evaluation is also one of the few in which interpretation is best with knowledge of the coronary anatomy and the specific questions the healthcare professionals are most interested in. This is in contrast to most of nuclear cardiology in which the test is performed prior to catherization rather than after. Often the questions are revascularization of one or more specific vessels, or even a decision between PCI vs CABG depending upon viability results. Communication and discussion with the referring team is extremely important to maximize outcomes. One interesting aspect of the FDG viability research was that outcomes for patients were best when the referring physicians followed the findings of the FDG study in terms of viability vs nonviability, rather than ignoring the results.[1] Thus, a full discussion of the results with the clinical team is critical. While the interpreting nuclear cardiologist cannot make clinical decisions for a particular study, he/she can be instrumental in providing a clear recommendation regarding viability/nonviability for a particular vascular territory(s). This will optimize the test and patient outcomes.

Reference for Editor's Perspective

1. Shukla T, Nichol G, Wells G, et al. Does FDG PET-assisted management of patients with left ventricular dysfunction improve quality of life? A substudy of the PARR-2 trial. *Can J Cardiol.* 2012;28(1):54-61.

SECTION

6

CURRENT STATUS OF ASSESSMENT OF CARDIOVASCULAR INFLAMMATION AND INFECTION IMAGING

CHAPTER 12

Current Status of Assessment of Cardiac Sarcoid and Cardiac Amyloid with PET/CT Imaging

Dillenia Rosica and Sharmila Dorbala

CARDIAC SARCOIDOSIS

Clinical Need: Current Assessment and Supportive Data

Sarcoidosis is a multisystem inflammatory disease of unknown etiology that affects young men and women, typically before the age of 50 years.[1] The incidence of sarcoidosis varies based on a variety of factors including race, gender, and geography with incidence ranging from 0.73 per 100,000 in Japanese males,[2] 10 per 100,000 age- and gender-adjusted in a predominantly white cohort in the United States[1] and 71 per 100,000 in African American females.[3]

Cardiac sarcoidosis (CS) has been reported to involve approximately 2%-5% of patients with systemic sarcoidosis.[1] It can also be the only manifestation of sarcoidosis. The clinical presentation is nonspecific and includes sudden cardiac death, ventricular arrhythmias, progressive heart failure, and conduction disturbances. Despite its low reported prevalence, CS accounts for 13%-25% of sarcoidosis-related deaths.[4]

Current diagnostic criteria for CS include the Japanese Ministry of Health and Welfare (JMWH) criteria[5] and the Heart Rhythm Society Consensus (HRS).[6] The gold standard for CS is endomyocardial biopsy, which has a low diagnostic yield owing to heterogeneous and patchy involvement of the myocardium. 2-Deoxy-2-[F-18]Fluoro-D-glucose (^{18}F-FDG) PET-CT is the best advanced imaging tool to evaluate myocardial inflammation in patients with suspected CS. It has a reported sensitivity of up to 85%-100% with more variable specificity of 39%-100%.[7–10] The low specificity is likely due in part to using the JMHW criteria as a gold standard and the difficulty of a definitive diagnosis.

In the HRS guidelines,[6] clinical diagnosis of CS is probable if there is histological proof of extra CS and one or more advanced imaging findings of CS or unexplained decreased systolic function or arrhythmias when other causes have been reasonably excluded (Table 12-1).

Given the rarity of overt diagnosis of this disease, most of the available literature comes from small observational or retrospective studies and large prospective randomized trials are challenging. Much of the guidance for CS is based on consensus statements from major medical societies. Recent statements are the Joint SNMMI-ASNC Expert Consensus Document on the Role of PET/CT in Cardiac Sarcoid Detection and Therapy Monitoring[11] and a joint procedural position statement on imaging in CS from the European Association of Nuclear Medicine, the European Association of Cardiovascular Imaging, and the American Society of Nuclear Cardiology.[12]

The joint SNMMI-ASNC expert consensus document details specific scenarios where cardiac PET/CT may be helpful and these include: patients with

Table 12-1

Diagnostic Criteria for Cardiac Sarcoidosis

Japanese Ministry of Health and Welfare (JMHW 2006)[45]	Heart Rhythm Society (HRS 2014)[6]
Histological diagnosis	**Histological diagnosis**
Confirmed by endomyocardial biopsy, and histologic or clinical diagnosis of extra cardiac sarcoidosis	Noncaseating granuloma on endomyocardial biopsy with no alternative cause identified
Clinical diagnosis	**Clinical diagnosis**
Histologic or clinical diagnosis of extra cardiac sarcoidosis and two or more major criteria OR one major criterion and two or more minor criteria	Probable diagnosis of cardiac sarcoid exists if There is histologic diagnosis of extra cardiac sarcoid and one or more of the following is present (and other causes of cardiac manifestations are excluded):
Major Criteria	Cardiomyopathy or atrioventricular block responsive to immunosuppressive treatment
Advanced atrioventricular block	Unexplained reduced LVEF (<40%)
Basal thinning of intraventricular septum	Unexplained ventricular tachycardia
^{67}Ga uptake in heart	Mobitz II 2nd- or 3rd-degree heart block
Depressed LVEF (<50%)	Patchy ^{18}F-FDG uptake on cardiac PET consistent with cardiac sarcoid
Minor Criteria	Late gadolinium enhancement on CMR consistent with cardiac sarcoid
Electrocardiography: ventricular tachycardia, premature ventricular contractions, right bundle branch block, abnormal axis, abnormal Q wave	Cardiac ^{67}Ga uptake
Echocardiography: structural or wall motion abnormality	
Nuclear medicine: perfusion defect, ^{201}Tl, ^{99m}Tc	
CMR: late gadolinium enhancement	
Endomyocardial biopsy: moderate fibrosis or monocyte infiltration	

LVEF = left ventricular ejection fraction; Ga = gallium; Tl = thallium; Tc = technetium; PET = positron emission tomography; CMR = cardiac magnetic resonance imaging Reproduced with permission from hareonthaitawee P, Beanlands RS, Chen W, et al: Joint SNMMI-ASNC expert consensus document on the role of 18F-FDG PET/CT in cardiac sarcoid detection and therapy monitoring. J Nucl Cardiol. 2017;58(8):1341–1353.

histologic evidence of extra CS and abnormal screening of CS; unexplained, new onset of significant conduction system disease; idiopathic SVT and proven CS to follow response to treatment.[11] (Table 12-2 is reproduced with permission from SNMMI-ASNC expert consensus document.)

Perfusion defects and mismatch between perfusion and ^{18}F-FDG images can result from coronary artery disease. Hence, prior to performing ^{18}F-FDG PET/CT for sarcoidosis, significant coronary artery disease (CAD) must be excluded using noninvasive ischemia testing with radionuclide imaging, echocardiography, or cardiac magnetic resonance imaging or coronary angiography with CT or catheterization.

Assessment of Risk and Therapies: Timing, Indications

Immunosuppressive therapy and implantable cardiac devices (ICD) along with standard heart failure therapy are the mainstays of treatment for CS. Current indications for immunosuppressive therapy

Table 12-2

Clinical Scenarios in Which Cardiac PET May Be Useful in Suspected or Known Cardiac Sarcoidosis

Scenario	Specifics
Patients with histologic evidence of extraCS, and abnormal screening for CS, defined as one or more of the following	Abnormal electrocardiography findings of complete left or right bundle branch block or the presence of unexplained pathologic Q waves in two or more leads
	Echocardiography with findings of regional wall motion abnormality, wall aneurysm, basal septum thinning or LVEF <-50%
	Holter findings of sustained or nonsustained ventricular tachycardia
	Cardiac MRI findings suggestive of CS
	Unexplained palpitations or syncope
Young patients (<60y) with unexplained, new onset, significant conduction system disease (such as sustained second- or third-degree atrioventricular block)	
Patients with idiopathic sustained ventricular tachycardia, defined as not fulfilling any of the following criteria:	Typical outflow tract tachycardia
	Fascicular ventricular tachycardia
	Ventricular tachycardia secondary to other structural heart disease (coronary artery disease or any cardiomyopathy other than idiopathic)
Patients with proven CS as adjunct to follow response to treatment	

PET = positron emission tomography; LVEF = left ventricular ejection fraction; y = years; CS = cardiac sarcoidosis. Reproduced with permission from hareonthaitawee P, Beanlands RS, Chen W, et al: Joint SNMMI-ASNC expert consensus document on the role of 18F-FDG PET/CT in cardiac sarcoid detection and therapy monitoring. J Nucl Cardiol. 2017;58(8):1341–1353

include: LV systolic dysfunction, ventricular arrhythmias, evidence of inflammation on ^{18}F-FDG-PET, conduction defects, late gadolinium enhancement (LGE), or CMR or right ventricular dysfunction in the absence of pulmonary hypertension.[13] ICD is indicated if LVEF remains <35% after immunosuppressive therapy (Class I) or if LGE is present in patients with LVEF 35%-49% after immunosuppression (Class IIb).[6]

While the optimal timing for repeat ^{18}F-FDG -PET/CT is not known, current recommendations are to repeat it 4–6 months after initiation of immunosuppression.[12] Observational studies have shown decreased intensity and extent of ^{18}F-FDG uptake correlating with improved LVEF following initiation of treatment,[14] suggesting that ^{18}F-FDG-PET/CT may help guide the duration of treatment. In one longitudinal study of 23 patients who had serial ^{18}F-FDG PET-CT scans for CS, a quantitative decrease in intensity and extent of ^{18}F-FDG uptake correlated with improvement in ejection fraction, suggesting a role for ^{18}F-FDG PET-CT in guiding immunosuppressive therapy[14] (Figure 12-1). Both visual and quantitative evaluation using standardized uptake value (SUV) and volume of inflamed myocardium based on an SUV threshold is recommended to increase detection of partial response, which may not be apparent with qualitative/visual analysis. Prospective randomized clinical trials are needed to further assess the role of imaging in guiding immunosuppressive therapy.

With regard to prognosis, focal uptake in the right ventricle, abnormal myocardial perfusion, abnormal myocardial ^{18}F-FDG uptake, or both (Figure 12-2) and reduced ejection fraction have been found to correlate with worse survival free of ventricular tachycardia

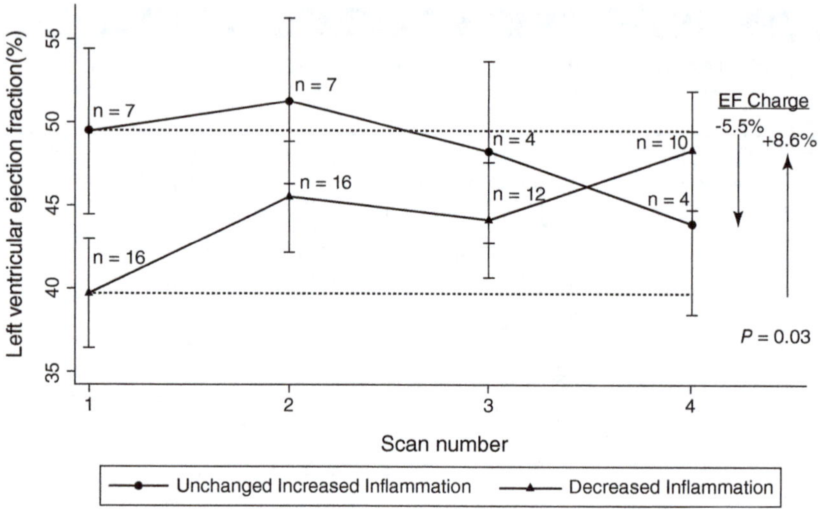

FIGURE 12-1 Changes in LVEF as a Function of Changes in Myocardial ^{18}F-FDG Uptake on Baseline Compared to 6-Month Scans. Patients with significant improvement in inflammation on serial scans (solid triangles) showed improvement in LVEF. LVEF = left ventricular ejection fraction. Reproduced with permission from Osborne MT, Hulten EA, Singh A, et al. Reduction in ^{18}F-fluorodeoxyglucose uptake on serial cardiac positron emission tomography is associated with improved left ventricular ejection fraction in patients with cardiac sarcoidosis, J Nucl Cardiol. 2014 Feb;21(1):166-174

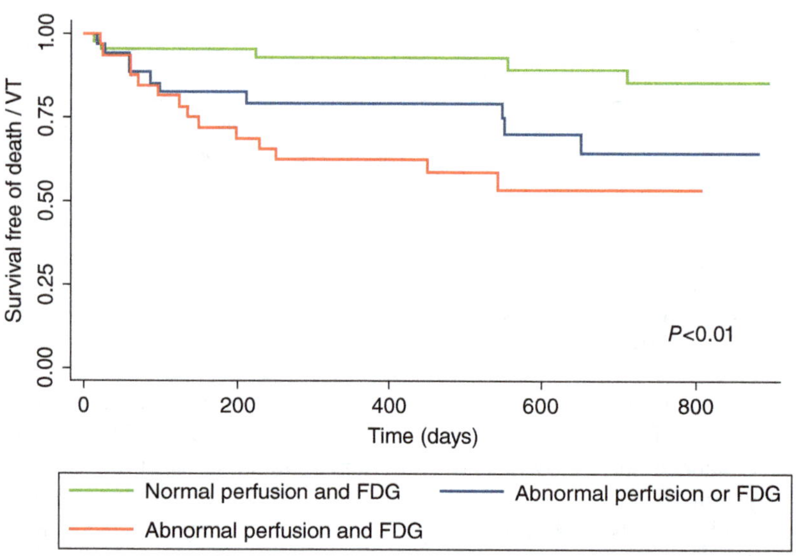

FIGURE 12-2 Prognostic Value of Myocardial Perfusion and ^{18}F-FDG PET/CT Imaging in Sarcoidosis. Patients with both normal perfusion and no myocardial ^{18}F-FDG uptake (green line) showed the best prognosis, while those with both abnormal perfusion and abnormal ^{18}F-FDG uptake (red line) showed the worst survival free of death or ventricular tachycardia. FDG = fluorodeoxyglucose. Reproduced with permission from Blankstein R, Osborne M, Naya M, et al. Cardiac positron emission tomography enhances prognostic assessments of patients with suspected cardiac sarcoidosis, J Am Coll Cardiol. 2014 Feb 4;63(4):329-336

and death.[14,15] Furthermore, recent studies suggest that quantitative measures of extent and severity of perfusion and ^{18}F-FDG metabolic mismatch as well as the coefficient of variation of ^{18}F-FDG uptake provides incremental prognostic value in CS.[16]

Patient Preparation

The key aspect of patient preparation for ^{18}F-FDG PET-CT for CS assessment is suppression of physiological myocardial glucose metabolism. This can be done through several approaches, all of which share a common goal of shifting myocardial metabolism from glucose to fatty acid use. Current SNMMI/ASNC/SCCT guidelines recommend a high-fat, zero-carbohydrate diet for 12–24 hours, followed by fasting for 12–18 hours and optional IV unfractionated heparin (single dose of 50 IU/kg) 15 minutes prior to radiotracer injection.[17]

The best approach remains somewhat controversial. One meta-analysis showed that the diagnostic odds ratio of ^{18}F-FDG PET-CT was affected by fasting time and heparin administration but not with a high-fat low-carbohydrate diet[18] whereas other studies have shown that fasting alone is inferior to a high-fat low-carbohydrate diet.[19] Also, the appropriate amount of fat or carbohydrate intake has not been standardized. Some suggest more than 35 g of fat and less than 5 g of carbohydrates for at least two meals.[20,21] A high-fat beverage given right before administration of ^{18}F-FDG, in addition to the diet, has not been shown to have an added benefit.[22–24] There have also been studies showing longer duration of high-fat, high-protein, very low carbohydrate diet of up to 72 hours, can increase diagnostic accuracy of the scan.[25]

For vegetarians, eggs are an option. Oil and butter can also be used for people on a vegan diet or for those who cannot eat solid foods. For diabetic patients, those on insulin should continue the basal rate and avoid rapid acting insulin if possible. Patients with diabetes on oral hypoglycemic agents, should avoid these medications while fasting and on the day of the exam.

As with standard ^{18}F-FDG PET-CT for other indications, preparation includes avoiding strenuous activity for at least 24 hours. Despite adequate preparation, the rate of incomplete or unsuccessful myocardial suppression has been reported to be 20%.[21]

How to Perform the Procedure

^{18}F-FDG PET-CT is performed in conjunction with rest myocardial perfusion imaging. Ideally, obstructive CAD should be ruled out prior to performing sarcoid protocol ^{18}F-FDG scan. If stress testing with imaging is necessary to exclude CAD, it is preferably performed a day prior to ^{18}F-FDG PET-CT. Myocardial perfusion imaging should ideally be performed with PET ^{82}Rubidium PET or ^{13}N-ammonia PET using standard protocols. However, if PET is not available, ^{99m}Tc-SPECT is an acceptable alternative. This is followed by injection of 5-15 mCi of ^{18}F-FDG for either 3D or 2D PET, respectively. Recommended uptake time is 90 minutes (minimum 60 minutes), during which there should be no food intake or exercise. Dedicated cardiac PET-CT is then performed followed by limited PET-CT of at least the thorax and upper abdomen to assess for extra cardiac sarcoid involvement. If available, hybrid PET/CT is preferable to dedicated PET, because the CT obtained for attenuation correction (AC) enables better localization of ^{18}F-FDG uptake to the myocardium versus lung or mediastinal lymph nodes. If PET-CT is not available, PET-only imaging is an alternative. Images are processed and reviewed with standard cardiac displays (short axis, horizontal and vertical long axis) and standard nuclear medicine display for PET/CT. Cardiac images are normalized to the maximum counts per pixel of the respective data set.

Value of Cardiac MRI (CMR)

CMR has an upfront role in diagnosis and is the first line of imaging in patients with suspected CS. Focal myocardial hyperenhancement on delayed contrast enhanced images (LGE) is the most common finding in CS with initial reported sensitivity of 100% and specificity of 78%.[26] LGE on CMR showed similarly high diagnostic accuracy (sensitivity 96.9%, specificity 100%) and risk stratification for major adverse cardiac events (cardiac death, heart failure hospitalization, ventricular tachyarrhythmia, or cardiac transplantation) in another study.[27] Furthermore, a recent meta-analysis, including 694 patients from 7 studies, showed that LGE increases the risk of ventricular tachyarrhythmia and cardiovascular death.[28] However, LGE does not distinguish between myocardial fibrosis and active inflammation. Because disease-modifying therapy is directed by the presence, extent, and severity of myocardial inflammation, following a CMR suspicious for sarcoidosis, ^{18}F-FDG PET-CT can be performed for evaluation of active inflammation.[12] In a subset of patients who either have non-MR-compatible implanted devices or are unable to obtain a CMR for other reasons, ^{18}F-FDG PET-CT then becomes the initial imaging test to aid in diagnosis.[28]

Combining the high spatial resolution of MRI with the high sensitivity of ^{18}F-FDG PET for inflammation could improve diagnostic accuracy with the use of hybrid PET/MRI imaging. This can potentially show both the extent of scarring and active inflammation. There are a few case reports in the literature that demonstrate the added value of ^{18}F-FDG PET/MR imaging.[29]

Following diagnosis of cardiac sarcoid and initiation of immunosuppressive therapy, ^{18}F-FDG PET-CT is the recommended test for assessment of treatment response (Figure 12-3).

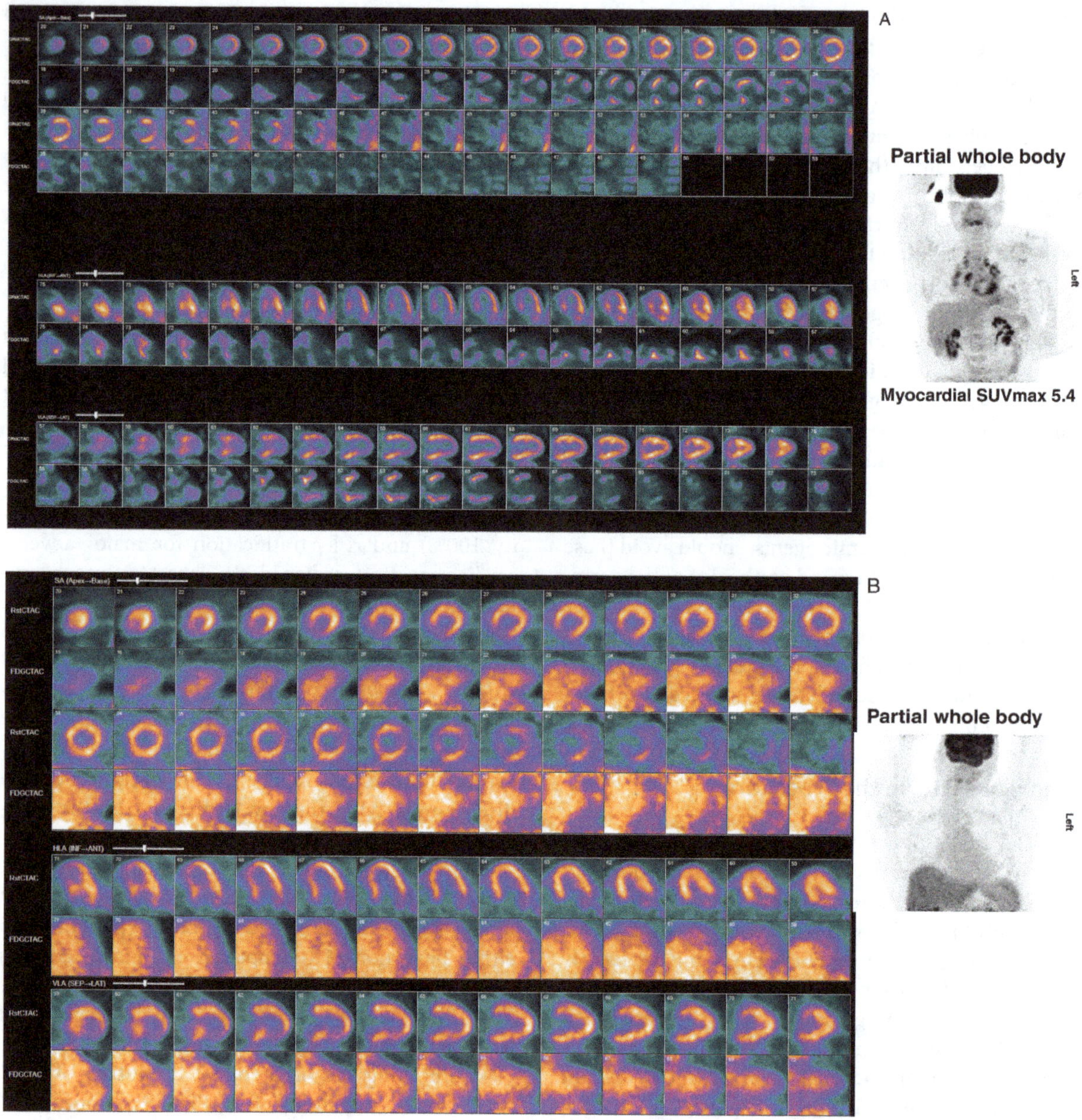

FIGURE 12-3 Assessment of Response to Therapy in Cardiac Sarcoidosis Using ^{18}F-FDG. Figures 12-3A and 12-3B are arranged in standard cardiac projections (short axis, horizontal long axis, and vertical long axis) with myocardial perfusion in the top rows and FDG in the bottom rows. The far-right image is the maximum intensity projection image (MIP). Figure 12-3A is a baseline scan showing myocardial perfusion defect in the mid- to distal inferoseptal segments with corresponding ^{18}F-FDG uptake in this area consistent with active myocardial inflammation. SUVmax in the myocardium was 5.4. MIP images also demonstrate evidence of active extracardiac sarcoidosis with ^{18}F-FDG avid bilateral hilar and mediastinal lymph nodes. Figure 12-3B is a follow-up scan after corticosteroid treatment showing complete resolution of ^{18}F-FDG uptake in the myocardium. Myocardial SUVmax was similar to blood pool. MIP images also demonstrate resolution of FDG uptake in the hilar and mediastinal lymph nodes. SUV = standardized uptake value; FDG = fluorodeoxyglucose; PET = positron emission tomography.

Interpretation and Reporting of Cardiac Sarcoid and Amyloid Studies with Case Examples

^{18}F-FDG is a nonspecific marker of myocardial glucose uptake. In inflammation, infection, and malignancy the high glycolytic activity of inflamed cells as well as glucose utilization of activated macrophages and cancer cells leads to increased uptake of ^{18}F-FDG. Notably, patients with sarcoidosis are at increased risk of hematological and solid malignancy, making it even more challenging to interpret ^{18}F-FDG uptake solely as inflammation in these cases.

Interpretation of the perfusion and ^{18}F-FDG images involves: (1) assessment of resting myocardial perfusion, (2) assessment of quality of the ^{18}F-FDG PET/CT for interpretation, (3) assessment of cardiac and extra cardiac ^{18}F-FDG uptake, (4) correlation with myocardial perfusion data, and (5) comparison with prior ^{18}F-FDG scan or CMR or echocardiography findings, if available, for assessment of treatment response.

Assessment of resting myocardial perfusion: This is the same as for standard myocardial perfusion imaging. Evaluate for the size, location, and severity of perfusion defects. If gated acquisition was performed, assess for wall motion abnormalities.

Assessment of quality of ^{18}F-FDG PET/CT for interpretation: It is critical to determine whether myocardial ^{18}F-FDG uptake was adequately suppressed. In general, diffuse ^{18}F-FDG uptake throughout the myocardium usually means suppression was inadequate, as discussed in the next section. It is important to remember that suppression can also be incomplete, particularly if the area of ^{18}F-FDG uptake does not have a matching perfusion defect or LGE on CMR. If clinical suspicion remains high, repeating the ^{18}F-FDG PET study can be considered with rigorous adherence to the diet and perhaps a longer fasting period.

Assessment of cardiac ^{18}F-FDG uptake: Uptake within the myocardium from CS is a marker of active inflammation and appears patchy and does not follow a vascular territory. It is important to note that absence of ^{18}F-FDG uptake does not exclude fibrosis from CS, only that there is no active inflammation.

Patterns of myocardial ^{18}F-FDG uptake can be classified into four categories: (1) no ^{18}F-FDG uptake, (2) diffuse ^{18}F-FDG uptake, (3) focal ^{18}F-FDG uptake, and (4) focal on diffuse ^{18}F-FDG uptake. Categories (3) and (4) are considered abnormal, while (2) is nonspecific and can be attributed to incomplete myocardial suppression.[15]

Correlation with myocardial perfusion data: Correlation with myocardial perfusion is helpful because it can significantly increase the specificity of the findings. The key correlation patterns are shown in Figure 12-4 (A-E) and listed as follows:[15,30]

A. Normal perfusion and normal ^{18}F-FDG scan (no uptake in the myocardium) = normal study (Figure 12-4A)
B. Normal perfusion with diffuse myocardial ^{18}F-FDG uptake = likely failure to suppress normal myocardial FDG uptake (Figure 12-4B)
C. Normal perfusion with focal abnormal ^{18}F-FDG uptake = early disease (Figure 12-4C). Note that this pattern may represent a normal variant (incomplete suppression) particularly in the lateral wall, unless there is corresponding LGE on CMR.
D. Abnormal perfusion with a defect corresponding to a site of ^{18}F-FDG uptake ("mismatch pattern") = active CS (Figure 12-4D)
E. Abnormal perfusion with a defect with no abnormal ^{18}F-FDG uptake = scar from chronic sarcoidosis or other causes (eg, infarct) (Figure 12-4E)
F. Other patterns: Abnormal perfusion with a focal defect/defects and focal on diffuse patchy ^{18}F-FDG uptake that is of greater extent than the perfusion defect may represent active inflammation with likely areas of incomplete suppression, or extensive disease. Abnormal perfusion with a focal defect/defects and ^{18}F-FDG uptake in a different site may indicate the presence of both scar and inflammation in different segments

Quantitative Analysis

Quantitative metrics that have been used in the literature include SUV, SUV_{max} in the myocardium,[31] SUV_{mean} in each of the 17 segments,[32] SUV_{total} of all segments,[8] heart-to-blood pool ratio (SUV_{max} of myocardium: SUV_{max} of aorta),[33] coefficient of variance (standard deviation of uptake divided by average uptake in 17 segments),[5] and volume of ^{18}F-FDG avid voxels above a certain SUV threshold.[14,31] Although

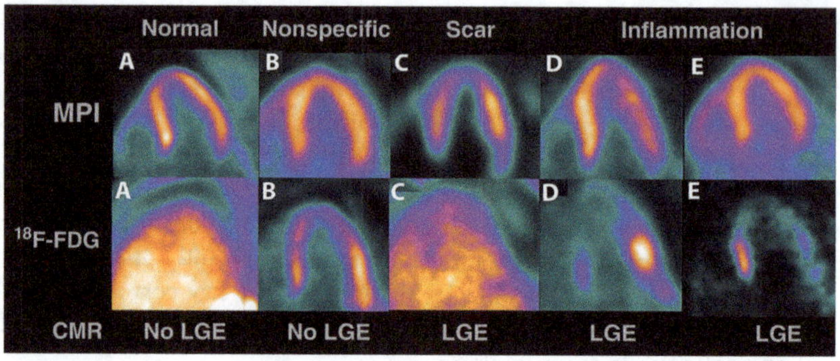

FIGURE 12-4 Patterns of Myocardial Perfusion and ^{18}F-FDG Imaging. Myocardial perfusion images are depicted in the first row, ^{18}F-FDG images in the second row, and expected CMR patterns in the third row. Distinct patterns of perfusion and metabolism can identify normal myocardium to nonspecific changes, inflammation, and scar. Note that absence of myocardial uptake of ^{18}F-FDG (A and E, showing blood pool activity) may indicate normal myocardium or scar; perfusion imaging findings can differentiate between the two entities. CMR = cardiac magnetic resonance imaging; LGE = late gadolinium enhancement; FDG = ^{18}F-fluorodeoxyglucose.

there is no accepted standard for quantification, SUV has been shown to be more reproducible than qualitative assessment alone, especially when imaging parameters and ^{18}F-FDG uptake period are standardized. The volume of metabolically active myocardium (ie, pixels above a certain SUV threshold) is a better tool to identify disease extent and for assessment of response to therapy since SUV_{max} alone may fail to accurately identify the extent of inflammation.

Assessment of Extra Cardiac Uptake

Extra cardiac uptake can be helpful to assess other sites of active disease or to determine a potential biopsy site if the diagnosis has not yet been established. Common extra cardiac findings in sarcoidosis include symmetric mediastinal and hilar hypermetabolic lymphadenopathy, cervical, axillary, and upper abdominal lymph nodes, lung consolidations. Less common findings on PET/CT include hepatic uptake, splenic uptake, and osseous uptake. Osseous uptake often has no CT correlate.

Pitfalls in Interpretation

It is important to recognize that normalization of images on the cardiology display systems can make it difficult to assess the absolute intensity of ^{18}F-FDG uptake. When assessing response to therapy, semiquantitative analysis, such as SUV_{max}, volume of metabolically active myocardium above a certain SUV threshold,[14] total SUV of the heart,[8] SUV_{mean} of the heart,[32] heart-to-blood pool SUV ratios,[33] coefficient of variance of SUVs[5] may be helpful to assess subtle changes. At the time of writing, these methods have not yet been rigorously compared. Studies should only be compared in a quantitative manner if they were performed with the same protocol (including patient preparation for myocardial suppression) on the same scanner.

Conversely, low background uptake can cause relatively mild ^{18}F-FDG uptake to appear more intense in the normalized images. As mentioned earlier, semiquantitative analysis may be helpful as well.

Cardiac devices such as ICDs can cause issues owing to artifactual uptake from AC. Metal artifact reduction feature can help with this. However, when this feature is not routinely available, it is important to review the nonattenuation corrected (NAC) images to confirm if the uptake is real (ie, if uptake on AC images persist on NAC, this is likely to represent true ^{18}F-FDG uptake).

Other radiotracers: ^{67}Gallium-SPECT imaging has been used in the past for imaging systemic and CS, including assessment of response to therapy.[34] However, in addition to the long test time (interval between injection of tracer and imaging 48-72 hours), ^{67}Ga SPECT has limited sensitivity, lower spatial resolution, and lower yield for extracardiac lesions compared to ^{18}F-FDG PET.[35] Hence, ^{18}F-FDG PET has for the most part replaced gallium SPECT for sarcoidosis imaging in clinical practice. Also, clinical trials are ongoing for ^{68}Gallium-labeled PET tracers of somatostatin receptor agonists (^{68}Ga 68-DOT-ANOC, ^{68}Ga 68-DOTA) for imaging sarcoidosis (ClinicalTrials.gov identifier: NCT01729169). Small studies have been published of ^{68}Ga-DOTANOC for imaging sarcoidosis showing high specificity in relation to ^{18}F-FDG PET.

CARDIAC AMYLOIDOSIS

Clinical Need: Current Assessment and Supportive Data

Amyloidosis is a systemic protein misfolding disease characterized by deposition of fibrils with a beta pleated sheet structure in various organs. Cardiac involvement in systemic amyloidosis is a primary determinant of prognosis in these patients. There are multiple types of cardiac amyloidosis, the two main subtypes light chain amyloid (AL) and transthyretin amyloid (ATTR) affect the heart and are compared in Table 12-3.

Given the differences in mortality and treatment approaches for AL and ATTR cardiac amyloidosis, diagnosis, and differentiation between the two types is important. Diagnosis can be established directly by endomyocardial biopsy or indirectly by echocardiographic/CMR evidence of amyloidosis and histologic confirmation of extra cardiac amyloid. However, the diagnostic yield may be limited, particularly in early stages of the disease, and endomyocardial biopsy is associated with risks of complications including myocardial perforation and tamponade.

Noninvasive techniques to image cardiac amyloidosis include echocardiography and CMR. While both can identify amyloidosis, neither modality can distinguish between the two subtypes, AL from ATTR amyloidosis. In contrast, bone compound imaging agents ^{99m}Tc-pyrophospate (PYP) and ^{99m}Tc-3, 3-diphosphono-1, 2-propranodicarboxylic acid (DPD) have been shown to identify ATTR amyloidosis with high sensitivity and specificity (see Table 12-4).

Table 12-3

Major Subtypes of Cardiac Amyloidosis[46–49]

Light chain amyloid (AL)	Transthyretin amyloidosis (ATTR)
Amyloid fibril composition/Cause	***Amyloid fibril composition/Cause***
Predominantly light chain fragments formed from immunoglobulin light chains produced by clonal population of plasma cells	Misfolded monomers and dimers from either mutant or wild type TTR deposit as fibrils in the myocardium ATTRm (mutant type): autosomal dominant disorder ATTRwt (wild type): associated with aging (senile amyloidosis)
Mortality	***Mortality***
Median survival, if untreated, is <12 months after heart failure onset	**ATTRm:** median survival, if untreated, is 25 months after heart failure onset **ATTRwt:** median survival, if untreated, is 75 months after heart failure onset
Treatment	***Treatment***
High dose chemotherapy Autologous stem cell transplant Heart transplant (controversial)	Supportive care Novel therapies include drugs that inhibit TTR synthesis, stabilize TTR or degrade proteins ATTRm: orthotopic liver transplantation +/- heart transplantation ATTRwt: heart transplant (uncommon)

AL = light chain amyloid; TTR = transthyretin amyloidosis

Table 12-4

Diagnostic Performance of Bone Compound Radionuclide Imaging Agents for TTR Cardiac Amyloidosis

^{99m}Tc-PYP	Sensitivity	Specificity
Bokhari, et al[39]	97%	100%
Castano, et al[44]	91%	92%
Gillmore, et al[50]	>99%	86%
^{99m}Tc-DPD		
Perugini, et al[51]	100%	100%
Hutt, et al[52]	91%	82%
Gillmore, et al[50]	>99%	85%

ATTR = transthyretin amyloidosis Tc = technetium; PYP = pyrophosphate; DPD = ^{99m}Tc-3, 3-diphosphono-1, 2-propranodicarboxylic acid

Several PET agents are currently being investigated for cardiac amyloid imaging including ^{18}F-florbetapir, ^{18}F-florbetaben, and ^{18}F-sodium fluoride. None are in routine clinical use at this time. ^{18}F compounds have the potential for routine clinical use because they would not require an on-site cyclotron for synthesis. Table 12-5 summarizes literature on the ^{18}F compounds.

The current role of ^{99m}Tc-PYP/DPD imaging is in the diagnosis of ATTR cardiac amyloidosis in the following situations[36,37]:

- Suspected cardiac amyloidosis with echocardiography findings classic for cardiac amyloid and no evidence of plasma cell dyscrasia
- Individuals with heart failure and unexplained increase in left ventricular wall thickness
- African Americans over the age of 60 years with heart failure, unexplained or with increased left ventricular wall thickness (>12 mm)
- Individuals over the age of 60 years with unexplained heart failure with preserved ejection fraction
- Individuals, especially elderly males, with unexplained neuropathy, bilateral carpal tunnel syndrome or atrial arrhythmias in the absence of usual risk factors, and signs/symptoms of heart failure
- Evaluation of cardiac involvement in individuals with known or suspected familial amyloidosis
- Diagnosis of cardiac ATTR in individuals with CMR or echocardiography consistent with cardiac amyloidosis

Table 12-5

^{18}F Compounds for Detection of Cardiac Amyloidosis

^{18}F-florbetapir
Dorbala, et al. *Eur J Nucl Med Mol Imaging.* 2014[53] • left and right ventricular uptake in all amyloid patients and none in controls • myocardial retention higher in AL vs ATTR amyloidosis
Osborne, et al. *Front Cardiovasc Med.* 2015[54] • describes quantitative protocol using SUV and SUV ratios in the septal wall to identity cardiac amyloidosis
^{18}F-florbetaben
Law, et al. *J Nucl Med.* 2016[55] • uptake and percent myocardial retention was able to differentiate cardiac amyloid patients from hypertensive controls • percent myocardial retention was an independent determinant of myocardial dysfunction
^{18}F-sodium fluoride
Morgenstern, et al. *J Nucl Card* 2017[56]
• uptake present in ATTR patients and absent in controls and AL patients

SUV = standardized uptake value; AL = light chain amyloidosis; ATTR = transthyretin amyloidosis

- Patients with suspected cardiac ATTR amyloidosis and contraindications to CMR, such as renal insufficiency or an implantable cardiac device

A patient with a strongly positive ^{99m}Tc-PYP/DPD scan in these situations can be considered to have ATTR amyloidosis and a biopsy may not be necessary. Notably, a negative scan, however, does not exclude AL amyloidosis.

Assessment of Therapies: Timing, Indications

^{99m}Tc-PYP/DPD scans have not been found to be useful in monitoring response to therapy. One study of serial ^{99m}Tc-PYP studies showed no significant changes in uptake in ATTR patients despite clinical progression.[38] Whether this reflects the limitations of the technique (ie, SPECT with limited quantitation) or the lack of highly effective disease modifying therapies or a combination of both is unclear.

Patient Preparation

No special preparation is necessary for either ^{99m}Tc-PYP/DPD scintigraphy or any of the ^{18}F PET-CT studies for evaluation of cardiac amyloidosis.

How to Perform the Procedure

^{99m}Tc-PYP/DPD Scintigraphy

This can be performed with either planar or SPECT/SPECT-CT or SPECT/SPECT-CT only imaging. For either approach, 20-25 mCi of ^{99m}Tc-PYP is injected intravenously followed by a minimum of 60-minute uptake time. Planar imaging is performed in anterior, lateral, and LAO projections (LEHR collimator, 256 x 256 matrix, 1.46 zoom factor. Protocol options include: (1) both planar and SPECT/SPECT-CT routinely; (2) start with planar imaging followed by SPECT/SPECT-CT only if there is abnormal uptake on planar imaging; or (3) just doing SPECT/SPECT-CT and foregoing planar imaging. (LEHR, minimum 64 x 64 matrix, 1.46 zoom factor, Butterworth filter cut off 0.50 and order of 5.00.)[39] An example of a negative (Figure 12-5) and a positive (Figure 12-6) ^{99m}Tc-PYP scan for evaluation of heart failure from suspected cardiac transthyretin amyloidosis is shown.

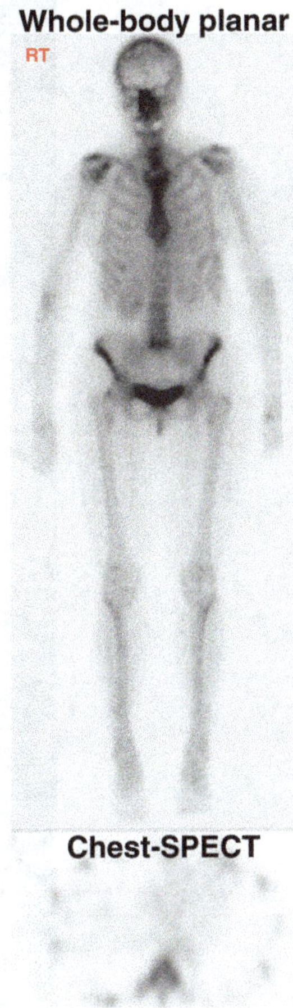

FIGURE 12-5 Negative ^{99m}Tc-PYP Scan. Anterior planar whole body image with no significant myocardial uptake. There is physiologic renal excretion. Distribution in the osseous structures is similar to what is expected with ^{99m}Tc-MDP with increased uptake in areas of osteoblastic activity, such as the joints. Tc = technetium. PYP = pyrophosphate; MDP = medronic acid.

^{18}F-Florbetapir/Florbetaben/Sodium Fluoride PET-CT

Protocols can be found in the references from Table 12-5. PET-CT for cardiac amyloidosis is not currently in routine clinical use. The two major advantages of the amyloid PET compounds are that they are quantitative, and are the only radiotracers that can image AL amyloid in the heart.

Value of CMR

CMR findings suggesting cardiac amyloidosis generally manifest in the more advanced stage of disease. Increased wall thickness, bi-atrial enlargement, pericardial/pleural effusions, varying patterns of LGE (subendocardial, diffuse, focal, global), atrial LGE, difficulty nulling the myocardium or classic pattern of myocardial nulling prior to blood pool nulling on the inversion time scout images suggest amyloidosis.[31,37,40] Although certain CMR features are fairly typical for amyloidosis, none of the features can definitively distinguish AL from ATTR amyloidosis. Hence, in cases where the clinical suspicion is high for ATTR amyloidosis, a bone compound imaging study can be considered to type amyloidosis and potentially avoid endomyocardial biopsy. LGE on CMR and native T1 mapping[41] as well as extracellular volume expansion[42] indicate more advanced disease phenotype and portend worse prognosis.[43]

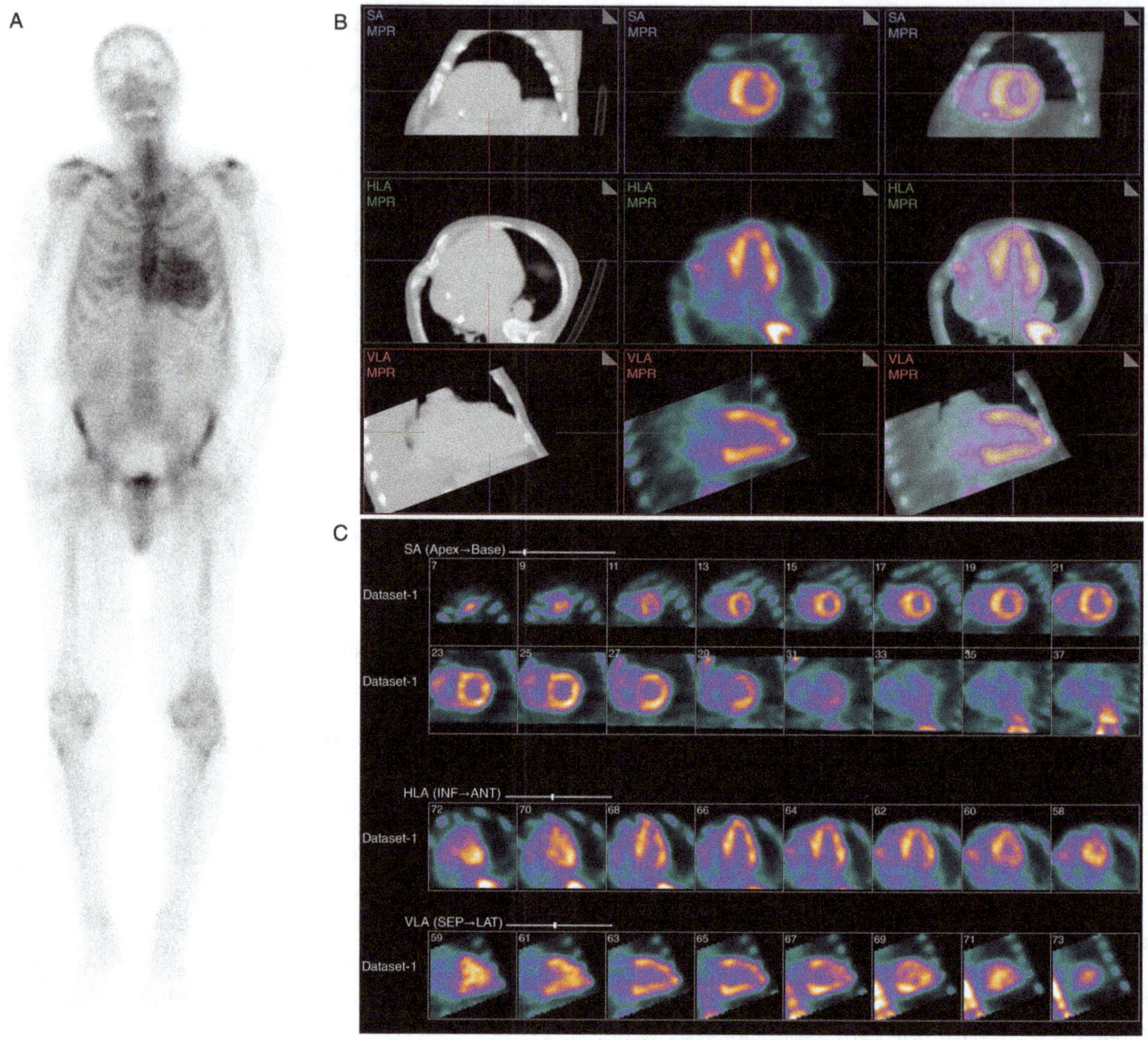

FIGURE 12-6 Positive ^{99m}Tc-PYP Scan. (A) Whole body anterior planar image, (B) SPECT standard cardiac projections (first two rows: short axis, third row: vertical long axis, fourth row: horizontal long axis), and (C) SPECT/CT images (first column: attenuation correction CT, second and third columns: fused SPECT/CT images) shows diffuse myocardial uptake. SPECT = single photon emission computed tomography.

Interpretation and Reporting of Cardiac Amyloid Studies with Case Examples

^{99m}Tc-PYP/DPD Scintigraphy

Images can be assessed in a semi-quantitative and quantitative manner. Semi-quantitative assessment involves scoring the degree of uptake visually in comparison to bone uptake with scores as follows: 0 = no cardiac uptake, 1 = mild uptake (less than bone), 2 = moderate uptake (equal to bone), 3 = high (greater than bone). Quantitative uptake involves circular region of interest around the heart and in the contralateral chest and taking the ratio of total cardiac counts over total counts in the contralateral chest (H/CL ratio).[39] A semi-quantitative score of 2 or greater and a H/CL ratio of greater than 1.5 indicate ATTR amyloidosis.[44]

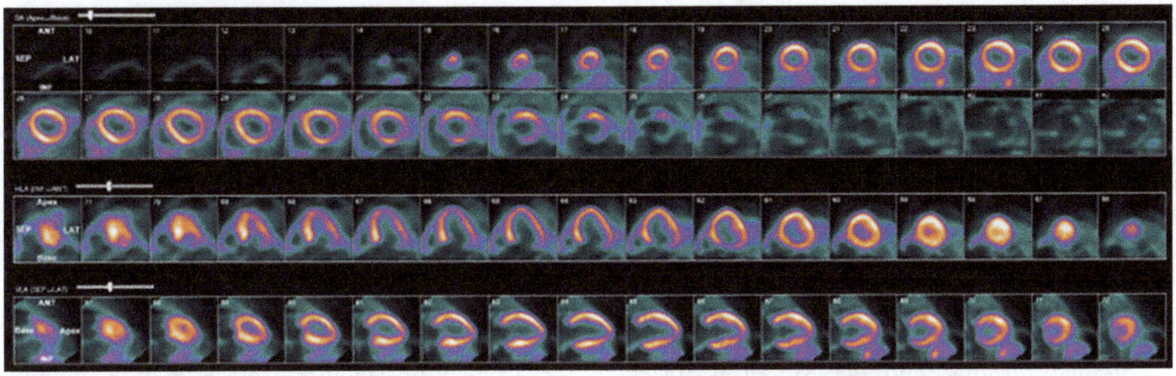

FIGURE 12-7 Positive ^{18}F-florbetapir PET Scan. ^{18}F-florbetapir PET images in standard cardiac projections (as described in Figure 12-6B) demonstrate diffuse myocardial ^{18}F-florbetapir uptake. PET = positron emission tomography.

^{18}F-Florbetapir/Florbetapen/Sodium Fluoride PET-CT

Uptake is assessed both visually and through various quantitative methods, including myocardial SUV, myocardial to background SUV ratio, myocardial to liver SUV ratio, and myocardial retention. An example of a positive ^{18}F-florbetapir scan in a patient with light chain cardiac amyloidosis is shown in Figure 12-7.

CONCLUSIONS

Cardiovascular PET radionuclide imaging plays a major role in the evaluation and management of CS and amyloidosis. Quantitative imaging methods, particularly with PET radiotracers, may provide information on disease extent, and severity and allow for detection of changes in response to therapy. When compared to structural imaging methods like echocardiography and CMR, targeted radionuclide imaging methods offer the potential to guide new drug development.

REFERENCES

1. Ungprasert P, Carmona EM, Utz JP, Ryu JH, Crowson CS, Matteson EL. Epidemiology of sarcoidosis 1946–2013: a population-based study. *Mayo Clin Proc.* 2016;91:183–188.
2. Morimoto T, Azuma A, Abe S, et al. Epidemiology of sarcoidosis in Japan. *Eur Respir J.* 2008;31:372–379.
3. Cozier YC, Berman JS, Palmer JR, Boggs DA, Serlin DM, Rosenberg L. Sarcoidosis in black women in the United States: data from the Black Women's Health Study. *Chest.* 2011;139:144–150.
4. Silverman KJ, Hutchins GM, Bulkley BH. Cardiac sarcoid: a clinicopathologic study of 84 unselected patients with systemic sarcoidosis. *Circulation.* 1978;58:1204–1211.
5. Tahara N, Tahara A, Nitta Y, et al. Heterogeneous myocardial FDG uptake and the disease activity in cardiac sarcoidosis. *JACC Cardiovasc Imaging.* 2010;3:1219–1228.
6. Birnie DH, Sauer WH, Bogun F, et al. HRS expert consensus statement on the diagnosis and management of arrhythmias associated with cardiac sarcoidosis. *Heart Rhythm.* 2014;11:1305–1324.
7. Ohira H, Tsujino I, Ishimaru S, et al. Myocardial imaging with 18F-fluoro-2-deoxyglucose positron emission tomography and magnetic resonance imaging in sarcoidosis. *Eur J Nucl Med Mol Imaging.* 2008;35:933–941.
8. Okumura W, Iwasaki T, Toyama T, Iso T, Arai M. Usefulness of fasting [1] F-FDG PET in identification of cardiac sarcoidosis. *J Nucl Med.* 2004:1989–1998.
9. Yamagishi H, Shirai N, Takagi M, et al. Identification of cardiac sarcoidosis with $^{13}N\text{-}NH_3/^{18}F$-FDG PET. *J Nucl Med.* 2003;44:1030–1036.
10. Youssef G, Leung E, Mylonas I, et al. The use of ^{18}F-FDG PET in the diagnosis of cardiac sarcoidosis: a systematic review and metaanalysis including the Ontario experience. *J Nucl Med.* 2012;53:241–248.

11. Chareonthaitawee P, Beanlands RS, Chen W, et al. Joint SNMMI-ASNC expert consensus document on the role of ^{18}F-FDG PET/CT in cardiac sarcoid detection and therapy monitoring. *J Nucl Cardiol.* 2017;58(8):1341–1353.
12. Slart RHJA, Glaudemans AWJM, Lancellotti P, et al. A joint procedural position statement on imaging in cardiac sarcoidosis: from the Cardiovascular and Inflammation & Infection Committees of the European Association of Nuclear Medicine, The European Associtionof Cardiovascular Imaging, and the American Society of Nuclear Cardiology. *Eur Heart J Cardiovasc Imaging.* 2017;18(10):1073–1089.
13. Hamzeh NY, Wamboldt FS, Weinberger HD. Management of cardiac sarcoidosis in the United States: a Delphi study. *Chest.* 2012;141:154–162.
14. Osborne MT, Hulten EA, Singh A, et al. Reduction in ^{18}F-fluorodeoxyglucose uptake on serial cardiac positron emission tomography is associated with improved left ventricular ejection fraction in patients with cardiac sarcoidosis. *J Nucl Cardiol.* 2014;21:166–174.
15. Blankstein R, Osborne M, Naya M, et al. Cardiac positron emission tomography enhances prognostic assessments of patients with suspected cardiac sarcoidosis. *J Am Coll Cardiol.* 2014;63:329–336.
16. Sperry BW, Tamarappoo BK, Oldan JD, et al. Prognostic impact of extent, severity, and heterogeneity of abnormalities on ^{18}F-FDG PET scans for suspected cardiac sarcoidosis. *JACC Cardiovasc Imaging.* 2017;11(2 Pt 2):336–345.
17. Dilsizian V, Bacharach SL, Beanlands RS, et al. ASNC imaging guidelines/SNMMI procedure standard for positron emission tomography (PET) nuclear cardiology procedures. *J Nucl Cardiol.* 2016;23:1187–1226.
18. Tang R, Wang JT, Wang L, et al. Impact of patient preparation on the diagnostic performance of 18F-FDG PET in cardiac sarcoidosis: a systematic review and meta-analysis. *Clin Nucl Med.* 2016;41:e327-e339.
19. Harisankar CNB, Mittal BR, Agrawal KL, Abrar ML, Bhattacharya A. Utility of high fat and low carbohydrate diet in suppressing myocardial FDG uptake. *J Nucl Cardiol.* 2011;18:926–936.
20. Cheng VY, Slomka PJ, Ahlen M, Thomson LEJ, Waxman AD, Berman DS. Impact of carbohydrate restriction with and without fatty acid loading on myocardial ^{18}F-FDG uptake during PET: a randomized controlled trial. *J Nucl Cardiol.* 2010;17:286–291.
21. Osborne MT, Hulten EA, Murthy VL, et al. Patient preparation for cardiac fluorine-18 fluorodeoxyglucose positron emission tomography imaging of inflammation. *J Nucl Cardiol.* 2017;24:86–99.
22. Demeure F, Hanin FX, Bol A, et al. A randomized trial on the optimization of ^{18}F-FDG myocardial uptake suppression: implications for vulnerable coronary plaque imaging. *J Nucl Med.* 2014;55:1629–1635.
23. Kobayashi Y, Kumita S-i, Fukushima Y, Ishihara K, Suda M, Sakurai M. Significant suppression of myocardial ^{18}F-fluorodeoxyglucose uptake using 24-h carbohydrate restriction and a low-carbohydrate, high-fat diet. *J Cardiol.* 2013;62: 314–319.
24. Wykrzykowska J, Lehman S, Williams G, et al. Imaging of inflamed and vulnerable plaque in coronary arteries with ^{18}F-FDG PET/CT in patients with suppression of myocardial uptake using a low-carbohydrate, high-fat preparation. *J Nucl Med.* 2009;50:563–568.
25. Lu Y, Grant C, Xie K, Sweiss NJ. Suppression of myocardial ^{18}F-FDG uptake through prolonged high-fat, high-protein, and very-low-carbohydrate diet before FDG-PET/CT for evaluation of patients with suspected cardiac sarcoidosis. *Clin Nucl Med.* 2017;42:88–94.
26. Smedema J-P, Snoep G, van Kroonenburgh MPG, et al. Evaluation of the accuracy of gadolinium-enhanced cardiovascular magnetic resonance in the diagnosis of cardiac sarcoidosis. *J Am Coll Cardiol.* 2005;45:1683–1690.
27. Kouranos V, Tzelepis GE, Rapti A, et al. Complementary role of CMR to conventional screening in the diagnosis and prognosis of cardiac sarcoidosis. *JACC Cardiovasc Imaging.* 2017;10:1437–1447.
28. Hulten E, Agarwal V, Cahill M, et al. Presence of late gadolinium enhancement by cardiac magnetic resonance among patients with suspected cardiac sarcoidosis is associated with adverse

cardiovascular prognosis: a systematic review and meta-analysis. *Circ Cardiovasc Imaging.* 2016;9:e005001.
29. Schneider S, Batrice A, Rischpler C, Eiber M, Ibrahim T, Nekolla SG. Utility of multimodal cardiac imaging with PET/MRI in cardiac sarcoidosis: implications for diagnosis, monitoring and treatment. *Eur Heart J.* 2014;35:312.
30. Skali H, Schulman AR, Dorbala S. 18F-FDG PET/CT for the assessment of myocardial sarcoidosis. *Curr Cardiol Rep.* 2013;15:352–352.
31. Ahmadian A, Brogan A, Berman J, et al. Quantitative interpretation of FDG PET/CT with myocardial perfusion imaging increases diagnostic information in the evaluation of cardiac sarcoidosis. *J Nucl Cardiol.* 2014;21:925–939.
32. McArdle BA, Birnie DH, Klein R, et al. Is there an association between clinical presentation and the location and extent of myocardial involvement of cardiac sarcoidosis as assessed by 18F-fluorodoexyglucose positron emission tomography? *Circ Cardiovasc Imaging.* 2013;6:617–626.
33. Langah R, Spicer K, Gebregziabher M, Gordon L. Effectiveness of prolonged fasting ^{18}F-FDG PET-CT in the detection of cardiac sarcoidosis. *J Nucl Cardiol.* 2009;16:801–810.
34. Okayama K, Kurata C, Tawarahara K, Wakabayashi Y, Chida K, Sato A. Diagnostic and prognostic value of myocardial scintigraphy with thallium-201 and gallium-67 in cardiac sarcoidosis. *Chest.* 1995;107:330–334.
35. Nishiyama Y, Yamamoto Y, Fukunaga K, et al. Comparative evaluation of 18F-FDG PET and ^{67}Ga scintigraphy in patients with sarcoidosis. *J Nucl Med.* 2006;47:1571–1576.
36. American Society of Nuclear Cardiology. ^{99m}Technetium-pyrophosphate imaging for transthyretin cardiac amyloidosis. *ASNC Practice Points* 2016;2017.
37. Falk RH, Quarta CC, Dorbala S. How to image cardiac amyloidosis. *Circ Cardiovasc Imaging.* 2014;7:552–562.
38. Castaño A, DeLuca A, Weinberg R, et al. Serial scanning with technetium pyrophosphate (^{99m}Tc-PYP) in advanced ATTR cardiac amyloidosis. *J Nucl Cardiol.* 2016;23:1355–1363.
39. Bokhari S, Castaño A, Pozniakoff T, Deslisle S, Latif F, Maurer MS. ^{99m}Tc-pyrophosphate scintigraphy for differentiating light-chain cardiac amyloidosis from the transthyretin-related familial and senile cardiac amyloidoses. *Circ Cardiovasc Imaging.* 2013;6:195–201.
40. White JA, Kim HW, Shah D, et al. CMR imaging with rapid visual T1 assessment predicts mortality in patients suspected of cardiac amyloidosis. *JACC Cardiovasc Imaging.* 2014;7:143–156.
41. Fontana M, Banypersad SM, Treibel TA, et al. Native T1 mapping in transthyretin amyloidosis. *JACC Cardiovasc Imaging.* 2014;7:157–165.
42. Banypersad SM, Sado DM, Flett AS, et al. Quantification of myocardial extracellular volume fraction in systemic AL amyloidosis: an equilibrium contrast cardiovascular magnetic resonance study. *Circ Cardiovasc Imaging.* 2013;6:34–39.
43. Banypersad SM, Fontana M, Maestrini V, et al. T1 mapping and survival in systemic light-chain amyloidosis. *Eur Heart J.* 2015;36:244–251.
44. Castano A, Haq M, Narotsky DL, et al. Multicenter study of planar technetium 99m pyrophosphate cardiac imaging: predicting survival for patients with ATTR cardiac amyloidosis. *JAMA cardiology.* 2016;1:880–889.
45. Hiraga H, Yuwai K, Hiroe M. Diagnostic standard and guidelines for sarcoidosis. *Japanese J Sarcoid Granul Disorders.* 2007;27:89–102.
46. Ruberg FL, Berk JL. Transthyretin (TTR) cardiac amyloidosis. *Circulation.* 2012;126:1286–1300.
47. Rapezzi C, Merlini G, Quarta CC, et al. Systemic cardiac amyloidoses: disease profiles and clinical courses of the 3 main types. *Circulation.* 2009;120:1203–1212.
48. Falk RH, Alexander KM, Liao R, Dorbala S. AL (light-chain) cardiac amyloidosis: a review of diagnosis and therapy. *J Am Coll Cardiol.* 2016;68:1323–1341.
49. Dubrey SW, Cha K, Skinner M, LaValley M, Falk RH. Familial and primary (AL) cardiac amyloidosis: echocardiographically similar diseases with distinctly different clinical outcomes. *Heart.* 1997;78:74–82.
50. Gillmore JD, Maurer MS, Falk RH, et al. Nonbiopsy diagnosis of cardiac transthyretin amyloidosis. *Circulation.* 2016;133:2404–2412.

51. Perugini E, Guidalotti PL, Salvi F, et al. Noninvasive etiologic diagnosis of cardiac amyloidosis using ^{99m}Tc-3,3-diphosphono-1,2-propanodicarboxylic acid scintigraphy. *J Am Coll Cardiol.* 2005;46:1076–1084.
52. Hutt DF, Quigley AM, Page J, et al. Utility and limitations of 3,3-diphosphono-1,2-propanodicarboxylic acid scintigraphy in systemic amyloidosis. *Eur Heart J Cardiovasc Imaging.* 2014:1289–1298.
53. Dorbala S, Vangala D, Semer J, et al. Imaging cardiac amyloidosis: a pilot study using ^{18}F-florbetapir positron emission tomography. *Eur J Nucl Med Mol Imaging.* 2014;41:1652–1662.
54. Osborne DR, Acuff SN, Stuckey A, Wall JS. A routine PET/CT protocol with streamlined calculations for assessing cardiac amyloidosis using ^{18}F-florbetapir. *Front Cardiovasc Med.* 2015;2:23–23.
55. Law WP, Wang WY, Moore PT, Mollee PN, Ng AC. Cardiac amyloid imaging with ^{18}F-florbetaben PET: a pilot study. *J Nucl Med.* 2016;57:1733–1739.
56. Morgenstern R, Yeh R, Castano A, Maurer MS, Bokhari S. ^{18}Fluorine sodium fluoride positron emission tomography, a potential biomarker of transthyretin cardiac amyloidosis. *J Nucl Cardiol.* 2017:1–9.

EDITOR'S PERSPECTIVE

Timothy M. Bateman

This chapter covers in detail two growth opportunities for cardiovascular PET/CT imaging. PET/CT for active cardiac sarcoidosis has no imminent competitors, but nonetheless has deficiencies that can hopefully be addressed in the future. PET/CT for cardiac amyloidosis has formidable competitors in Tc-99m pyrophosphate planar and SPECT scintigraphy, which have limitations but are less expensive. What is so exciting about both of these topics, however, is that subspecialists who traditionally have not looked to nuclear cardiology to address their clinical challenges are doing so now.

In the case of cardiac sarcoidosis, clinical cardiologists, electrophysiologists, congestive heart failure specialists, echocardiographers, cardiac magnetic resonance subspecialists, and pulmonologists are now thinking about this relatively rare but potentially devastating cardiac inflammatory condition. Echocardiography and cardiac magnetic resonance imaging play a role in screening for the likelihood of cardiac sarcoidosis, but currently only F18-FDG PET can identify the presence of *active* cardiac sarcoidosis. As such, referrals are growing and labs must respond. While increased demand is a good problem to have, here is a partial list of near-term requirements for the overall value of FDG sarcoid imaging:

- Development of appropriate use criteria for screening for cardiac sarcoidosis, as the positivity rate is currently low.
- An agreement regarding patient selection.
- Development of best-practice preparation protocols for diabetics and non-diabetics undergoing FDG sarcoid imaging.
- Guidelines to assist in the integration of traditional cardiac cold-spot detection tools with radiology hot-spot tools, in order to optimize interpretations.
- Development of structured reporting formats.
- Billing codes are currently non-existent but are essential, as in the current era many patients needing this test have to pay out of pocket.
- Quantification criteria for extent and severity of inflammation are needed, both for initial assessment and for follow-up. For example, what is a successful therapeutic response?
- Either structured registries or prospective studies in order to overcome the limitations of the current single-center, relatively small populated studies.
- Ideally, a new specifically targeted tracer to avoid the challenges when cardiac sarcoidosis is suspected in patients with co-existent coronary artery disease.

In the case of cardiac amyloidosis, the new referral specialists include clinical cardiologists, heart failure subspecialists, gerontologists, and specialists in hematology/oncology. Referral specialists are another clinical need arising from the large and growing population of patients with congestive heart failure. Several potential treatments for the most common form, transthyretin amyloidosis (ATTR), are undergoing evaluation. If (and when) an effective therapy is approved, it is likely that imaging referrals will grow dramatically. Combined planar and SPECT Tc-99m pyrophosphate is the current standard, but new PET tracers show even greater promise for more complete assessment.

FDG PET/CT for Imaging Cardiovascular Device Infection

CHAPTER 13

Wengen Chen and Vasken Dilsizian

INTRODUCTION

There has been a worldwide increase in implantation of cardiovascular devices, including cardiac implantable electronic devices (CIED), valve prostheses, left ventricular assist devices (LVAD), and vascular grafts. CIEDs, including pacemakers and implantable cardioverter defibrillators (ICDs) are the major devices installed. Almost one-half of the world's cardiac device installation is performed in the United States.[1] Infection is a major complication after device installation, and, unfortunately, the increasing number of cardiac device procedures is exceeded by an even higher rate of increasing cases of device infection, mainly because of older age of the new device recipients with longer hospital stays and multiple comorbidities.[2,3] Approximately 20%-30% of patients with CIED require device extraction and reinstallation, mainly due to infection,[4] which is a major societal and medical burden. Infection of a foreign body device is also associated with a high risk of mortality. It has been reported that 12-week all-cause mortality was 35% in patients with a confirmed cardiac device infection, especially for those with methicillin-resistant *S. aureus* infection.[5] One-year mortality was reported as high as 17% in endovascular infection patients even after device removal.[6] Thus, early and accurate diagnosis of cardiac device infection is critical for prompt clinical decision making, such as intravenous antibiotics alone or device removal in a timely manner before significant damage occurs. Diagnosis of cardiac device infection remains a challenge for current diagnostic radiology tools. For example, CT or MRI suffers from metal artifacts and findings are nonspecific for infection. Transthoracic echocardiography (TTE) or transesophageal echocardiography (TEE) is limited to identification of intracardiac infection, and not useful for extracardiac source of infection. Although radiolabeled autologous white blood cell (WBC) scintigraphy has been used for infection evaluation, its sensitivity for device infection is variable.[7,8] Thus, a scan with high sensitivity and accuracy is needed to facilitate the prompt and accurate diagnosis of cardiac device infection.

^{18}F-fluoro-2-deoxyglucose positron emission tomography/computed tomography (FDG PET/CT) is a functional imaging tool that targets the body's glucose utilization. Clinically it is mainly used for cancer staging, restaging, and posttreatment effect evaluation, as malignant cells have increased glucose uptake. On the other hand, preexisting inflammatory cells (macrophages, neutrophils, and lymphocytes) at an infection site also overexpress glucose transporters and could accumulate FDG. Bacteria at the infection site also rely on glucose as an energy source. FDG uptake in both inflammatory cells and bacteria at an infection site can then be detected by PET with high sensitivity. Compared to radiolabeled WBC scintigraphy, FDG PET/CT has the advantages of high spatial resolution with superior tomographic images, short procedure time (less than 2 hours, compared to 24 hours with WBC scan), less labor- intensive and lower radiation exposure. Prospectively conducted studies have shown that FDG PET/CT has a better accuracy in detecting infection for patients with joint prostheses than the WBC scan.[9,10] Although most of the published results regarding the role of FDG PET/CT for cardiac device infection are from retrospective studies, case reports, or even incidental findings without a well-designed multicenter prospective study, current data in the literature support the application of FDG PET/CT for earlier detection of cardiac device infection, particularly for complicated and difficult cases, before morphological changes occur.[11] An additional benefit of FDG PET/CT is its ability to identify other sites of infection given the whole body scan nature, which could be the original source of infection. Noninfectious inflammation remains a challenge for the FDG PET/CT to image infection and could be a false positive source, but it can be potentially differentiated from true infection by careful evaluation of imaging patterns, and clinical history, such as timing of device implant.

This chapter discusses the roles of FDG PET/CT in diagnosing infection of four major cardiac devices: CIED, valve prosthesis, LVAD, and vascular graft.

IMAGING PROTOCOL AND DATA ACQUISITION

Although the heart preferentially utilizes fatty acid as its energy source, based on the nutritional supply, it can also use other substrates such as glucose, ketones, or amino acids. With the current FDG PET/CT imaging protocol for cancer evaluation, it is common for the heart to accumulate FDG uptake after a simple 4-hour fasting. This may not be a major issue for cancer imaging as it is rare to have cardiac primary or metastatic malignancy, but would definitely hinder evaluation of cardiac device infection, for example, lead vegetation or valve prosthesis infection, leading to a false positive study. Thus, it is critical to suppress physiological myocardial FDG uptake when performing PET/CT for cardiac device infection. In addition, cardiac and respiratory motion can also affect visualization of FDG uptake, particularly in a small infected lesion, such as vegetation. Currently, there is no standardized imaging protocol for cardiac device infection diagnosis with FDG PET/CT. As a general rule, the following procedures work well in the authors' clinical practice. It is highly recommended that a standardized protocol be used once it is published.

Dietary Preparation

The most critical portion of the scan is dietary preparation to completely suppress the physiological myocardial FDG uptake. A high-fat and low-carbohydrate diet has been shown to decrease myocardial FDG uptake.[12] Despite this, a commonly agreed protocol has not been defined in terms of the amount and timing of high- fat, low- carbohydrate diet for cardiac infection imaging. It is generally suggested that patient should start a high- fat and low- carbohydrate diet one day before or at least the prior dinner before the scheduled FDG PET/CT scan. The patient should then fast for at least 4 hours before the injection of FDG. If a scan is scheduled in the late morning or early afternoon, a continued high- fat and low- carbohydrate breakfast would improve the suppression. Although prolonged fasting (18 hours) would generate fatty acids due to the metabolic switch to fat, its effect on myocardial FDG uptake is not complete and consistent.[13] In addition, long- time fasting is a compliance challenge for some patients.

Heparin

Heparin can increase serum free fatty acid level by inducing lipolysis of lipoprotein particles. Thus, intravenous unfractionated heparin injection before the scan has been used alone or in combination with a high- fat and low- carbohydrate diet preparation to suppress myocardial uptake. However, the effect of heparin on myocardial FDG uptake suppression has not been well established. Further, the optimal dose and timing of heparin injection has not been defined. Heparin is not applied in our own practice.

Imaging Acquisition Time After FDG Injection Shows

For routine cancer evaluation, PET/CT data are acquired 1 hour after FDG injection. Studies on atherosclerosis imaging suggested that delayed acquisitions at 2 or 3 hours after FDG injection increased plaque visualization.[14] It is unknown whether delayed PET imaging would improve infection diagnosis or not, though both target inflammatory macrophages and neutrophils (which is different from cancer imaging). In our practice, imaging acquired at 1 hour after FDG injection shows good results for injection evaluation. An uptake interval of 60 minutes is recommended, but delayed imaging at 90–120 minutes can be considered.

Although most of the cardiac devices are located in the chest, acquiring whole-body PET/CT scan in order to assess extracardiac infection source is highly recommended. The images can be reconstructed and reviewed according to procedure guidelines for oncology PET/CT imaging. The registered PET/CT images can be displayed on a standard workstation in the axial, coronal, and sagittal planes as well as a rotating maximum-intensity projection (MIP) image. It is important that PET images with and without attenuation correction should be reviewed for device infection evaluation, given the attenuation artifact from the metal device. Respiratory motion correction has not been shown significant improvement and is not essential. The interpretation criteria will be incorporated in the following each of the devices.

CARDIAC IMPLANTABLE ELECTRONIC DEVICE INFECTION

CIEDs, mainly implantable cardioverter defibrillators and pacemakers, are the most widely used cardiac devices. No matter its type, a CIED consists of a pocket that is usually placed in the upper chest wall subcutaneous region and leads that are placed intravascularly or in the epicardial area of the heart (Figure 13-1). Infection can occur at any part of a CIED with different clinical significances. Infection limited to the superficial soft tissue of a CIED pocket may be treated by local debridement or by antibiotics alone, while infection deep to a pocket or along the leads requires complete extraction of the entire device. Given its tomographic imaging, FDG PET/CT is capable of localizing the site of infection and guiding clinical management.

Performance of FDG PET/CT for CIED Infection

While it appears straightforward to diagnose pocket infection in the presence of severe local

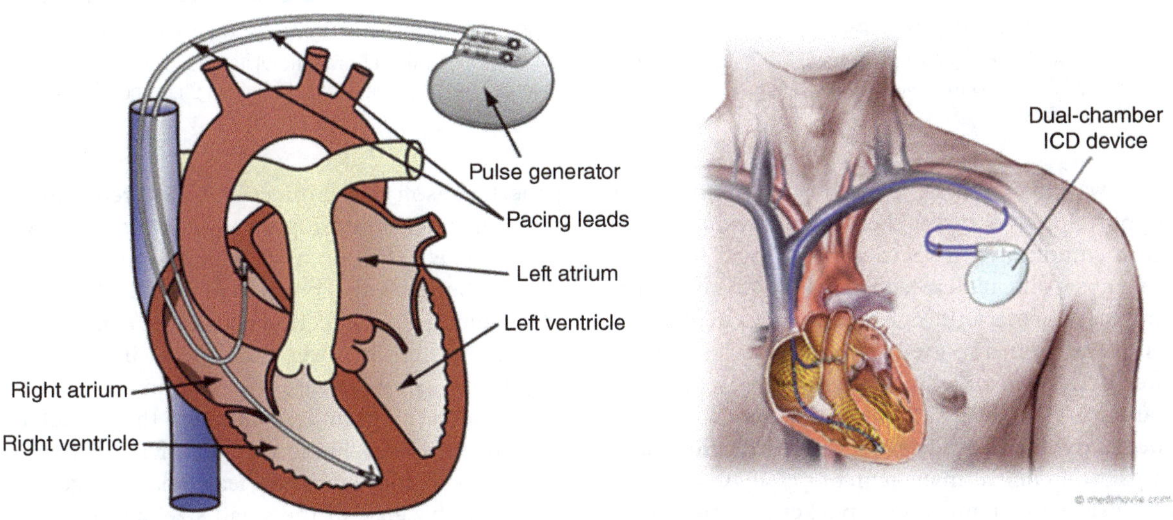

FIGURE 13-1 Illustrations of a pacemaker (left), and a dual-chamber defibrillator (right).

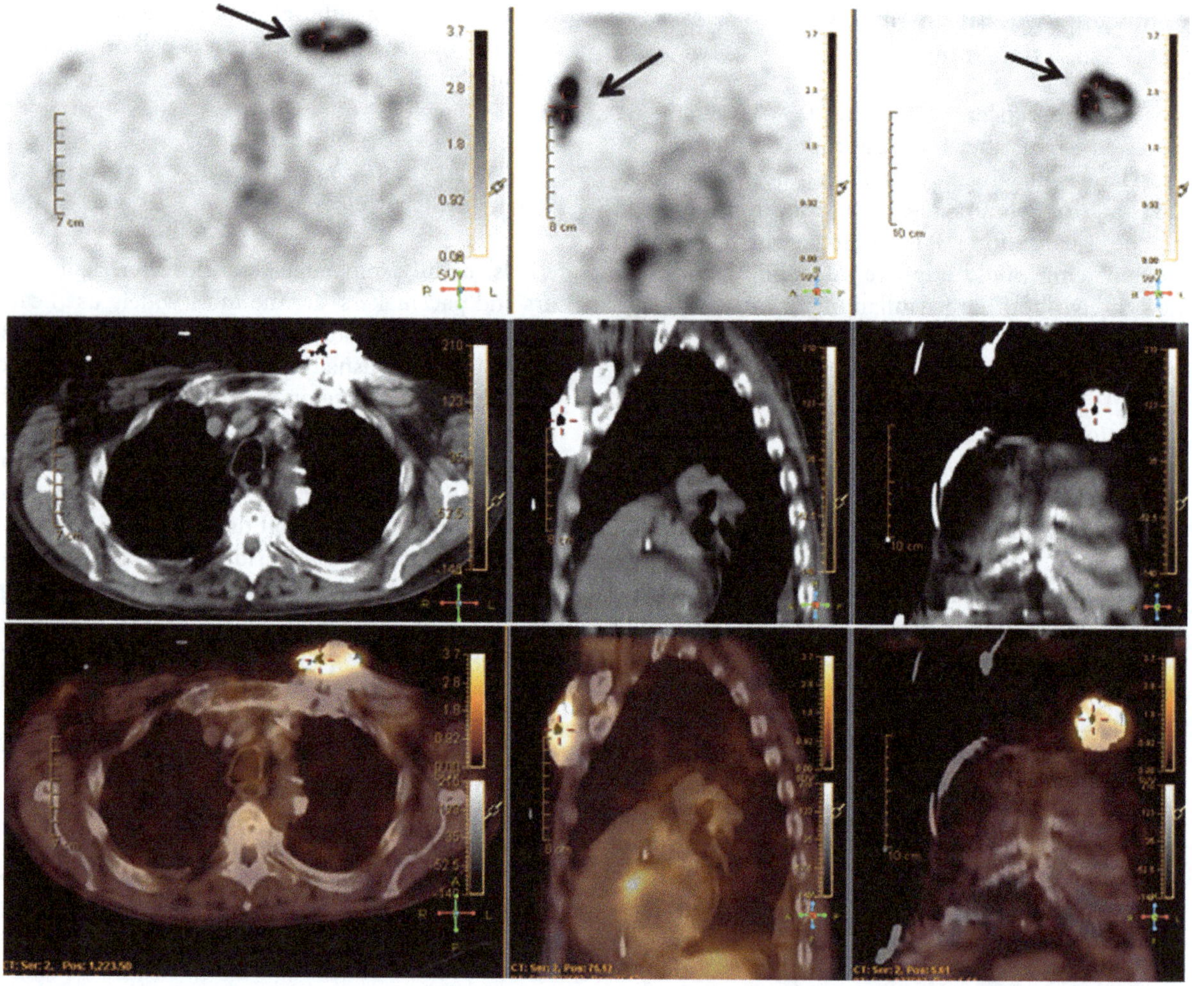

FIGURE 13-2 A Case With Deep Pocket Infection. There was intense FDG uptake around the deep portion of the pocket in the left upper chest wall on PET (upper row, arrow), CT (middle row, arrow), and fused PET/CT (lower row, arrow) images, with axial (left), sagittal (middle), and coronal views (right), compatible with deep pocket infection. (Used with permission from Chen and Dilsizian, unpublished data)

chest wall infection signs, such as skin redness or suppuration over the pocket, real clinical cases are more complicated if there are equivocal findings. For those difficult cases, FDG PET/CT can provide incremental information for accurate diagnosis. It has been reported that with device culture after extraction or clinical follow-up as the gold standard, FDG PET/CT has a high sensitivity and specificity for diagnosis of CIED infection, and impact on clinical management.[15,16] FDG PET/CT can clearly distinguish deep pocket infection from superficial soft tissue infection which requires different managements. Figure 13-2 shows a case with deep pocket infection, with a focus of intense FDG uptake beneath the pocket. FDG PET/CT could also detect lead infection along its course, with sensitivity slightly lower than pocket infection.[15,16] Figure 13-3 shows a case with lead infection in the subcutaneous region. In contrast to the pocket and lead infection evaluation, FDG PET/CT may be less sensitive for identifying lead-related vegetation infection, because of the small size and motion of

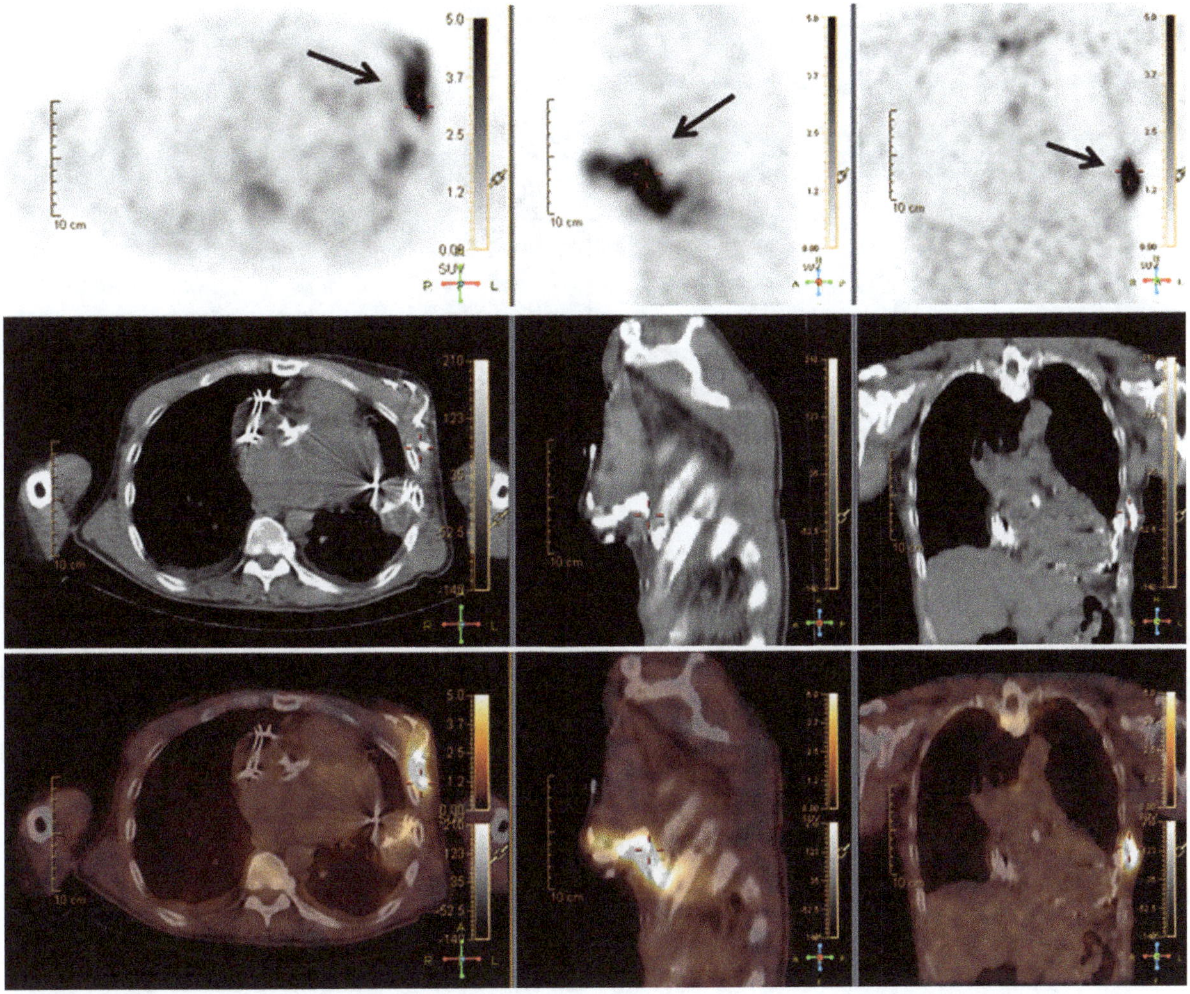

FIGURE 13-3 A Case With CIED Lead Infection. There was focal FDG uptake in the left lateral chest wall along the course of the lead seen on PET (upper row, arrow), CT (middle row, arrow), and fused PET/CT (lower row, arrow) images, with axial (left), sagittal (middle), and coronal views (right), compatible with lead infection. (Used with permission from Chen and Dilsizian, unpublished data)

the vegetation during a cardiac cycle. Figure 13-4 shows a focus of uptake corresponding to the tip of lead in the left ventricle, indicating infection, although vegetation is not clearly seen on the CT portion of the PET.

Differentiation of Infection from Inflammation

FDG is a nonspecific tracer and can accumulate in any cells with increased glucose utilization. Thus, it is critical to address the significance of FDG uptake related to noninfectious inflammation, which could create a potential false positive diagnosis. Quantitative measurement of metabolic activity as assessed by standard uptake value (SUV) on PET scan has not been demonstrated reliable for differentiation between inflammation and true infection. There is overlapping of SUV between the two conditions. Visual or semi-quantification (compared to the liver uptake) remains the most reliable way for the differentiation. Infection tends to show focal and

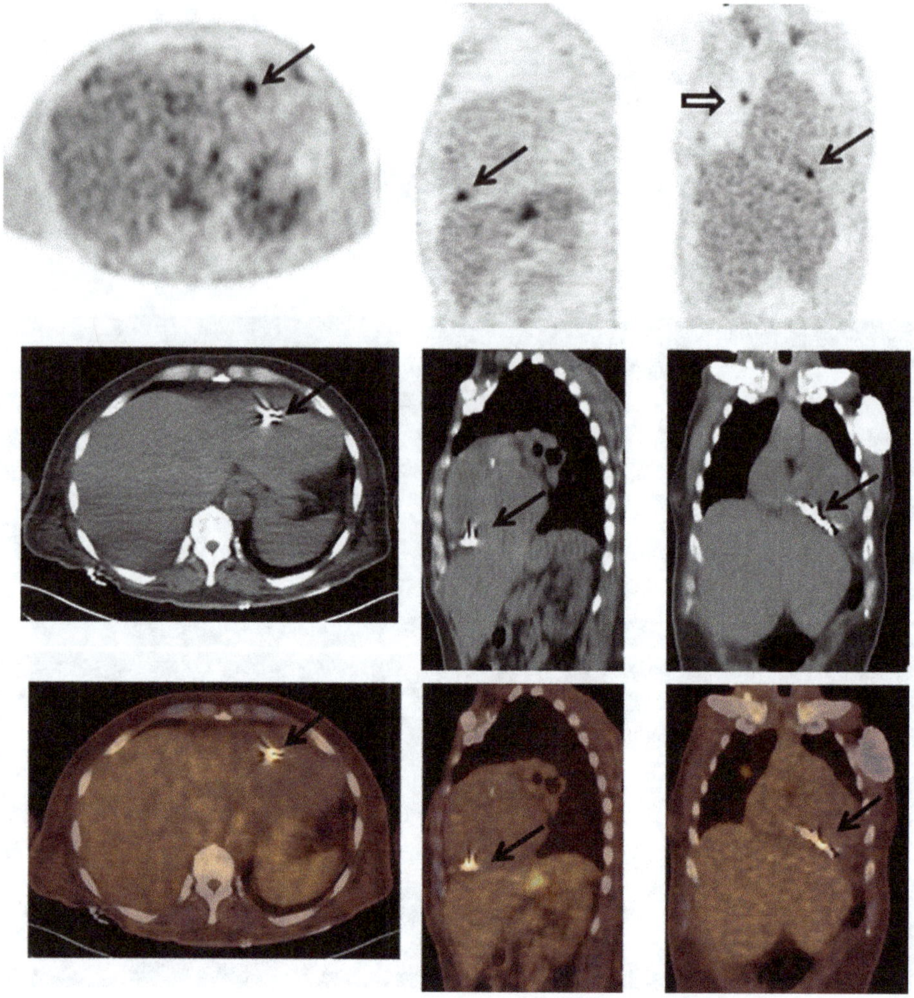

FIGURE 13-4 A Case With CIED Lead Vegetation Infection. There was a focal uptake corresponding to the tip of lead in the right ventricle on PET (upper row, arrow), CT (middle row, arrow), and fused PET/CT (lower row, arrow) images, with axial (left), sagittal (middle), and coronal views (right). The finding was compatible with lead vegetation infection, although TEE was negative for vegetation (not shown). There was also a focal uptake in the right lung region (open arrow on coronal PET view, right upper), corresponding to an infectious embolism in the lung. (Used with permission from Chen and Dilsizian, unpublished data)

intense FDG uptake within or immediately adjacent to the CIED pocket or along the lead, while FDG uptake in inflammatory area is mild, and in a diffuse/homogenous pattern along the entire pocket, rather than limited to a focal area.[17] Clinical history is also helpful, that inflammatory change occurs in recently implanted devices (less than 8 weeks). Figure 13-5 shows a case with postsurgical inflammation without evidence of infection, which demonstrates a different pattern as infection (Figures 13-2 and 13-3).

Clinical Significance of FDG PET/CT for CIED Infection

In addition to providing incremental information for accurate diagnosis of CIED infection, FDG PET/CT findings could guide subsequent clinical management

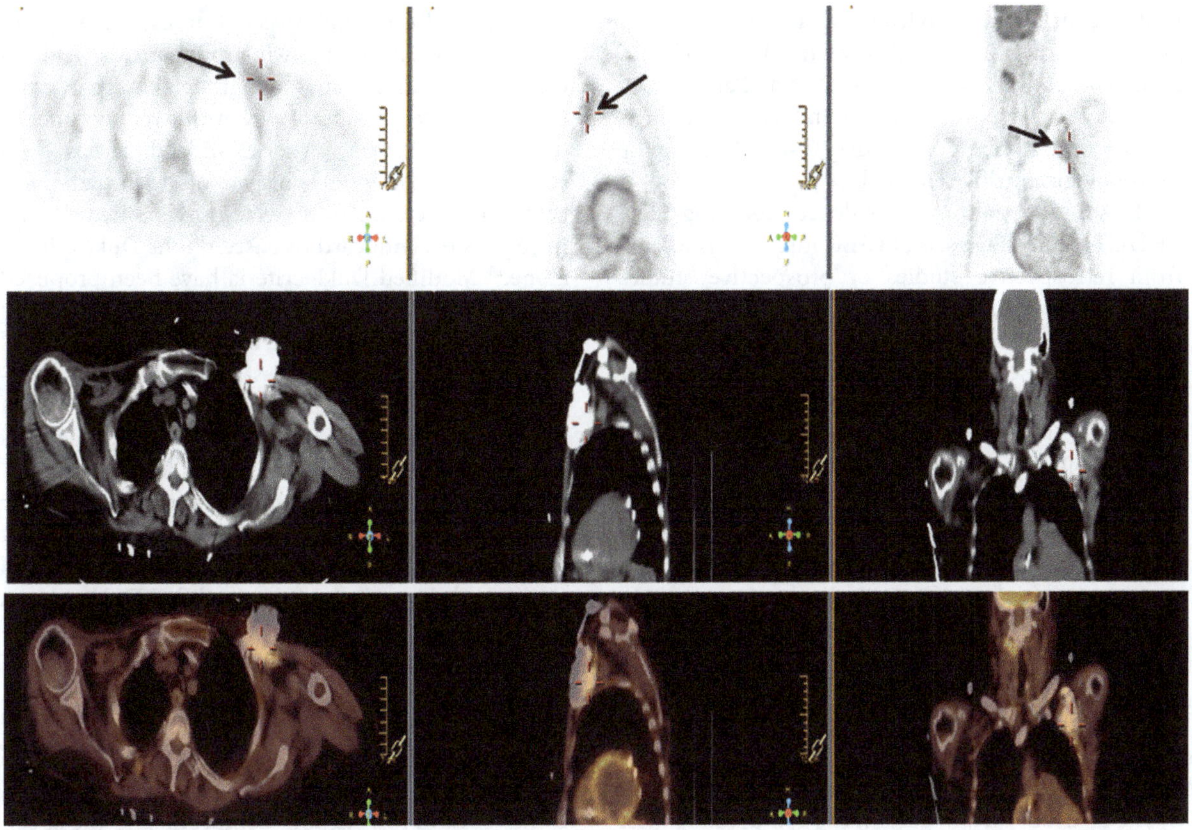

FIGURE 13-5 A Case With CIED Noninfectious Inflammation. There was mild activity around the pocket in the left upper chest wall on PET (upper row, arrow), CT (middle row, arrow), and fused PET/CT (lower row, arrow) images, with axial (left), sagittal (middle), and coronal views (right). The device was implanted 6 weeks ago before the PET/CT. (Used with permission from Chen and Dilsizian, unpublished data)

of these cases. Despite clinical suspicion of infection, if an FDG PET/CT scan is negative, then the device system can be left in place, without objective signs of disease progression during follow-up.[15] On the other hand, if PET is positive for a deep pocket or lead infection, then the entire system should be extracted. Superficial tissue infection as seen on PET/CT without abnormal uptake in the rest of the pocket and leads can be managed by antibiotics. Overall, studies have shown that FDG PET/CT positive cases correlate well with device extraction culture results. FDG PET/CT negative cases correlate well with clinical follow up without device extraction.[16,17] The results suggest that FDG PET/CT findings can guide the clinical decision making for difficult cases with clinically suspected but not confirmed cardiac device infection.[16]

Pitfalls and Mimics

A CIED infection treated with intensive intravenous antibiotics, or a less severe infection may not be definitely detected by FDG PET/CT (false negative). The possible underlying mechanism may include the less migration of WBCs to the infection site due to decreased secretion of cytokines by bacteria after antibiotics. Nevertheless, as mentioned earlier, studies have shown that if FDG PET/CT is negative, then the device can be left in place with good clinical outcome after a course of antibiotics alone without device extraction, even if the diagnosis is a false negative. On the other hand, a false positive diagnosis can be caused by inflammation, which can be differentiated by clinical history, pattern of uptake, and intensity as mentioned earlier. Attenuation correction artifact from the metals can also lead to a false positive diagnosis. Thus, it is important to review FDG PET/CT images on both the attenuation-corrected and nonattenuation-corrected images. Thrombus formation is also a source of false positive diagnosis, which can be morphologically differentiated.

In summary, although evidence regarding FDG PET/CT in the diagnosis of CIED infection is mainly from retrospective studies or prospective studies with a small cohort of patients, data advocate the role of FDG PET/CT in diagnosing CIED infection, particularly for cases with equivocal anatomical imaging findings. Importantly, FDG PET/CT correlates well with clinical outcome, that is, a positive PET correlates well with device extraction culture, while a negative PET correlates well with clinical follow up without extraction. It is essential to standardize the imaging protocol, including patient preparation, data acquisition processes (for example, the time of imaging after FDG injection), and, more importantly, imaging interpretation. Aggressive dietary preparation is always required to suppress the physiological myocardial glucose utilization for better evaluation of intracardiac lead infection, such as vegetation. Noninfectious inflammation is better differentiated by the distribution and pattern of FDG uptake rather than the intensity. A focal uptake favors a true infection while mild diffuse activity along the device or the lead is more likely inflammation.

PROSTHESIS VALVE ENDOCARDITIS

In addition to hemolysis and thrombosis, infection is a major complication of valve prosthesis implantation. Diagnosis of prosthesis valve endocarditis remains a challenge. If not treated promptly, mortality from endocarditis is high.[18] The final diagnosis of endocarditis is made based on the Duke Endocarditis Service criteria,[19] which are mainly based on blood culture and TEE or TTE findings. Unlike a native valve, a prosthetic valve is more challenging for TEE or TTE to detect vegetation due to acoustic shadowing from the metal ring.[20] On the other hand, TEE may prompt a false-positive diagnosis related to thickened valve, nodular valve, or calcifications.[19] The yield of a positive blood culture can be affected by many factors like blood sampling, or antibiotic treatment, and a positive culture result does not necessarily point to the source of infection. Owing to inconclusive blood culture and TEE findings, a high percentage of cases with clinically suspected endocarditis remain unconfirmed by the Duke criteria. Indeed, it has been reported that up to 24% of patients with pathologically proven endocarditis were misclassified as having a possible endocarditis based on the Duke criteria alone.[21] Modified Duke criteria have been proposed and are the current gold standard for diagnosis of endocarditis.[22] It should be noted that the modified Duke criteria were initially established for epidemiological study of endocarditis, classified at the end of the disease. It may not be optimal for early diagnosis of endocarditis in an acute clinical setting. In addition, the criteria have a lower accuracy for prosthetic valve endocarditis than native endocarditis. Thus, it is a plausible goal to develop a new imaging tool to facilitate and supplement the modified Duke criteria for early diagnosis of prosthetic valve endocarditis.

An important finding regarding the role of FDG PET/CT for prosthetic valve endocarditis is that inclusion of abnormal FDG uptake at the prosthetic valve on PET/CT scan as a novel major criterion can increase the sensitivity of the modified Duke criteria from 70% to 97%, without compromising the specificity.[23] The improvement of sensitivity is mainly because of a significant reduction in cases classified as "possible" by the modified Duke criteria after inclusion of FDG PET/CT findings. Thus, the European Society of Cardiology (ESC) has included FDG PET/CT findings in its new version of the guidelines for the diagnosis and management of infectious endocarditis.[24] Figure 13-6 shows a case with infection in an aortic prosthesis valve.

Similar to CIED infection diagnosis, focal intense uptake higher than the liver on both attenuation- and nonattenuation-corrected images is the most reliable method to diagnose prosthetic valve endocarditis, particularly if the uptake is twice of that in the liver.[25] There is always overlapping of SUV_{max} between the prosthetic valve endocarditis patients and controls as seen in most of the studies, and there is no clear cut-off threshold of SUV for differentiation, although a few studies showed that SUV_{max} is statistically higher in endocarditis patients than controls.[26]

Peri-annular extension (abscess/mycotic aneurysm) is a common complication of prosthetic valve

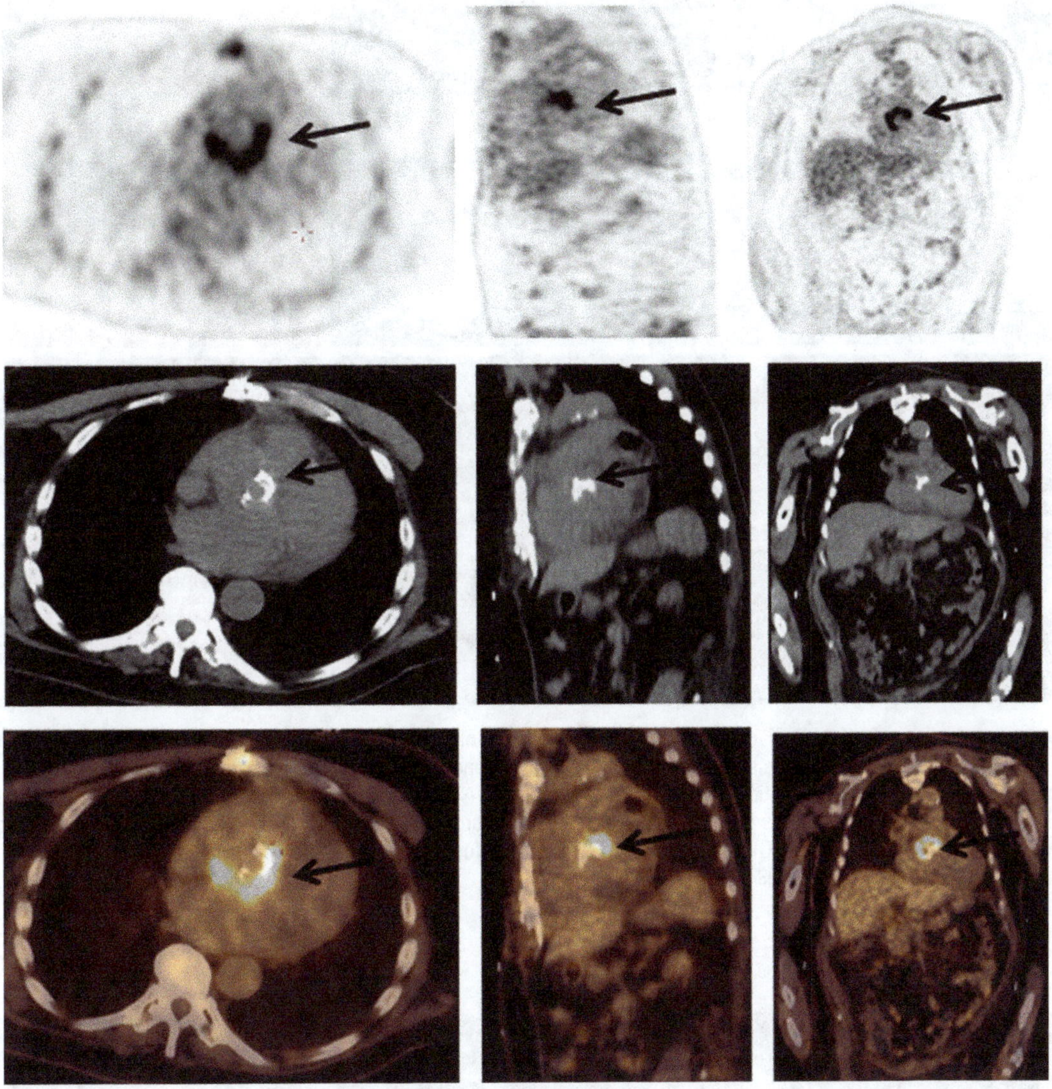

FIGURE 13-6 A Case With Aortic Prosthesis Valve Infection. There was a focal abnormal uptake around the aortic prosthesis on PET (upper row, arrow), CT (middle row, arrow), and fused PET/CT (lower row, arrow) images, with axial (left), sagittal (middle), and coronal views (right), compatible with aortic prosthetic valve endocarditis. (Used with permission from Chen and Dilsizian, unpublished data)

endocarditis, which warrants immediate surgical extraction.[20] It has been shown that FDG PET/CT can detect endocarditis complication earlier than surgical exploration and anatomical imaging findings in certain circumstances.[27] As shown in Figure 13-7, there are foci of abnormal FDG uptake around the aortic prosthetic valve (B) indicating infection. However, there is no abnormal finding on ECG-gated computed tomography angiography (CTA) (A), and even open surgical exploration (C). Eight days later, a repeated CTA showed mycotic aneurysm (D, arrow) and also abscess on the TEE. Subsequent surgery showed severe infection (F). The findings emphasize the power of FDG PET/CT in early diagnosis of prosthetic endocarditis complication before anatomical damage occurs on the valve.

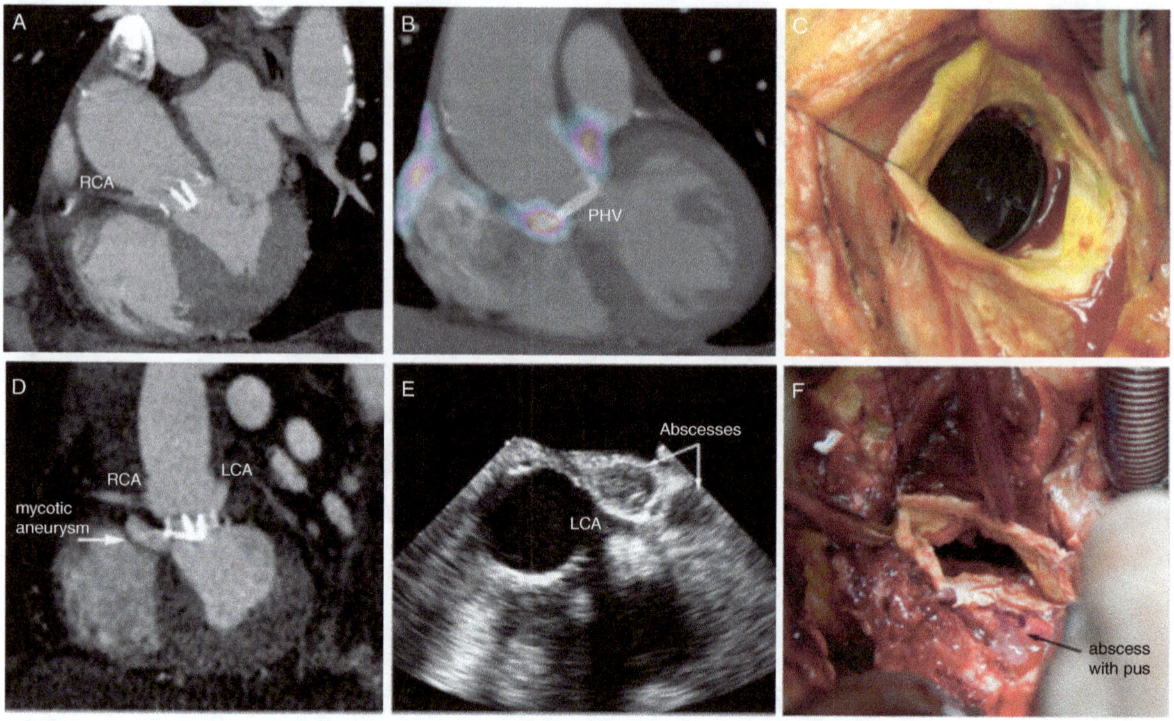

FIGURE 13-7 An Example of Early Diagnosis of Periannular Extension of Aortic Valve Endocarditis by PET/CT. There was intense focal uptake around the aortic prosthesis valve on PET (B, fused image) indicating infection. However, CTA (A) and open surgical inspection (C) did not reveal abnormalities. Eight days later, repeated CTA revealed a mycotic aneurysm beneath the RCA origin (D), and TEE (E) showed abscess around the LCA, which were confirmed by urgent reoperation (F). (Reproduced with permission from Tanis W, Scholtens A, Habets J, et al: CT angiography and ^{18}F-FDG-PET fusion imaging for prosthetic heart valve endocarditis, JACC Cardiovasc Imaging. 2013 Sep;6(9):1008-1013)

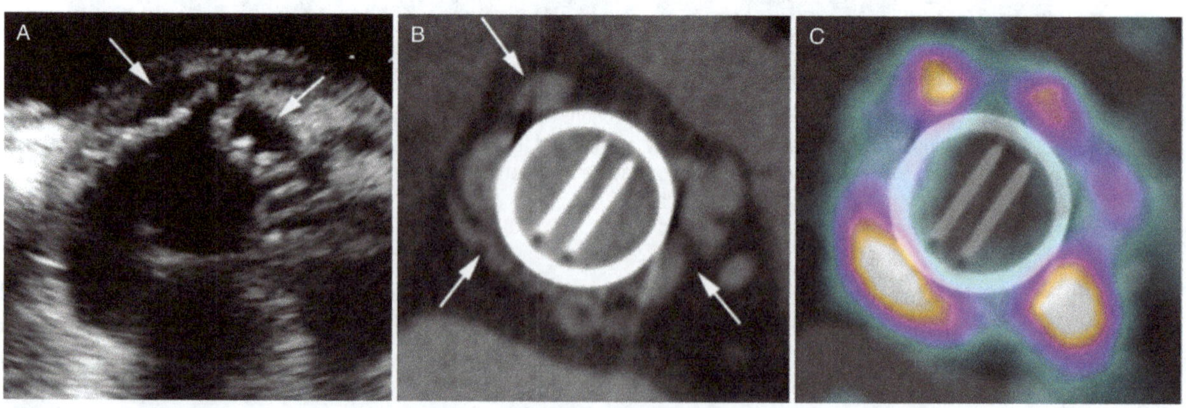

FIGURE 13-8 An Example of Valve Prosthesis Infection Confirmed by FDG PET/CT. TEE (A) and CTA (B) showed abnormal changes, suspicious for endocarditis with complications. FDG PET/CT (C) showed corresponding foci of increased FDG uptake in corresponding areas, confirming the diagnosis of infection. (Reproduced with permission from Tanis W, Scholtens A, Habets J, et al: CT angiography and ^{18}F-FDG-PET fusion imaging for prosthetic heart valve endocarditis, JACC Cardiovasc Imaging. 2013 Sep;6(9):1008-1013)

In most of cases, FDG PET/CT provides confirmatory information to facilitate a final diagnosis.[27] As shown in Figure 13-8, TEE and CTA both showed abnormal changes, suspicious for endocarditis with complications, and FDG PET/CT also showed foci of increased FDG uptake in that areas, confirmed the diagnosis of infection.

It should be noted that physiologic cardiac FDG uptake and cardiac motion could hinder FDG PET/CT findings. On the other hand, inflammation related to surgery and particularly related to adhesive material used to seal the device can be a false-positive source.[28] Generally, a biological valve creates less inflammation compared to a metal one. Thus, careful evaluation of FDG PET/CT images and clinical history, such as time of surgery and prosthesis type, is important.

Given its whole body scan nature, FDG PET/CT can potentially identify extra cardiac infection, which could be the source of device infection. As shown in Figure 13-9, an intense uptake is seen in the left toe corresponding to a site of osteomyelitis.[27]

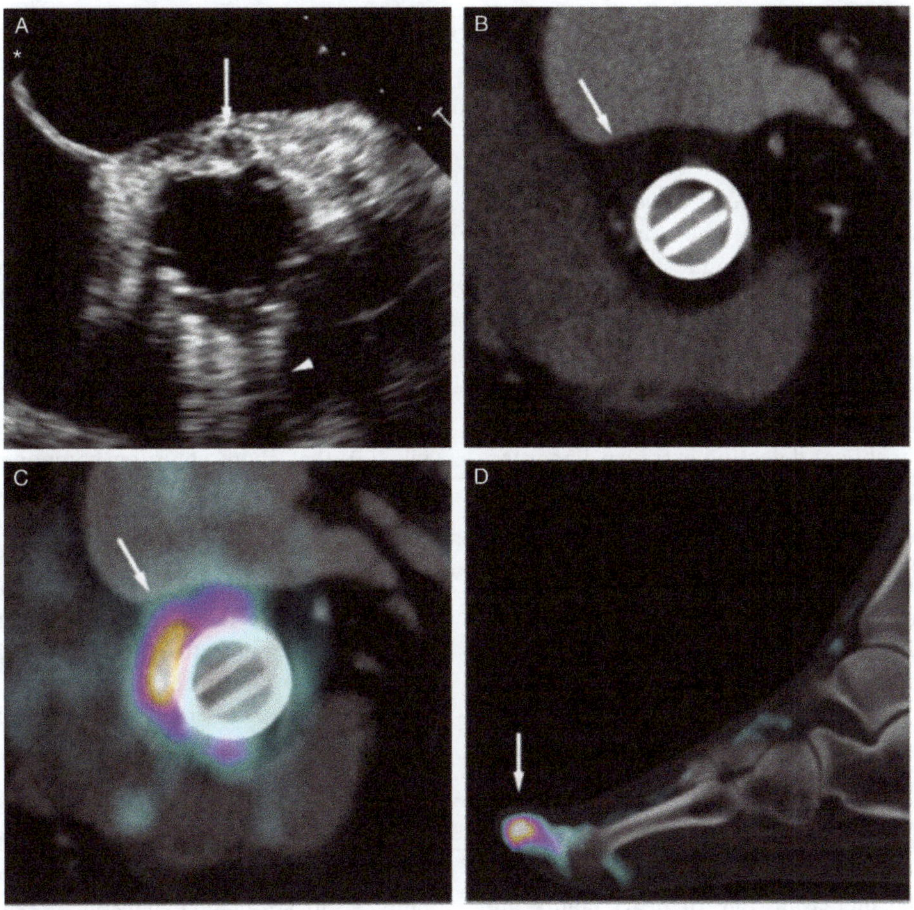

FIGURE 13-9 An Example of Extracardiac Infection Source Detected by FDG PET/CT, in a Patient With Proven Aortic Prosthesis Valve Endocarditis. There was the suggestion of an abscess (A, arrow, TEE). (B) CTA confirmed the TEE findings, showing a thickened aortic root (arrow) without significant contrast extravasations and no vegetation. Fusion of the CTA with FDG-PET (C) showed high metabolic activity (arrow) corresponding to the thickened aortic root, confirming abscess formation. There was an intense uptake in the left 4th toe corresponding to a site of osteomyelitis (D). (Reproduced with permission from Tanis W, Scholtens A, Habets J, et al: CT angiography and ^{18}F-FDG-PET fusion imaging for prosthetic heart valve endocarditis, JACC Cardiovasc Imaging. 2013 Sep;6(9):1008-1013)

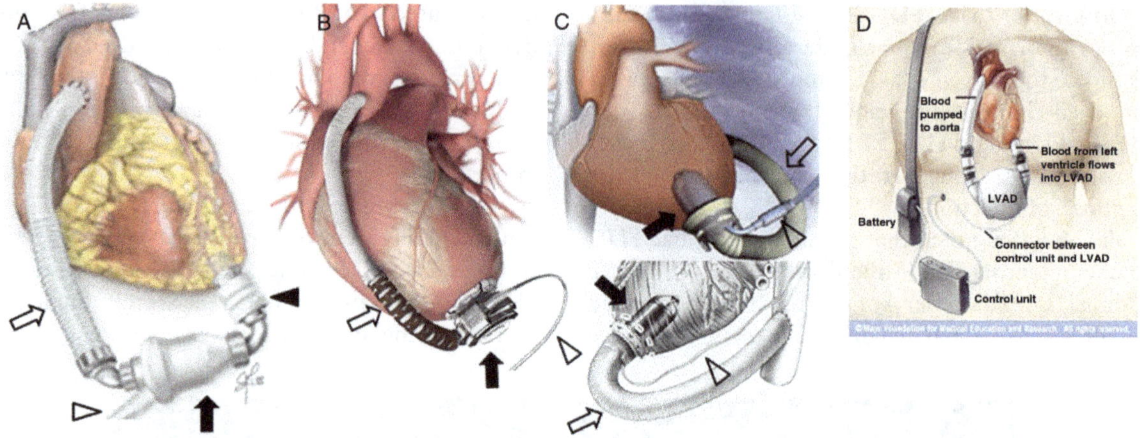

FIGURE 13-10 Types of LVAD. HeartMate II (A), HeartWare (B), and Jarvik (C), as well as illustration of the entire device of LVAD after installation (D).

In summary, for prosthetic valve endocarditis, FDG PET/CT can increase the sensitivity of the modified Duke criteria in diagnosing endocarditis without compromising specificity. In addition to confirming the findings of CTA and TEE for endocarditis complications, FDG PET/CT can potentially detect infection earlier than CTA and TEE before significant anatomical damages. FDG PET/CT is also capable of detecting extra cardiac infection source, which is critical for clinical management of endocarditis. Although these results are encouraging, FDG PET/CT is not advocated as a "first-line" imaging study for detecting prosthetic valve endocarditis. Rather, it should be reserved for cases with clinical and microbiological suspicion of endocarditis but indeterminate or negative TEE.[29]

LEFT VENTRICULAR ASSIST DEVICE INFECTION

Owing to the increasing rate of heart failure and shortage of donor hearts, LVAD has been increasingly installed in heart failure patients both as a bridge to heart transplantation and as a destination therapy.[30] Infection remains a major complication after LVAD implantation. It is reported that up to 30% patients experienced LVAD associated infection within 1 year after implantation.[31] LVAD infection is difficult to treat, with a high mortality.[32,33] Moreover, infection during LVAD therapy is associated with a worse 1-year posttransplant survival rate.[34] Thus, it is critical to accurately diagnose LVAD infection to guide clinical treatment including peri- and post heart transplant management.

There are several types of LVADs (Figure 13-10), such as HeartMate II (A), HeartWare (B), and Jarvik (C), that share common components of pump (made of Titanium) and flow tubes (made of Dacron or Gore-Tex). The pump is powered by a battery in a patient's back via a subcutaneous driveline exited at the abdominal wall (Figure 13-10 D). Infection is most commonly initiated at the percutaneous exit site of the driveline due to daily activity, progressing along the line to the central parts of the pump and flow tubes of the device. Infection limited to the exit site of a driveline can be managed by antibiotics. Once extended into the entire line and central components, the entire device needs to be extracted, and the patient may need an urgent heart transplantation. Thus, early detection of infection and, more importantly, its location and extension are critical for clinical management of the patients.

Systematic studies regarding the role of FDG PET/CT in LVAD infection evaluation is lacking due to the relatively small number of procedures compared to CIED. Perhaps the most important role of FDG PET/CT for LVAD is to assess the extent of infection into the central part of the device including the pump

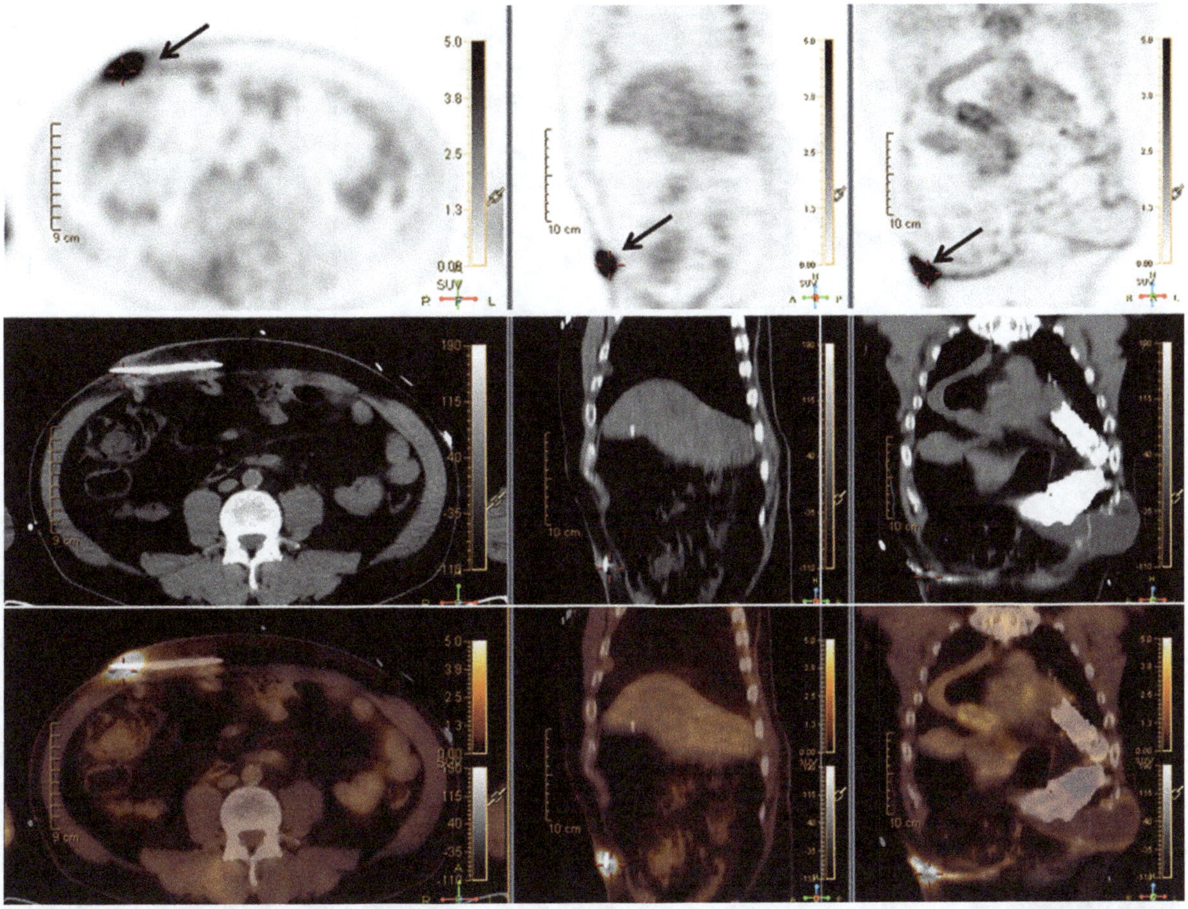

FIGURE 13-11 A Case With Driveline Exit Site Infection of LVAD. There was a focal intense activity confined to the percutaneous exit site of the driveline in the right lower abdominal wall on PET (upper row, arrow), CT (middle row, arrow), and fused PET/CT (lower row, arrow) images, with axial (left), sagittal (middle), and coronal views (right), compatible with driveline exit site infection. (Used with permission from Chen and Dilsizian, unpublished data)

housing.[35] A series of cases have demonstrated the ability of FDG PET/CT in detecting infection in different parts of LVAD.[36]

As shown in Figure 13-11, a focal intense activity is seen confined to the percutaneous exit site of the drive line in the right lower abdominal wall, compatible with infection. This can be differentiated from whole line infection as linear increased FDG uptake along the driveline and percutaneous exit, compatible with driveline infection (Figure 13-12). Figure 13-13 shows intense linear activity along the outflow tube attached to the ascending aorta, more prominent in the distal portion than the proximal metallic portion near the pump, consistent with outflow tube infection. Figure 13-14 shows abnormally increased FDG uptake corresponding to the pump pocket and cannula exterior (arrow head), compatible with central portion infection.

A recent study showed that FDG PET/CT can not only localize the site of infection as peripheral (percutaneous exit site and/or driveline) versus central (outflow tube and/or pump) infection, but also predict the survival of patients with suspected LVAD infection. Those who had central infection of LVAD had significantly shorter survival than the peripheral infection and noninfection patients (Figure 13-15).[37]

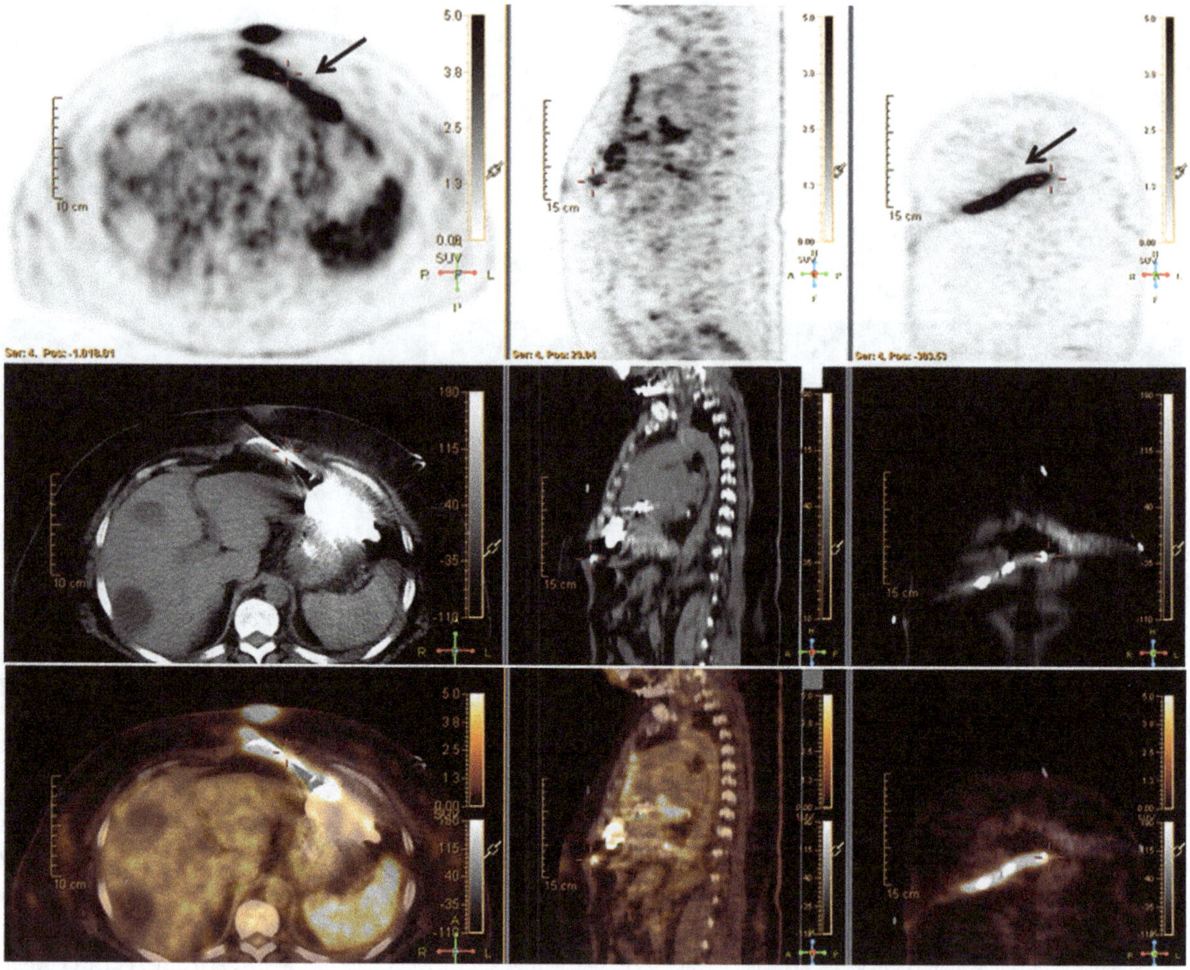

FIGURE 13-12 A Case With Driveline Line Infection of LVAD. There was intense linear increased FDG activity along the entire driveline in the left upper abdominal wall on PET (upper row, arrow), CT (middle row, arrow), and fused PET/CT (lower row, arrow) images, with axial (left), sagittal (middle), and coronal views (right), compatible with driveline infection. (Used with permission from Chen and Dilsizian, unpublished data)

VASCULAR GRAFT INFECTION

Vascular graft infection is a rare but life- threatening complication. It is estimated to occur in a 0.5% to 5% range, depending on the locations.[38] Delayed treatment of an infected graft can lead to limb amputation and death due to sepsis or hemorrhage.[39] CT is the procedure of choice currently for graft infection evaluation, and the diagnosis is straight forward if an obvious perigraft abscess is seen in a patient with clinically suspected infection.[40] However, CT findings, such as soft tissue attenuation, fluid collection with air are nonspecific, particularly in patients with a low- grade graft infection, and accuracy of CT decreases significantly.[41] For those non acute or low- grade infection cases with equivocal clinical and CT findings, FDG PET/CT is particularly useful for further differential diagnosis to confirm or exclude infection,[42] which is critical for appropriate treatment of vascular graft infection, to achieve a long-term eradiation of infection and limb preservation in the patients with this medical issue.

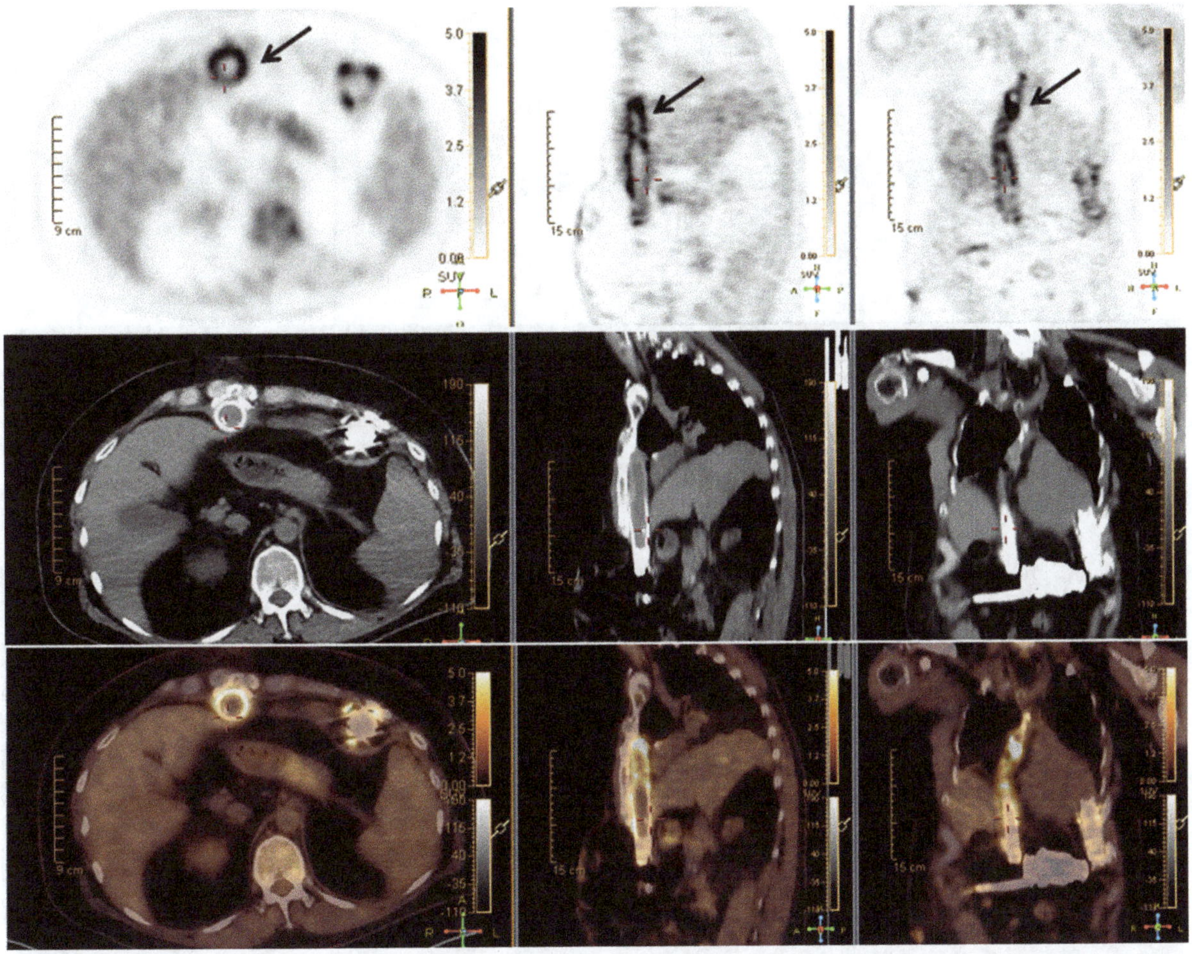

FIGURE 13-13 A Case With Outflow Tube Infection of LVAD. There was intense linear activity along the outflow tube attached to the ascending aorta, more prominent in the distal portion than the proximal metallic portion near the pump on PET (upper row, arrow), CT (middle row, arrow), and fused PET/CT (lower row, arrow) images, with axial (left), sagittal (middle), and coronal views (right), compatible with outflow tube infection. (Used with permission from Chen and Dilsizian, unpublished data)

In a relatively large cohort of study[43] regarding the role of FDG PET/CT for nonacute or suspected lower graft infection, 76 patients (a total of 96 prosthetic grafts) who did not require urgent surgery were enrolled. Patients with fulminant sepsis, anastomotic abscess, bleeding or prosthesoenteric fistula were excluded. The results showed that focal intense FDG uptake was specific for graft infection in 92.7% of cases (Figure 13-16), with a very high positive prospective value (PPV) of 93.5%. No focal FDG uptake excludes infection with a very high specificity of 96.9% (Figure 13-17), with a low rate of 1.8% of false-negative PET rate. Meanwhile, in nearly one-fifth of prostheses, FDG uptake was inhomogeneous and considered as nondiagnostic (Figure 13-18), which is a diagnostic challenge. Nevertheless, mild inhomogeneous FDG uptake either represents very-low-grade infection or noninfectious inflammation related to reaction to the graft or postsurgical change. Overall, the study shows that FDG PET/CT is a useful imaging tool for difficult cases with equivocal clinical and CT findings.

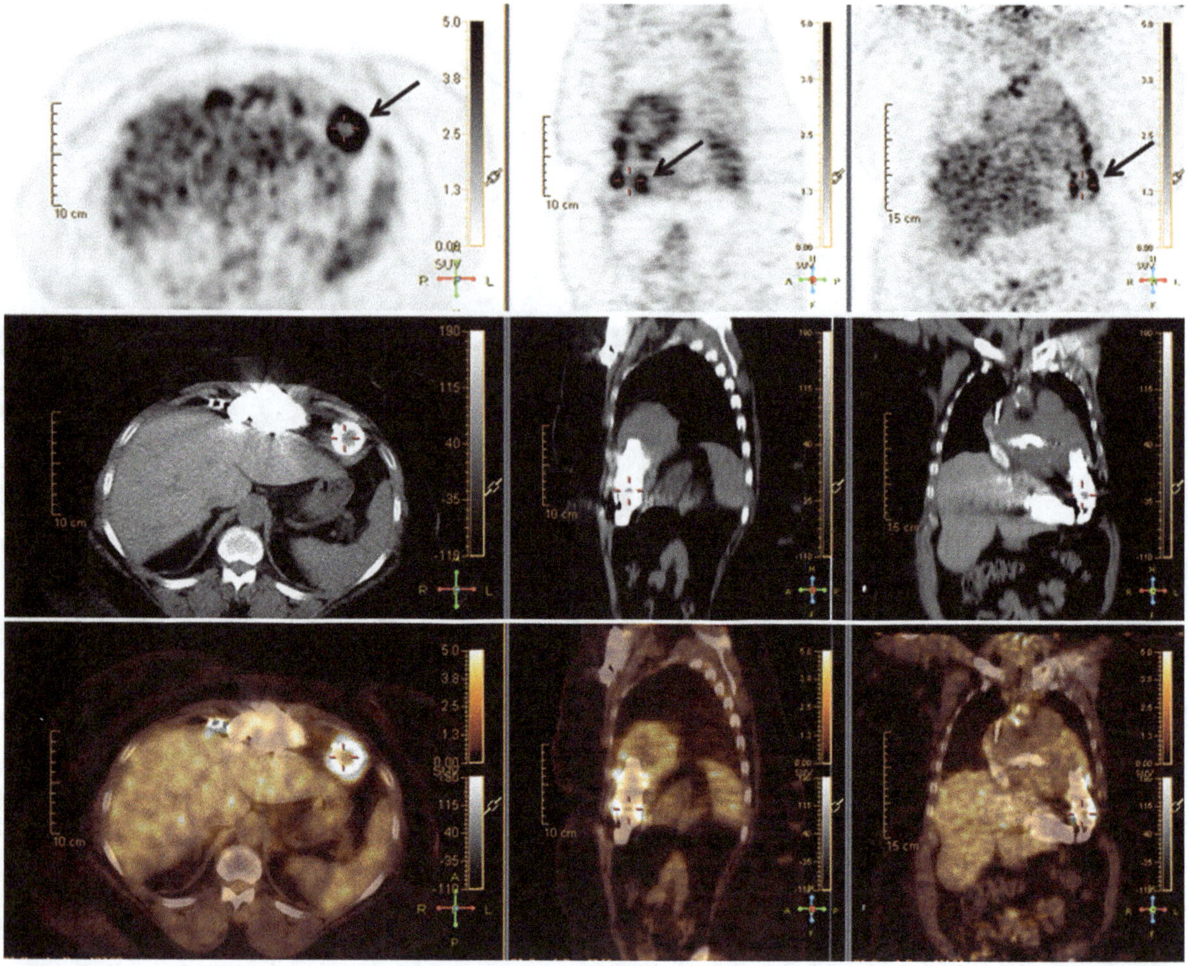

FIGURE 13-14 A Case With Pump Infection of LVAD. There was abnormally increased FDG uptake corresponding to the pump pocket on PET (upper row, arrow), CT (middle row, arrow), and fused PET/CT (lower row, arrow) images, with axial (left), sagittal (middle), and coronal views (right), compatible with pump infection. (Used with permission from Chen and Dilsizian, unpublished data)

CONCLUSION

FDG PET/CT is a promising tool for early and accurate diagnosis of cardiac devices infection. It is particularly useful for difficult cases with equivocal clinical and anatomical imaging findings. For CIED, FDG PET/CT can accurately localize the site and extension of pocket infection, such as superficial versus deep pocket, although its sensitivity is relatively lower for evaluation of lead vegetation infection. FDG PET/CT findings can guide clinical management. A positive PET requires CIED device extraction, whereas a negative case can be managed clinically by intravenous antibiotics without adverse clinical outcome on follow-up. FDG PET/CT can detect prosthetic valve endocarditis earlier than anatomical tools, and, in most of cases, provide incremental and confirmatory information for final accurate diagnosis. Adding PET findings as a new major criterion can increase the sensitivity of modified Duke criteria for valve endocarditis diagnosis without compromising the specificity. Similarly, FDG PET/CT can identify the site of LVAD infection and extension, which is critical for clinical management in the heart failure patients, and

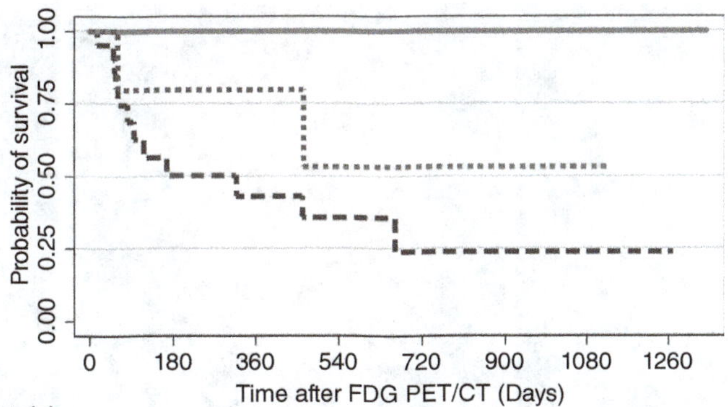

Number at risk

noninfection	7	5	4	4	3	2	2	1
central infection	23	8	6	5	2	1	1	1
peripheral infection	5	4	3	2	1	1	1	0

central infection — noninfection — peripheral infection

FIGURE 13-15 Kaplan-Meier Survival Curves in LVAD Patients. Patients were grouped according to central and peripheral infection or noninfection on the basis of FDG PET/CT diagnosis. There was a significantly higher mortality in FDG-avid central versus peripheral infection groups. None of the noninfected patients died. (Reproduced with permission from Kim J, Feller ED, Chen W, et al: FDG PET/CT for Early Detection and Localization of Left Ventricular Assist Device Infection: Impact on Patient Management and Outcome, JACC Cardiovasc Imaging. 2018 Mar 9. pii: S1936-878X(18)30135-9).

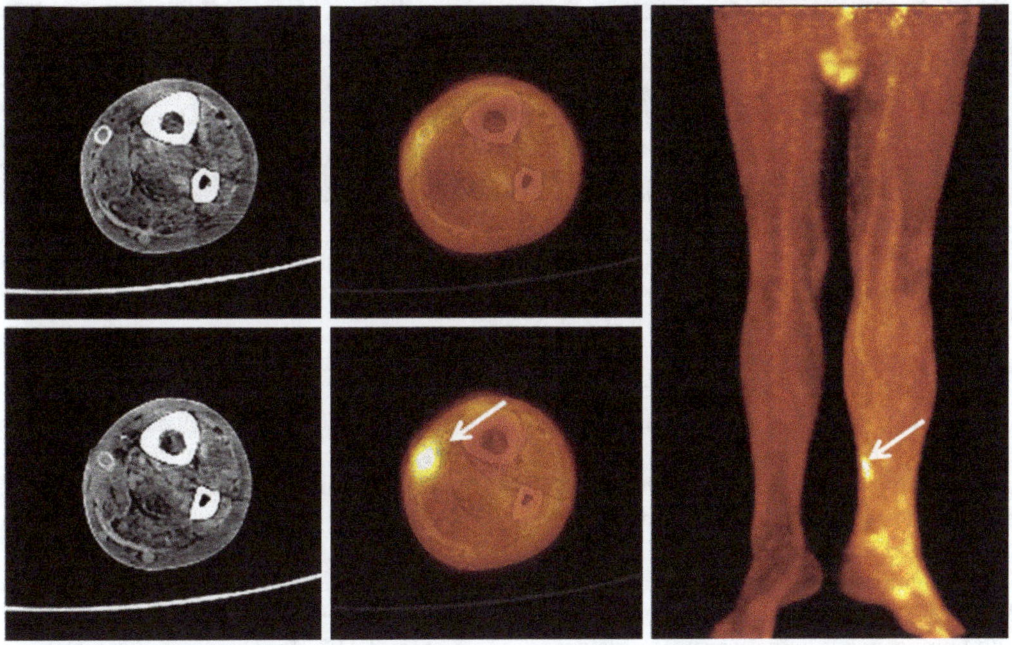

FIGURE 13-16 An Example of Lower Extremity Vascular Graft Infection. There was a focal FDG uptake and irregularity of the boundary of the distal portion of the left femorotibial bypass 6 months after grafting (arrow on the axial slice in the *lower row* and maximum intensity projection on the right). There was a normal finding 15 mm above this focus (*upper row*). (Reproduced with permission from Spacek M, Belohlavek O, Votrubova J, et al: Diagnostics of "non-acute" vascular prosthesis infection using ^{18}F-FDG PET/CT: our experience with 96 prostheses, Eur J Nucl Med Mol Imaging. 2009 May;36(5):850-858)

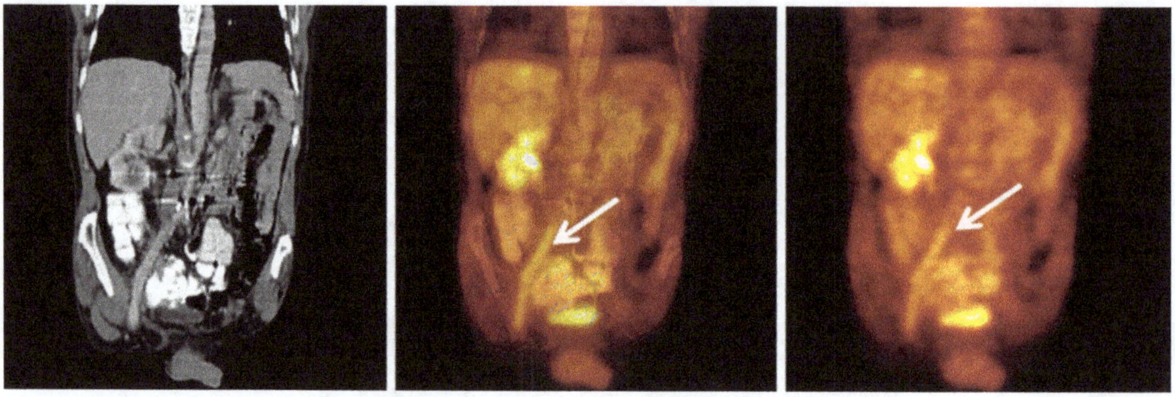

FIGURE 13-17 An Example of Noninfectious Inflammatory Change. Mild homogeneous FDG uptake (arrow) without any focal accumulation in the course of the right iliofemoral bypass 23 months after grafting. A further 18 months of clinical follow-up did not reveal any infection. (Reproduced with permission from Spacek M, Belohlavek O, Votrubova J, et al: Diagnostics of "non-acute" vascular prosthesis infection using ^{18}F-FDG PET/CT: our experience with 96 prostheses, Eur J Nucl Med Mol Imaging. 2009 May;36(5):850-858)

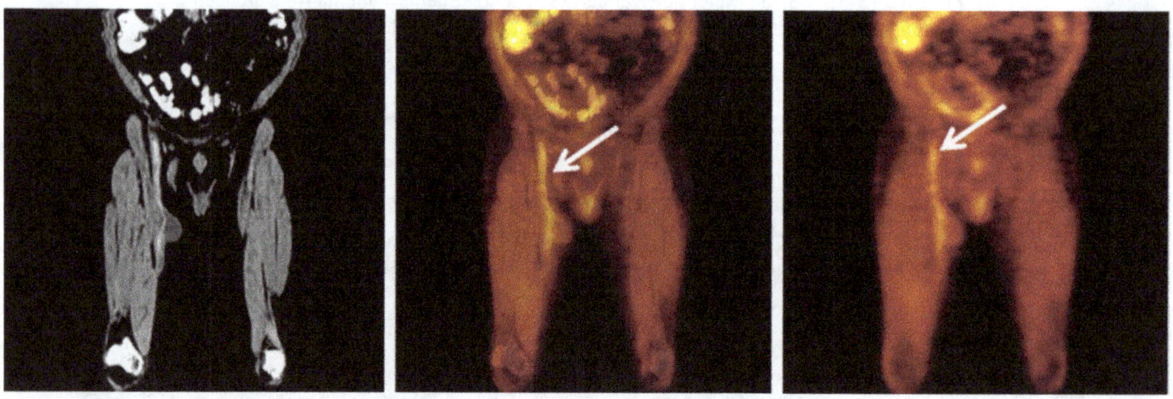

FIGURE 13-18 An Example of Nondiagnostic Graft Infection Case. Mild, but in homogeneous FDG uptake without corresponding liquid collection in the course of right femoropopliteal bypass 6 months after grafting. (Reproduced with permission from Spacek M, Belohlavek O, Votrubova J, et al: Diagnostics of "non-acute" vascular prosthesis infection using ^{18}F-FDG PET/CT: our experience with 96 prostheses, Eur J Nucl Med Mol Imaging. 2009 May;36(5):850-858)

further predict the patient's outcome. For vascular graft infection, FDG PET/CT is particularly useful for nonacute, low-grade infectious cases, which is a challenge for CT. Visual evaluation of FDG PET/CT findings on both attenuation corrected and nonattenuation corrected images remains the most reliable method for diagnosis: focal intense uptake associated with a device structure is suggestive of infection, while mild homogeneous activity around a device is more likely noninfectious inflammation. Nevertheless, a consensus needs to be established as regards to a standardized imaging protocol including patient preparation (to suppress physiological cardiac FDG uptake), time of imaging after FDG injection, data acquisition (cardiac gating), data processing (attenuation and nonattenuation correction), and, most importantly, imaging interpretation criteria.

REFERENCES

1. Mond HG, Proclemer A. The 11th world survey of cardiac pacing and implantable cardioverter-defibrillators: calendar year 2009: a World Society of Arrhythmia's project. *Pacing Clin Electrophysiol.* 2011;34(8):1013–1027.

2. Greenspon AJ, Patel JD, Lau E, et al. 16-year trends in the infection burden for pacemakers and implantable cardioverter-defibrillators in the United States 1993 to 2008. *J Am Coll Cardiol.* 2011;58(10):1001–1006.
3. Kurtz SM, Ochoa JA, Lau E, et al. Implantation trends and patient profiles for pacemakers and implantable cardioverter defibrillators in the United States: 1993–2006. *Pacing Clin Electrophysiol.* 2010;33(6):705–711.
4. Baddour LM, Epstein AE, Erickson CC, et al. Update on cardiovascular implantable electronic device infections and their management: a scientific statement from the American Heart Association. *Circulation.* 2010;121(3):458–477.
5. Chu VH, Crosslin DR, Friedman JY, et al. Staphylococcus aureus bacteremia in patients with prosthetic devices: costs and outcomes. *Am J Med.* 2005;118(12): 1416.e19–1416.e24.
6. Tarakji KG, Chan EJ, Cantillon DJ, et al. Cardiac implantable electronic device infections: presentation, management, and patient outcomes. *Heart Rhythm.* 2010;7(8):1043–1047.
7. Hyafil F, Rouzet F, Lepage L, et al. Role of radiolabelled leucocyte scintigraphy in patients with a suspicion of prosthetic valve endocarditis and inconclusive echocardiography. *Eur Heart J Cardiovasc Imaging.* 2013;14(6):586–594.
8. Erba PA, Sollini M, Conti U, et al. Radiolabeled WBC scintigraphy in the diagnostic workup of patients with suspected device-related infections. *JACC Cardiovasc Imaging.* 2013;6(10): 1075–1086.
9. Pill SG, Parvizi J, Tang PH, et al. Comparison of fluorodeoxyglucose positron emission tomography and (111)indium-white blood cell imaging in the diagnosis of periprosthetic infection of the hip. *J Arthroplasty.* 2006;21(6 Suppl 2):91–97.
10. Basu S, Kwee TC, Saboury B, et al. FDG PET for diagnosing infection in hip and knee prostheses: prospective study in 221 prostheses and subgroup comparison with combined (111)In-labeled leukocyte/(99m)Tc-sulfur colloid bone marrow imaging in 88 prostheses. *Clin Nucl Med.* 2014;39(7):609–615.
11. Chen W, Kim J, Molchanova-Cook OP, et al. The potential of FDG PET/CT for early diagnosis of cardiac device and prosthetic valve infection before morphologic damages ensue. *Curr Cardiol Rep.* 2014;16(3):459–466.
12. Williams G, Kolodny GM. Suppression of myocardial 18F-FDG uptake by preparing patients with a high-fat, low-carbohydrate diet. *AJR Am J Roentgenol.* 2008;190(2):W151-W156.
13. Manabe O, Yoshinaga K, Ohira H, et al. The effects of 18-h fasting with low-carbohydrate diet preparation on suppressed physiological myocardial (18)F-fluorodeoxyglucose (FDG) uptake and possible minimal effects of unfractionated heparin use in patients with suspected cardiac involvement sarcoidosis. *J Nucl Cardiol.* 2016;23(2):244–252.
14. Bucerius J, Hyafil F, Verberne HJ, et al. Position paper of the Cardiovascular Committee of the European Association of Nuclear Medicine (EANM) on PET imaging of atherosclerosis. *Eur J Nucl Med Mol Imaging.* 2016;43(4):780–792.
15. Ploux S, Riviere A, Amraoui S, et al. Positron emission tomography in patients with suspected pacing system infections may play a critical role in difficult cases. *Heart Rhythm.* 2011;8(9):1478–1481.
16. Bensimhon L, Lavergne T, Hugonnet F, et al. Whole body [(18) F]fluorodeoxyglucose positron emission tomography imaging for the diagnosis of pacemaker or implantable cardioverter defibrillator infection: a preliminary prospective study. *Clin Microbiol Infect.* 2011;17(6): 836–844.
17. Sarrazin JF, Philippon F, Tessier M, et al. Usefulness of fluorine-18 positron emission tomography/computed tomography for identification of cardiovascular implantable electronic device infections. *J Am Coll Cardiol.* 2012;59(18):1616–1625.
18. Baddour LM, Wilson WR, Bayer AS, et al. Infective endocarditis in adults: diagnosis, antimicrobial therapy, and management of complications: a scientific statement for healthcare professionals from the American Heart Association. *Circulation.* 2015;132(15):1435–1486.
19. Durack DT, Lukes AS, Bright DK, et al. New criteria for diagnosis of infective endocarditis: utilization of specific echocardiographic findings. Duke Endocarditis Service. *Am J Med.* 1994;96(3):200–209.

20. Hill EE, Herijgers P, Claus P, et al. Abscess in infective endocarditis: the value of transesophageal echocardiography and outcome: a 5-year study. *Am Heart J.* 2007;154(5):923–928.
21. Habib G, Hoen B, Tornos P, et al. Guidelines on the prevention, diagnosis, and treatment of infective endocarditis (new version 2009): the Task Force on the Prevention, Diagnosis, and Treatment of Infective Endocarditis of the European Society of Cardiology (ESC). Endorsed by the European Society of Clinical Microbiology and Infectious Diseases (ESCMID) and the International Society of Chemotherapy (ISC) for Infection and Cancer. *Eur Heart J.* 2009;30(19): 2369–2413.
22. Li JS, Sexton DJ, Mick N, et al. Proposed modifications to the Duke criteria for the diagnosis of infective endocarditis. *Clin Infect Dis.* 2000;30(4): 633–638.
23. Saby L, Laas O, Habib G. Positron emission tomography/computed tomography for diagnosis of prosthetic valve endocarditis: increased valvular 18F-fluorodeoxyglucose uptake as a novel major criterion. *J Am Coll Cardiol.* 2013;61(23): 2374–2382.
24. Habib G, Lancellotti P, Antunes MJ, et al. 2015 ESC Guidelines for the management of infective endocarditis: the Task Force for the Management of Infective Endocarditis of the European Society of Cardiology (ESC). Endorsed by: European Association for Cardio-Thoracic Surgery (EACTS), the European Association of Nuclear Medicine (EANM). *Eur Heart J.* 2015;36(44):3075–3128.
25. Jiménez-Ballvé A, Pérez-Castejón MJ, Delgado-Bolton RC, et al. Assessment of the diagnostic accuracy of 18F-FDG PET/CT in prosthetic infective endocarditis and cardiac implantable electronic device infection: comparison of different interpretation criteria. *Eur J Nucl Med Mol Imaging.* 2016;43(13):2401–2412.
26. Fagman E, van Essen M, Fredén Lindqvist JJ, et al. 18F-FDG PET/CT in the diagnosis of prosthetic valve endocarditis. *Int J Cardiovasc Imaging.* 2016;32(4):679–686.
27. Tanis W, Scholtens A, Habets J, et al. CT angiography and ^{18}F-FDG-PET fusion imaging for prosthetic heart valve endocarditis. *JACC Cardiovasc Imaging.* 2013;6(9):1008–1013.
28. Schouten LR, Verberne HJ, Bouma BJ, et al. Surgical glue for repair of the aortic root as a possible explanation for increased F-18 FDG uptake. *J Nucl Cardiol.* 2008;15(1):146–147.
29. Brinker J. Imaging for infected cardiac implantable electronic devices: a new trick for your pet. *J Am Coll Cardiol.* 2012;59(18):1626–1628.
30. Kirklin JK, Naftel DC, Kormos RL, et al. Second INTERMACS annual report: more than 1,000 primary left ventricular assist device implants. *J Heart Lung Transplant.* 2010; 29(1):1–10.
31. Kirklin JK, Naftel DC, Pagani FD, et al. Seventh INTERMACS annual report: 15,000 patients and counting. *J Heart Lung Transplant.* 2015;34(12): 1495–1504.
32. Koval CE, Thuita L, Moazami N, et al. Evolution and impact of drive-line infection in a large cohort of continuous-flow ventricular assist device recipients. *J Heart Lung Transplant.* 2014;33(11):1164–1172.
33. Gordon RJ, Weinberg AD, Pagani FD, et al. Prospective, multicenter study of ventricular assist device infections. *Circulation.* 2013;127(6): 691–702.
34. Healy AH, Baird BC, Drakos SG, et al. Impact of ventricular assist device complications on post-transplant survival: an analysis of the United network of organ sharing database. *Ann Thorac Surg.* 2013;95(3):870–875.
35. Dell'Aquila AM, Mastrobuoni S, Alles S, et al. Contributory role of fluorine 18-fluorodeoxyglucose positron emission tomography/computed tomography in the diagnosis and clinical management of infections in patients supported with a continuous-flow left ventricular assist device. *Ann Thorac Surg.* 2016;101(1): 87–94.
36. Kim J, Feller ED, Chen W, et al. FDG PET/CT imaging for LVAD associated infections. *JACC Cardiovasc Imaging.* 2014;7(8):839–842.
37. Kim J, Feller ED, Chen W, et al. FDG PET/CT for early detection and localization of left ventricular assist device infection: impact on patient management and outcome. *JACC Cardiovasc Imaging.* 2018; Mar 9, Epub ahead of print.
38. Seeger JM. Management of patients with prosthetic vascular graft infection. *Am Surg.* 2000;66(2):166–177.

39. Chang JK, Calligaro KD, Ryan S, et al. Risk factors associated with infection of lower extremity revascularization: analysis of 365 procedures performed at a teaching hospital. *Ann Vasc Surg.* 2003;17(1):91–96.

40. Orton DF, LeVeen RF, Saigh JA, et al. Aortic prosthetic graft infections: radiologic manifestations and implications for management. *Radiographics.* 2000;20(4):977–993.

41. Low RN, Wall SD, Jeffrey RB Jr, et al. Aortoenteric fistula and perigraft infection: evaluation with CT. *Radiology.* 1990;175(1):157–162.

42. Guenther SP, Cyran CC, Rominger A, et al. The relevance of 18F-fluorodeoxyglucose positron emission tomography/computed tomography imaging in diagnosing prosthetic graft infections post cardiac and proximal thoracic aortic surgery. *Interact Cardiovasc Thorac Surg.* 2015;21(4):450–458.

43. Spacek M, Belohlavek O, Votrubova J, et al. Diagnostics of "non-acute" vascular prosthesis infection using ^{18}F-FDG PET/CT: our experience with 96 prostheses. *Eur J Nucl Med Mol Imaging.* 2009;36(5):850–858.

EDITOR'S PERSPECTIVE

Timothy M. Bateman

There are several distinguishing features of this incredibly enlightening chapter on imaging cardiovascular device infection. First, this chapter is a virtual compendium of the current literature on this subject. Second, the excellent case examples deserve to be studied in detail by every reader. Third, the authors meticulously cover patient preparation and the rules of image acquisition and interpretation.

Structural cardiologists and surgeons, electrophysiologists, congestive heart failure specialists, and infectious disease specialists are facing a virtual epidemic of infections related to the increasing use of implanted cardiovascular hardware. Fortunately, it is often possible to make a diagnosis of site and severity of infection by relatively simple means such as physical exam, ultrasound, or transthoracic or transesophageal echocardiography. The more difficult cases, however, are being referred to PET/CT in increasing numbers. As imaging labs address these referrals, at least three challenges have become evident.

Currently there are no multisocietal guidelines focused specifically on device infections. Labs are left to develop their own patient preparation orders, dosing and acquisition protocols, image interpretation standards, and report formats. This chapter should be helpful until such guidelines appear.

The authors are distinguished nuclear medicine *and* nuclear cardiology specialists. They work in an environment where their training, experiences, and infrastructure permit the kind of excellent care needed when patients' problems cross over specialty lines. The authors are knowledgeable about the details of implanted devices, the kinds of infections that occur, and how their image interpretations translate directly into management such as device removal versus less invasive or even medication-only treatments. While a minority of facilities have this degree of expertise on staff, it is evident from this chapter how powerful the concept of dually-trained experts is when it comes to complex issues such as cardiovascular device-related infections.

Finally, there is the vexing issue for most labs of how to optimally care for patients whose problems cross specialty interests. Often in the case of device-related infections, decision-making is best approached by a team of experts all of whom should be involved in inspecting the images: specialists in nuclear medicine, cardiovascular imaging, infectious diseases, and CT experts. Guidelines specifying such team approaches would be helpful in moving disparate specialists into teams but, currently, the payment codes do not facilitate such teamwork. In some settings imaging gets parsed out in pieces, with two or more independent interpretations.

Hopefully, the urgency felt in the arena of cardiovascular device-related infections will hasten development of imaging guidelines, adoption of billing codes that address the realities of multisystem imaging, and either team approaches or cross-specialty trained experts. In the meantime, the authors of this chapter have provided an excellent and detailed overview of an important and rapidly evolving application of PET/CT imaging.

INDEX

D

Q

www.ingramcontent.com/pod-product-compliance
Lightning Source LLC
LaVergne TN
LVHW062158200926
848484LV00006B/1282
* 9 7 8 1 2 5 9 8 6 0 4 8 5 *